GUIDE TO
ECG
ANALYSIS

JOSEPH T. CATALANO, Ph.D., R.N., C.C.R.N.

ASSOCIATE PROFESSOR OF NURSING
EAST CENTRAL UNIVERSITY
ADA, OKLAHOMA

GUIDE TO
ECG
ANALYSIS

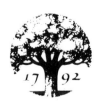

J.B. Lippincott Company
Philadelphia

Acquisitions Editor: David Carroll
Editorial Assistant: Patty L. Shear
Project Editor: Barbara Ryalls
Indexer: Victoria Boyle
Design Coordinator: Christopher Laird
Interior Design: Maria S. Karkucinski
Cover Designer: Larry Pezzato
Production Manager: Helen Ewan
Production Coordinator: Kathryn Rule
Compositor: Bi-Comp, Inc.
Printer/Binder: R.R. Donnelley & Sons Company
Cover Printer: John Pow

6   5   4   3   2   1

Library of Congress Cataloging-in-Publication Data

Catalano, Joseph T.
    Guide to ECG Analysis / Joseph T. Catalano
        p.   cm.
    Includes index.
    ISBN 0-397-55015-4
    1. Electrocardiography.   I. Title
    [DNLM: 1. Arrhythmia—diagnosis—nurses' instruction.
    2. Electrocardiography—methods—nurses' instruction.   3. Heart-
    -physiology—nurses' instruction.   WG 141 C357e]
    RC683.5.E5C29   1993
    616.1'207547—dc20
    DNLM/DLC
    for Library of Congress   92-49718
                                                           CIP

Any procedure or practice described in this book should be
applied by the healthcare practitioner under appropriate
supervision in accordance with professional standards of
care used with regard to the unique circumstances that
apply in each practice situation. Care has been taken to
confirm the accuracy of information presented and to
describe generally accepted practices. However, the
authors, editors, and publisher cannot accept any
responsibility for errors or omissions or for any
consequences from application of the information in this
book and make no warranty express or implied, with
respect to the contents of the book.

Every effort has been made to ensure drug selections and
dosages are in accordance with current recommendations
and practice. Because of ongoing research, changes in
government regulations and the constant flow of
information on drug therapy, reactions and interactions,
the reader is cautioned to check the package insert for each
drug for indications, dosages, warnings and precautions,
particularly if the drug is new or infrequently used.

To my loving wife, Pam, without whose support and encouragement this book would have been impossible; and to my girls, Sarah and Amanda, who keep the world a fresh and interesting place in which to live.

PREFACE

In the evolution of health care through the years, many skills and functions that were once considered to be strictly in the medical domain have gradually but inevitably moved into the nurse's realm of practice. No area has witnessed this migration of practice more than that of the Critical Care Unit. One of the last elements of critical care practice to move into the nurse's scope of practice is that of ECG interpretation. When nurses realized that there was nothing magical about ECG interpretation and that with a little study and practice they could become competent in this skill, the doors were opened.

One difficulty that nurses did find, and still do, in attempting to learn this skill is a lack of basic books that start at the beginning and proceed step-by-step through the process of learning the skills necessary to interpret ECG dysrhythmias. The majority of the books that deal with ECG interpretation start "in the middle" rather than at the beginning. The major reason for this tendency is that most people who write ECG books already know quite a bit about ECG interpretation and presume their readers do also. I became acutely aware of this problem some 10 years ago when I attempted to teach my first basic ECG dysrhythmia interpretation class to a group of senior (4th-year) nursing students at a Baccalaureate Degree nursing program. I fell quickly into the "start in the middle" trap, which, by the end of the semester, resulted in a group of confused and resentful students. Over the years of teaching this fairly complicated material to student nurses, EMTs, paramedics, and yes, even a few groups of physicians, I have developed a process and format that has met with a high degree of success. This book is a result of those efforts.

Guide to ECG Analysis starts at the beginning with very basic information concerning cardiac functioning and conduction principles. It presumes nothing on the part of the reader except an average level of intelligence and a willingness to learn. It has been my experience that the more basic the information concerning the functioning of the heart that is given to the student, the easier it will be for that student to analyze and interpret the various rhythm strips to be dealt with later. The book then provides an analysis format to be used on each rhythm strip encountered. In discussing the various dysrhythmias and rhythm problems, constant reference is made back to the physiologic origins of that problem in the conduction system of the heart. The book also includes such topics as bundle branch block, pre-excitation syndromes, and pacemakers, which are generally not found in basic ECG books but are common cardiac problems and often encountered by the novice nursing student.

In the writing of this book, I have attempted to avoid the pitfalls that many introductory ECG books suffer, especially being too elementary, not including enough information, and being *over*simplified or filled with half-truths or inaccuracies. In attempting to explain complicated material to a beginning group of learners, I have tried to walk the fine line between oversimplification and explanation. This book is for the beginner in ECG dysrhythmia interpretation, whether a nursing student, new graduate nurse, EMT, paramedic or medical student. I also have included enough advanced topics to make the book interesting and useful to the more experienced critical care practitioner.

The old adage that "practice makes perfect" is as true in learning ECG dysrhythmia interpretation as it is in learning any skill. To that end, I have included a large number of practice strips in this book, with their interpretations. To read about the principles or criteria of a particular dysrhythmia while looking at a sample strip is quite different from actually attempting to analyze a strip using the skills and knowledge learned. Practice also aids in the learning of the criteria that must be committed to memory at some point in the learning process.

If you are serious about learning how to analyze and interpret ECG rhythms and follow the step-by-step process in this book, you will master the skill. There is really no "easy" way to master this skill except by study, concentration, and practice. The reward of being able to perform this rather complicated skill will be well worth the effort. Although this book can be used for self-study, it is more appropriately used in conjunction with a tutor or in the classroom setting.

Through my years of teaching this material in the manner outlined above, my major source of satisfaction has been watching my students become proficient in the skills and seeing the sense of accomplishment they have derived from the ability. If this book makes mastery of this skill possible, then it has been a success.

Joseph T. Catalano, Ph.D., R.N., C.C.R.N.

ACKNOWLEDGMENTS

I wish to express my thanks to all the nursing students I have instructed over the past 12 years. Their probing questions and fresh insights have taught me more than a thousand books. I also wish to thank the dedicated monitor technicians who collected and saved for me many of the ECG strips in this book.

CONTENTS

GUIDE TO
ECG
ANALYSIS

1

STRUCTURES AND FUNCTIONS OF THE HEART

LEARNING OBJECTIVES

After studying this section, the learner will be able to:

1. Describe the general physiologic structures of the heart.
2. List and define the properties of cardiac muscle tissue.
3. Name the appropriate portions of the myocardium supplied by the various branches of the coronary arteries.
4. Name the parts of the electrical conduction system of the heart.
5. Describe polarization, depolarization, and repolarization in relationship to myocardial contraction.
6. Name the two branches of the autonomic nervous system and describe their effects on myocardial contraction.

The electrocardiogram (ECG) is just one of the many tools for assessing cardiac function available to health care providers. The ECG is a highly specialized and technical assessment method that is commonly used in health care today; it by no means provides a complete assessment of the heart. The ECG provides information about the electrical activity in the heart as it relates to both the conduction system of the heart and the normal or abnormal formation of electrical impulses. Other assessment methods of cardiac function ranging from invasive hemodynamic techniques, such as pulmonary artery catheters and central venous pressure (CVP) lines, to noninvasive measures, such as blood pressure, pulse determinations, and heart sounds, will aid in the assessment of the heart when used in conjunction with the ECG analysis.

A fundamental understanding of the structures and functions of the heart is necessary to effectively use any of the assessment techniques that are undertaken to determine myocardial function. Although the author firmly believes the more that is learned about how and why the heart functions, the easier it is to understand the use and the results of all assessment techniques, it is not within the scope of this text to provide detailed information about the structures and functions of the heart. Instead, basic information concerning cardiac function that is crucial to the understanding of ECG production and interpretation will be provided.

GENERAL FUNCTIONS OF THE HEART

The heart is a four-chambered, hollow muscular organ whose primary function is to create a pressure gradient in the vascular system of the body so that blood flows from areas of higher pressure to areas of lower pressure. A series of valves control the direction of the blood flow in the heart and the attached blood vessels so that unoxygenated blood flows through the heart to the lungs and oxygenated blood is circulated to the muscles, organs, and tissues of the body through the systemic circulation (Fig. 1-1).

The healthy heart in the adult is approximately the same size as the human fist. The heart is located in the midsternal and lower left side of the chest cavity.

FIG. 1–1. (A) CIRCULATION AND STRUCTURES IN THE HEART (FROM UNDERHILL ET AL. CARDIAC NURSING, PHILADELPHIA: JB LIPPINCOTT, 1982:4); **(B)** CORONARY CIRCULATION: ANTERIOR HEART; AND **(C)** CORONARY CIRCULATION: POSTERIOR HEART. (FROM UNDERHILL ET AL. CARDIAC NURSING, 2ND ED, PHILADELPHIA: JB LIPPINCOTT, 1989:22)

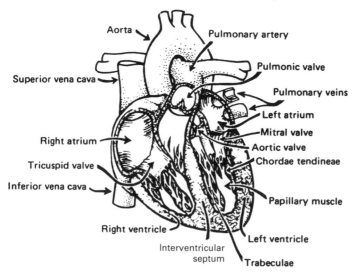

A

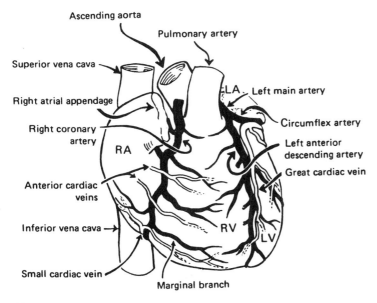

B

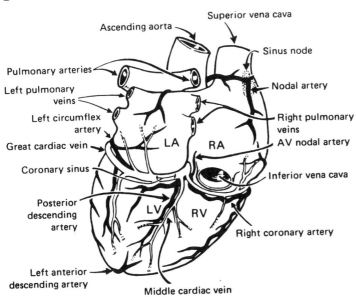

C

The bottom of the heart (the apex) is normally located between the fifth and sixth intercostal space on the left side of the chest. The top of the heart (the base) is normally located at the second intercostal space in the midsternal area. In this position, the heart "tips" to the left so that the right ventricle is facing the diaphragm of the lungs.

The main function of the heart is to pump blood through the vascular system of the body. Cardiac output (CO) is the amount of blood that is ejected (pumped out) by the left ventricle each minute. The right ventricle also has a CO that affects circulation of unoxygenated blood to the lungs. Right ventricular CO is extremely critical because the left ventricle can only pump the blood it receives from the right ventricle. Right ventricular CO is measured clinically by a pulmonary artery catheter.

Cardiac output is the product of two factors: the stroke volume (the amount of blood per contraction) and the heart rate. Any changes in either of these factors will affect the CO. Up to a point, increases in heart rate, given a normal conduction pattern of the ventricles, will increase CO. In general, abnormal contraction patterns of the ventricles will decrease the CO to some degree, although an increased rate may help compensate for that decrease. Both changes in heart rate and conduction pattern are detectable on the ECG and will provide an indirect indication of the CO. Also, certain abnormal ECG patterns are almost always accompanied by a decreased CO and require immediate intervention by the health care team.

STRUCTURES OF THE HEART

The internal structure of the heart, like most organs of the body, is composed of different layers and types of tissue. In addition, the heart is surrounded by a sac called the *pericardium*. The pericardium is composed of two types of tissue: an outer fibrous portion of heavy connective tissue and an inner lining of thin, smooth connective tissue called the *serous portion,* which is in contact with the external layer of tissue of the heart.

Although the pericardium is not absolutely necessary for the normal functioning of the heart, it performs several important duties. Primarily, it helps insulate the heart from the rest of the structures in the chest cavity, thereby preventing irritation of the heart and protecting the cardiac tissues from infection. A small amount of serous fluid (10–50 ml) is present in the pericardial space to act as a lubricant to prevent irritation between the pericardium and the heart. The pericardium also holds the heart in place since the heart is not attached to any structures in the chest cavity except the great blood vessels. In addition, the elastic nature of the pericardium helps in the contraction of the heart and will prevent sudden overdistention of the heart.

There are three layers of tissue present in the heart: the epicardium, the myocardium, and the endocardium.

The *epicardium* is the outermost layer of tissue; it is a type of connective tissue similar in structure to the serous portion of the pericardium. These flat, thin connective tissue cells glide over each other and prevent irritation of the cardiac tissue that occurs with the constant motion of the heart.

The *myocardium* is the muscle layer of the heart; it is the part of the heart that does the work of contracting and circulating the blood. The myocardium varies in thickness in the atria and ventricles. The myocardium in the atria is relatively thin because these chambers are normally low pressure and function mainly to complete the filling process of the ventricles. Although the myocardium in the right ventricle is thicker than the myocardium of the atria, it is still a relatively low pressure chamber. When the pressure is low, the workload demand on the muscle tissue is also low and can be accomplished with a reduced amount of myocardial tissue.

In contrast, the left ventricle is a high pressure chamber that requires a much thicker myocardium to meet the increased workload demands. The left ventricle contains the bulk of the cardiac muscle tissue of the heart and is vital to the maintenance of life because it produces systemic circulation. Correspondingly, it also requires the most oxygen of any of the cardiac tissues and is usually the chamber first affected by disruption of the internal myocardial blood supply.

Although it is a type of muscle tissue, myocardial tissue is different from the other two major types of muscle tissue found in the body both in structure and function. Striated or voluntary muscle tissue is found in the skeletal muscles, which are under direct control of the cerebrum of the brain. Smooth or involuntary muscle tissue is found in the internal organs of the body, as well as the blood vessels and such organs as the eyes. Smooth muscle tissue is controlled by the autonomic nervous system (ANS) in response to a variety of internal and external stimuli and is generally not under the control of the higher brain centers. Myocardial tissue, while it shares some of the involuntary properties of smooth muscle tissue and appears structurally similar to striated muscle, is unique and cannot be classified as either type.

One of the unique internal structures of myocardial tissues is an *intercalated disc*. In noncardiac muscle tissues, each individual muscle cell is surrounded by a cell membrane, which is of equal thickness all around. This cell membrane serves to insulate one cell from the next so that each fiber must receive a separate electrical innervation from a separate branch of a motor neuron to contract. Individual myocardial cells are also surrounded by a cell membrane. The myocardial cell membranes differ at the "ends" of the individual cells at the point where they come in contact with the next myocardial cell. At these points of contact, the cell membranes are much "thinner" than the membranes around the rest of the cell and do not act as an insulator to the conduction of electrical activity from one cell to the next. These contact points between the myocardial cells also form what is called a "tight junction," which increases the overall strength of the myocardium (Fig. 1-2). Under the microscope, these junctions between the muscle cells appear as dark lines or discs, hence the name, intercalated discs.

The *endocardium* is the third layer of tissue found in the heart. It is a thin connective tissue that lines the chambers of the heart and provides a smooth surface for the blood to pass over as it is pumped through the heart. It is continuous with the internal linings of the blood vessels and prevents clot formation in the heart.

PROPERTIES OF THE MYOCARDIUM

The myocardium has some unique properties and also shares some properties with other types of muscle tissue.

FIG. 1–2. CARDIAC MUSCLE TISSUE STRUCTURE
AND INTERCALATED DISCS.

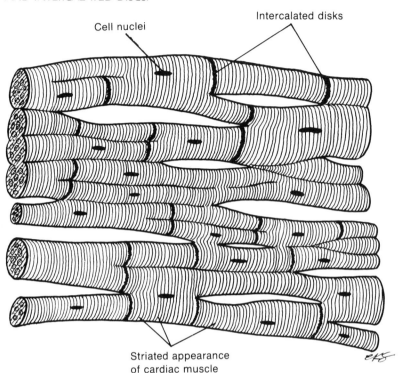

Cell nuclei

Intercalated disks

Striated appearance
of cardiac muscle
fibers

UNIQUE PROPERTIES OF MYOCARDIAL MUSCLE TISSUE

Automaticity is a unique property of cardiac muscle tissue that allows it to initiate an impulse without any external source of stimulation. This property is due, in part, to the relatively high degree of permeability of the cardiac cell membranes to potassium and sodium ions. When the concentration of these ions reaches a certain level, which varies from one part of the heart to another, a depolarizing impulse will automatically be initiated. Any part of the heart is capable of initiating an impulse except the atrioventricular (AV) node.

Rhythmicity is a unique property of cardiac muscle tissue that allows impulses to be formed at regular intervals. Again, this property is due to the permeability of the cell membranes.

A long refractory period in relation to other types of muscle tissue is an important property of cardiac muscle tissue. A long refractory period requires that the myocardial tissue recover completely before it contracts again. This property prevents the myocardium from going into spasm and also allows for filling of the chambers before the next contraction.

PROPERTIES MYOCARDIAL TISSUE SHARES
WITH OTHER TYPES OF TISSUE

Conductivity is a property that myocardial muscle tissue shares with nervous tissue. Once electrical impulses are initiated at any place in the myocardium, they travel quickly through the rest of the myocardium. The intercalated discs are the primary reason conductivity occurs. The rate of conduction in myocardial tissue is slower than what is found in the neurons because the myocardial tissue not only conducts but also contracts.

All-or-none response is a type of response to electrical stimulation in which all the cells respond completely or they do not respond at all. This property is also found in neurons. The all-or-none response causes the heart to contract as a unit, almost as a single cell, when it is stimulated. This unified contracting action produces the force and motion necessary to pump blood through the vascular system.

Contractility is a type of muscular activity that the myocardial tissues share with smooth muscle tissue, particularly smooth muscle tissue in the gastrointestinal tract. Because of the circular arrangement of the cardiac muscle tissue, when it contracts, it reduces the internal volume of the heart chambers and increases the pressure inside of the particular chamber that is being affected. This contracting action produces the pumping effect of the heart. To increase the strength of contraction, the cardiac muscle fibers must shorten even more, which reduces the internal volume so that more blood is pumped out under higher pressure.

In the normal, healthy adult heart functioning at rest, only about 70% of the total capacity of the heart is being used. A reserve capacity of about 30% remains. The heart can be made to contract more strongly through the effect of hormones, such as epinephrine and thyroxine. Increased physical activity will also increase the heart rate and allow for use of its reserve capacity. The hearts of infants and very young children function at near 100% capacity all the time so that they have little reserve capacity. Elderly patients also lose some of their cardiac reserve capacity as they age. This loss makes them less able to tolerate stressors that might increase demands on their hearts.

Excitability is a property of myocardial tissue that is shared with most other types of tissues in the body. Excitability is the ability of the heart to respond to outside stimuli. Not only can the heart initiate impulses internally on its own (automaticity), but it is affected by a number of neurotransmitters, hormones, and medications. The ANS and adrenal medulla produce the hormones epinephrine and norepinephrine that cause the heart to contract more strongly and at a faster rate (Table 1-1).

Hormones, such as thyroid hormone and growth hormone, also have an effect on the heart. A variety of medications can be used that will speed up the heart rate (*e.g.*, dopamine, atropine, aramine, and isoproterenol) or slow it down (*e.g.*, morphine sulfate, diazepam, and verapamil), increase the force of contraction (*e.g.*, digoxin, dobutamine, and glucagon) or decrease the force of contraction (*e.g.*, propranolol, diltiazem, and nifedipine).

The excitability of the heart can also be increased from internal damage to the myocardial cells from conditions such as myocardial infarction or hypoxic states from severe chronic obstructive pulmonary disease. This increased internal excitability of the myocardial tissue is often referred to as "irritability" and is a major cause of premature ectopic beats.

TABLE 1–1. SYMPATHETIC VERSUS PARASYMPATHETIC AUTONOMIC NERVOUS SYSTEM EFFECTS ON THE HEART

	Sympathetic (Adrenergic)	Parasympathetic (Cholinergic)
Neurotransmitters	Epinephrine Norepinephrine	Acetylcholine
Fibers		
Called:	Accelerators	Inhibitors
Origin	Superior, middle and inferior cervical ganglia	Cranial nerves and spinal nerve roots (Vagus nerve [Cranial Nerve X] is the primary branch)
Major Effects on the Heart	Affects all parts of heart—atria and ventricles	Affects primarily the right atrium, especially the sinus node and the AV node
Specific Effects		
Automaticity and Rate	Increases	Decreases
Contractility and		
Cardiac Output	Increases	Decreases
Conduction Rate	Increases	Decreases
Excitability	Increases	Decreases
Coronary Blood Vessels	Dilates	Constricts

Myocardial tissue *does not regenerate* once it is damaged. This property is shared with many other types of tissues in the body. If an area of the myocardium becomes necrotic from a myocardial infarction, that area goes through a 4- to 6-week healing process where it eventually becomes connective or scar tissue and never functions as cardiac tissue again. The electrical activity through this area of damaged tissues is altered and can be detected on an ECG. The 12 lead ECG is most effective for locating a particular area of damage. In the healing process, the damaged cells become more permeable to sodium and potassium ions with an increased internal excitability or irritability. Ectopic beats and rhythms are not uncommon during the first days after a myocardial infarction.

BLOOD SUPPLY TO THE HEART

The heart needs its own circulatory system to supply it with nutrients and oxygen. All the blood that passes through the heart daily provides little or no nourishment to the muscle layers of the heart. The coronary artery circulation provides this necessary blood supply to the myocardial tissues.

Keep in mind also that the heart is the organ in the body most sensitive to oxygen. The heart uses approximately 70% of the oxygen delivered to it through the coronary artery system; such organs as the brain, liver, and kidneys use only about 40% of the oxygen delivered to them. The coronary artery system receives its blood supply while the heart is in diastole (the resting or noncontraction phase of the cardiac cycle). Diastole is the part of the cycle that becomes proportionally shorter when the heart rate increases. If the heart rate is very fast, the coronary artery system does not have time to "fill" adequately and the heart will become hypoxic. One of the most common and earliest symptoms of low oxygen supply to the heart is the feeling of pressure or pain in the anterior chest.

The coronary artery system of the heart varies somewhat from individual to individual. While most individuals have the major subdivisions that are characteristic of the coronary artery system, as they subdivide, the variations increase. Detailed knowledge of the coronary artery system is not necessary for learning ECG analysis and interpretation; the following general information is presented about this system.

There are two main coronary arteries, which are the first vessels that branch off from the aorta near the aortic valve of the heart.

The right coronary artery divides into: (1) the posterior descending artery, which supplies the right atrium, the anterior wall of the right ventricle, and the posterior wall of the left ventricle; and (2) the marginal artery, which supplies the right ventricle and the right atrium including the sinoatrial (SA) node (in 55% of persons) and AV node (in 90% of persons).

The left coronary artery divides into: (1) the anterior descending and diagonal arteries, which supply the anterior wall of the left ventricle and the ventricular septum; and (2) the circumflex artery, which supplies the left atrium and the lateral and posterior walls of the left ventricle, the SA node (in 45% of persons), and the AV node (in 10% of persons).

The coronary artery system overlaps in its circulation of blood to the myocardial tissues. The left ventricle normally receives a rich supply of blood because of the work it does.

CONDUCTION SYSTEM OF THE HEART

The electrical conduction system of the heart (Fig. 1-3) is the most important aspect of the heart's anatomy and physiology to master when learning the analysis and interpretation of the ECG. The ECG supplies information about how well the conduction system of the heart is functioning. All of the dysrhythmias, conduction abnormalities, and ectopic beats are directly related to one or more of the parts of the cardiac conduction system. The identification and classification of the various dysrhythmias are organized around the specific part of the conduction system that is affected.

The cardiac conduction system is composed of myocardial tissue, which has become specialized so that its primary function is to conduct rather than to contract. In the rest of the body, the neurons serve the conduction function. The modified myocardial tissue in the conduction system of the heart has two important advantages over nervous tissue. First, the conduction rate is slower than the conduction rate of the neurons. This slower rate permits the heart to function as two separate pumps: one for the atria and one for the ventricles. Second, the recovery rate or refractory period of myocardial conduction tissue is much longer than neurons. This prevents spasms of the myocardial muscle tissue

FIG. 1–3. CONDUCTION SYSTEM OF THE HEART.

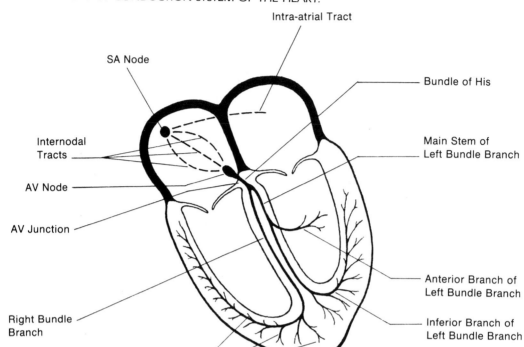

and permits a longer rest period between contractions so the muscle tissue can recover and the chambers can fill.

The following presentation of the conduction system of the heart follows the normal progression of impulses starting at the beginning and following the conduction system through the heart. The dysrhythmias presented later also follow this format because it seems the most logical way to approach abnormalities in the conduction system. Becoming familiar with the conduction system of the heart in sequence will help the reader master the analysis and interpretation of dysrhythmias.

SINOATRIAL NODE

The sinoatrial node (also called the SA node, Keith-Flack node, sinus node, and physiological pacemaker of the heart) is a small concentration of modified myocardial tissue, located in a cavity or sinus in the right atrial epicardium near the opening of the superior vena cava. It has the fastest inherent rate of impulse production of any other part of the heart and functions to initiate the impulses that depolarize the rest of the heart and produce contraction. It has an inherent rate of 60–100 beats per minute (BPM) in the adult. It is also affected by certain hormones that the body produces, as well as both branches of the ANS.

The SA node is an extremely reliable and regular pacemaker most of the time. It can be affected by internal conditions in the heart when abnormal contraction rates produced in other parts of the heart exceed the inherent rate of the SA node. The SA node's tendency is to stop producing impulses when the ectopic rate is faster than its normal inherent rate.

INTERNODAL TRACTS

While some experts deny that the internodal tracts (also called internodal pathways) exist as a separate part of the conduction system of the heart, there is enough evidence to identify at least three of these tracts. They are simply named: (1) anterior (superior) internodal tract; (2) middle internodal tract; and (3) posterior (inferior) internodal tract.

Their main function is to carry impulses from the SA node through the right atrium to the AV node. As the impulses pass along the internodal tracts, the right atrium usually contracts, pushing the blood it contains through the tricuspid valve into the right ventricle.

INTRA-ATRIAL TRACT

The intra-atrial tract (also called Bachman's Bundle) carries the impulse initiated by the SA node to the left atrium. This impulse then spreads through the muscle cells of the left atrium, usually resulting in contraction. The blood contained in the left atrium is pushed through the mitral valve into the left ventricle.

Any part of the conduction system of the atria as well as any part of the atrial muscle tissues has the ability to initiate impulses. These impulses can be initiated when the SA node fails to fire, in which case the atria act as a backup pacemaker. The inherent rate of the atria is very close to that of the SA node, usually between 60 and 80 BPM. The different form of the P waves can sometimes be used to determine when the atria are acting as a backup pacemaker site. More often, the atria become irritable and produce premature or fast rates that take over the pacemaker function from the SA node.

AV NODE

The AV node (also called atrioventricular node, and node of Tawara) (Fig. 1-4) is a relatively large bundle of modified myocardial conduction tissue located in the lower part of the right atrium near the intra-atrial septum. The AV node is connected to the SA node by the internodal tracts and receives the impulses from the SA node through these tracts. The AV node is a unique structure in the conduction system of the heart because of its internal structure. It contains two separate pathways, which have different internal conduction and recovery rates. The beta pathway has the fastest conduction rate and is the one through which the impulses normally travel. The alpha pathway has a slower conduction rate, although its recovery rate is somewhat faster than the beta pathway, and the impulses generally are prevented from passing through it. In the event of damage to the beta pathway, the alpha pathway would function as a backup to conduct the impulses to the ventricles.

The AV node serves two important functions. First, it delays the impulses

FIG. 1–4. STRUCTURE OF THE AV NODE, AV JUNCTION, AND THREE PARTS OF THE LEFT BUNDLE BRANCH.

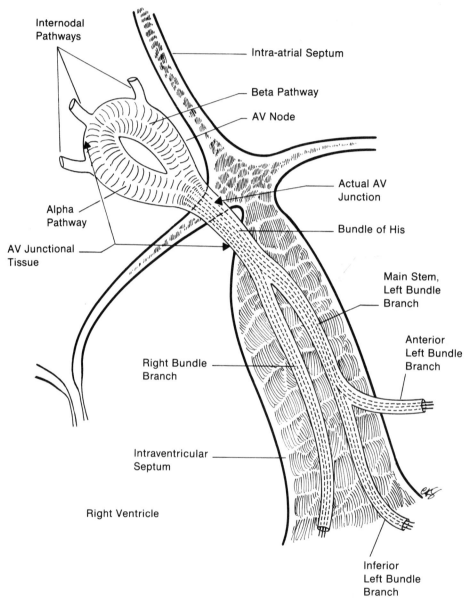

Internodal Pathways

Intra-atrial Septum

Beta Pathway

AV Node

Actual AV Junction

Alpha Pathway

Bundle of His

AV Junctional Tissue

Main Stem, Left Bundle Branch

Anterior Left Bundle Branch

Right Bundle Branch

Intraventricular Septum

Right Ventricle

Inferior Left Bundle Branch

from the SA node and atria for a fraction of a second (usually between 0.08 and 0.12 second). This delay permits the atria to complete their contraction and empty completely, thus, filling the ventricles. The ventricles will fill from 80% to 90% by themselves due to passive filling. The atria provide what is sometimes known as the "atrial kick," which finishes the filling process. Most individuals who have a healthy heart will not miss the 10% to 20% that comprise the atrial kick. Individuals who have a decreased CO caused by cardiac disease or injury will notice the lack of the atrial kick immediately because of a sudden drop in the blood pressure and a corresponding increase in heart rate. Certain dysrhythmias discussed below prevent the atria from emptying completely.

The second important function of the AV node is to prevent extra beats from being conducted to the ventricles. The atria, because of their smaller muscle mass and somewhat different structure, are capable of contracting up to 400 or more times per minute. The ventricles with their larger muscle mass and different arrangement of myocardium usually "top out" at approximately 250 contractions per minute. Because of the AV node's unique cell structure, it will prevent or filter out excessive atrial impulses from reaching the ventricles.

The AV node is the only part of the heart that cannot initiate impulses. For a long time, it was thought that the AV node did have this ability, but recent microelectrocardiology studies, which place extremely small electrodes in the various parts of the conduction system, have shown that the AV node cannot initiate impulses that will depolarize the rest of the heart.

AV JUNCTION

Some authors believe the structure called the AV junction (also called the atrioventricular junction, and junctional tissue; see Fig. 1-4) should include the AV node. However, the fibers immediately below the AV node and the bundle of His to the point of bifurcation of the bundle branches, the junction tissue where the atria join with the ventricles, is the actual AV junction. This part of the conduction system of the heart is composed of parallel tracts of modified myocardial conductive tissue, which primarily serves to carry impulses rapidly from the AV node to the lower conduction system of the ventricles.

Another main function of the AV junction is to serve as a backup pacemaker should the SA node or atria fail to initiate an impulse. As a backup pacemaker site, the AV junction produces regular impulses at a slower rate than the SA node. The usual rate for the AV junction is between 40 and 60 BPM. The AV junction is less reliable than the SA node in the production of impulses and has a tendency to just stop producing impulses at some point.

BUNDLE OF HIS

The bundle of His (pronounced "hiss"; also called atrioventricular bundle, and AV bundle) is a continuation of the AV junction. Located in the top left corner of the right ventricle and top of the intraventricular septum, it is composed of parallel tracts of specialized myocardial tissue. Its main function is to carry the impulses from the AV junction rapidly to the lower conduction system of the ventricles.

RIGHT BUNDLE BRANCH

The right bundle branch (RBB) is one of the major bifurcations or divisions of the bundle of His. Composed of parallel tracts of specialized myocardial tissue, it runs down the right side of the intraventricular septum and is responsible for conducting the depolarizing impulses to the muscle tissue in the right ventricle. Compared to the left bundle branch, it is relatively long and narrow and normally has a slightly longer repolarization time than the left bundle branch. In a normally functioning heart at a normal rate, this slight difference in repolarization times does not produce any noticeable changes in the ECG pattern.

LEFT BUNDLE BRANCH

The left bundle branch (LBB) is the second major bifurcation of the bundle of His. It is almost identical in structure to the right bundle branch except that it is a little thicker and slightly shorter. The LBB actually contains three separate parts (see Fig. 1-4).

The main stem LBB is that part of the LBB that bifurcates from the bundle of His. It is very short and soon divides into the other two parts of the LBB. It is located in the top portion of the intraventricular septum and carries impulses from the AV junction to the lower conduction system of the left ventricle.

The anterior (or superior) branch of the LBB is the portion of the LBB that divides from the main stem LBB and runs down the left side of the intraventricular septum and across the upper portion of the left ventricle. This branch terminates in the left ventricular anterior, superior papillary muscle and has only one artery to supply it blood. Its function is to carry the impulses from the main stem LBB to the upper portion of the left ventricle.

The posterior (or inferior) branch of the LBB is the portion of the LBB that divides from the main stem LBB and runs down the left side of the intraventricular septum and across the lower portion of the left ventricle, terminating in the left ventricular inferior, posterior papillary muscle. This branch has a dual blood supply. It functions to carry impulses from the main stem LBB to the lower portion of the left ventricle. It is somewhat longer and thicker than the anterior portion of the LBB.

PURKINJE FIBERS

As both the right and left bundle branches subdivide into smaller and smaller fibers, spreading out across their respective ventricles, they eventually become very fine threadlike bundles of specialized myocardial tissue called the Purkinje fibers (also called the Purkinje system). The Purkinje fibers distribute the electrical impulse from the bundle branches to the individual muscle fibers of the heart. These fibers form the last part of the efficient conduction system of the ventricles. Impulses, once they have passed the AV node, travel rapidly through the ventricular conduction system and produce a very rapid contraction of the ventricles.

Any part of the Purkinje system, as well as any part of the ventricles themselves, can serve as a backup pacemaker should the higher pacemakers fail. Purkinje or ventricular pacemaker sites tend to be less regular and much less reliable than the higher pacemaker sites. The rate is also markedly reduced, with a normal range of between 20 and 40 BPM for these sites. These lower pacemaker sites also produce an abnormal contraction pattern of the ventricles that further reduces the CO. Purkinje and ventricular sites that are functioning as backup pacemaker sites often do not produce enough systemic circulation to keep the brain and other vital organs adequately perfused.

INHERENT RATES OF CONDUCTION FOR THE VARIOUS PARTS OF THE HEART

The heart lacks the large reserve capacity that other organs of the body, such as the lungs, brain, and liver, have that are critical for the maintenance of life. The heart does have a small reserve capacity, but its chief mechanism of defense is its backup pacemaker sites that allow it to continue to initiate impulses and contract even though severely damaged by disease or injury. To summarize backup pacemaker sites and their inherent rates:

1. SA node: 60–100 BPM
2. Atrial sites: 60–80 BPM
3. AV junction: 40–60 BPM
4. Ventricular sites (Purkinje system): 20–40 BPM

POLARIZATION/DEPOLARIZATION/ REPOLARIZATION

The ECG is designed to measure electrical activity in the heart. The electrical activity of the myocardial cells is the result of a complex electrochemical reaction that occurs in each fiber of the myocardium. The small electrical changes that occur in the individual myocardial fibers are not detectable on the ECG. However, when the millions of fibers of the heart react electrically to an impulse, a wave of electrical energy is created that can be detected by ECG equipment. This electrical activity produces the characteristic wave forms known as the *ECG pattern.*

While the actual production of electrical activity in the myocardial cells is a complex process involving a multitude of actions and reactions, the underlying principles are relatively easy to understand. The entire cycle that produces the contraction of myocardial tissue can be divided into three distinct phases of electrochemical activity. These three phases are the polarization phase, the depolarization phase, and the repolarization phase (Fig. 1-5).

POLARIZATION PHASE

In the polarization stage (also called the resting phase), the individual cells of the myocardium are ready to contract. The SA node in the polarization phase is ready to initiate the impulse. It is called polarization because the electrical charges associated with the cell membrane are separated into a positive pole and a negative pole. This difference in electrical charges is due to the various ions that arrange themselves both inside and outside of the cell. Ions are elements that have either a positive or negative electrical charge.

FIG. 1–5. THE REFRACTORY PERIODS IN RELATIONSHIP TO POLARIZATION/DEPOLARIZATION/REPOLARIZATION.

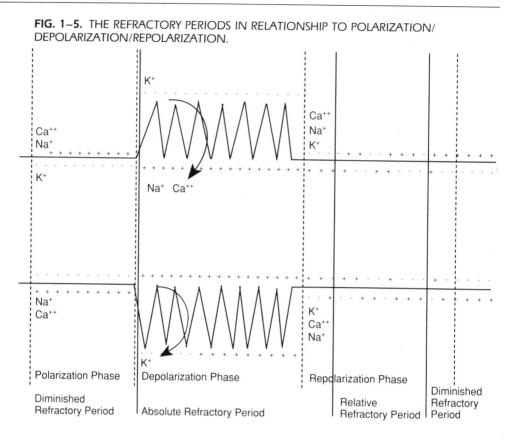

The primary extracellular ions, sodium and calcium, have a strong positive charge. The primary intracellular ion, potassium, has a relative weak positive electrical charge. This difference in the strength of the electrical charges creates a positive charge along the outside of the cell membrane and negative charge along the inside of the cell membrane. Nature will always attempt to balance polarized electrical charges so that an active mechanism must be present to create the electrical imbalance found along the cell membrane in the polarization phase. The mechanism that maintains the separation of the electrical charges along the cell membrane goes by several names but is generally referred to as the sodium pump, the sodium–potassium pump, or simply the cell membrane pump. Since this pump mechanism is fighting the tendency of nature to balance charges, it requires the use of a relatively high level of energy to maintain the separation of the charges.

The electrical charges gradually build up, and, at some point, the separation of the charges can no longer be maintained by the pump mechanism. The cell membranes of the myocardial cells play an important part in this process because they are more permeable to sodium and potassium ions than most other cell membranes in the body. This permeability to the various ions also produces the properties of automaticity and rhythmicity that are found in myocardial cells. When the polarization or separation of charges can no longer be maintained, the next phase in the process begins: depolarization.

DEPOLARIZATION PHASE

The depolarization phase is also called the discharge phase, action phase, contraction phase, and ventricular systole. During the depolarization phase, a major shift in the ion concentrations occurs across the cell membranes. The sodium ions quickly rush across the cell membrane into the cell, followed later by the slower calcium ions. These strongly charged positive ions displace and push the more weakly charged potassium ions out of the cell, so that the polarity of the cell actually reverses during this phase. The negative charge is now along the outside of the cell membrane and the positive charge is on the inside of the cell membrane.

Once the depolarization phase begins in one part of the heart, it is spread as a wave of electrical energy (wave of depolarization) to all other parts of the heart through the close contact between the individual cells from the presence of the intercalated discs. The depolarization of the heart occurs most quickly and efficiently if it follows the normal conduction system of the heart from the SA node down through the ventricles. When the depolarizing currents do not follow the normal conduction pathways or are initiated in an area of the heart other than the SA node, they travel more slowly and in an abnormal pattern, but they will eventually reach all parts of the heart and produce depolarization. This abnormal depolarization is detectable on the ECG.

In the modified myocardial cells of the conduction system of the heart, the depolarization process either initiates the impulse, especially in the SA node, or produces conduction of the impulse through the various parts of the conduction system of the heart. In the muscle fibers of the myocardium, the depolarization process results in shortening of the fibers and produces contraction of the various chambers of the heart. This contraction rapidly increases the pressure in the chambers, forcing the blood out and producing systole. There is a great deal of electrical activity being generated in the heart during the depolarization phase, and this electrical activity produces the characteristic wave forms found on the ECG. Because virtually all the myocardial tissue is involved in the depolarization process, a great deal of oxygen is required by the heart, making it very sensitive to decreases in the oxygen supplied by the coronary artery system.

REPOLARIZATION PHASE

Before depolarization of the cell can occur again, it must return to the polarization phase of the cycle. This intermediate phase between depolarization and polarization is called repolarization (also called recovery phase, and diastole). The sodium pump mechanism is important during the repolarization phase because it must pump out the sodium and calcium ions that have entered the cell during the depolarization phase and pump in the potassium ions to the inside of the cell so the electrical charge across the cell membrane is re-established. If repolarization does not occur, there can be no further depolarization in the cells.

In the early stages of repolarization, there is a mix of positive and negative charges along the cell membrane as the sodium and calcium ions begin to leave the cell and the potassium ions begin to return inside the cell. Gradually, the charges become more and more like they are in the polarization phase until they are again aligned in the outside positive and inside negative configuration. Rather than just ending, as the polarization phase does when the depolarization phase starts, the repolarization phase gradually progresses until at some point it blends into the polarization phase.

During the repolarization phase, the muscle fibers of the myocardium are relaxing and the individual fibers are lengthening so that they return to their precontraction state. Because this relaxation process decreases the pressure inside the vascular system of the body as well and allows the chambers of the heart to fill, it is referred to as diastole. The repolarization phase is also detectable on the ECG since there is electrical activity occurring.

REFRACTORY PERIODS OF THE CARDIAC CYCLE

Although a discussion of the various refractory periods of the heart in relationship to the ECG pattern will be presented in Chapter 2, it is important to understand the refractory period as it relates to the cellular activity of the heart (Fig. 1-5).

The term *refractory* is a general term that simply means resistant to change. When it is used in reference to the myocardial cells, it means resistant to depolarization of the cells. There are three refractory periods that more or less correspond to the three phases of the cardiac cycle: the absolute refractory period, the relative refractory period, and the diminished refractory period.

THE ABSOLUTE REFRACTORY PERIOD

The absolute refractory period (ARP) refers to that phase of the cardiac cycle during which no further depolarization can take place. No matter how strong a stimulus occurs during the absolute refractory period, the cardiac cells are not able to respond. The absolute refractory period starts at the beginning of the depolarization phase and extends into the very early part of the repolarization phase. Simply stated, while the myocardial cells are in a state of depolarization, they are unable to either depolarize again or to sustain a prolonged state of depolarization.

THE RELATIVE REFRACTORY PERIOD

The relative refractory period (RRP) refers to that phase of the cardiac cycle during which depolarization can occur if there is a strong enough stimulus. The relative refractory period is a small part of the cardiac cycle, which lasts from the early part to the middle part of the repolarization phase. The relative refractory period is a dangerous part of the cardiac cycle. During the relative refractory period, some of the myocardial cells are repolarized while other cells are still in various states of depolarization. A strong external stimulus, such as an electrical shock or blow to the chest, or a strong internal stimulus, such as an impulse discharged from a ventricular site occurring during the relative refractory period, can produce abnormal myocardial activity. The myocardial fibers that are already repolarized will depolarize again in response to this stimulus while the fibers that are still in depolarization from the previous impulse will not depolarize again. This type of sporadic depolarization of the myocardial fibers produces either a quivering of the cardiac muscle tissue or an abnormal rapid repeating depolarization of the ventricles effectively stopping all CO.

THE DIMINISHED REFRACTORY PERIOD

The diminished refractory period (DRP) refers to the phase of the cardiac cycle during which the myocardial cells are still resistant but depolarization can occur even with a relatively weak stimulus. The diminished refractory period is the largest portion of the cardiac cycle, beginning near the middle of the repolarization phase and extending through the polarization phase to the beginning of depolarization. During the diminished refractory period, the majority of the myocardial cells are repolarized so a stimulus that occurs at this time produces a unified depolarization and contraction of the heart. The contraction is premature because it occurs early in the cycle; most likely, it is abnormal in configuration because it is probably not following the normal conduction pathways through the heart. The CO produced by this type of depolarization is also less than normal because the chambers of the heart have not had enough time to fill completely.

EFFECTS OF THE AUTONOMIC NERVOUS SYSTEM ON CARDIAC FUNCTION

The ANS is the subdivision of the efferent nervous system that is responsible for the functions of the body that are generally not under the control of the cerebral cortex. The ANS carries impulses from the central nervous system to the smooth (involuntary) muscles of internal organs, blood vessels, and so on, to the various glands of the endocrine system, to organs such as the liver and pancreas, and to the cardiac tissues. The ANS is complex and affects all parts of the body in one way or another. Its control centers are located in the brain stem and the normal functioning of the ANS is absolutely necessary for the maintenance of life.

The ANS is divided into the sympathetic (adrenergic) system and the parasympathetic (cholinergic) system. These two systems have somewhat different effects on different parts of the body, depending on which system is dominant at a given time. In the heart, the effects of the ANS are very specific (Table 1-1). Normally, the sympathetic and parasympathetic systems tend to oppose each other to produce a homeostatic balance in the body in general and the heart in particular. In the heart, too much of one or too little of the other can produce dysrhythmias (Fig. 1-6).

The sympathetic system (also called the adrenergic system, thoracolumbar system, or activity responsive system) is responsible for increasing the activity of the heart. This system is one of the key protective systems of the body, which prepares it to respond to a variety of stressors ranging from fear and anxiety to major trauma or disease states. Stimulation of the sympathetic system can also be produced by a variety of medications. Suppression of the sympathetic system through medication therapy or severe brain stem injury has a tendency to slow the rate of the heart as well as reduce the blood pressure.

The fibers of the sympathetic system originate in the superior, middle, and inferior cervical ganglia. These sympathetic fibers are known as the *accelerator* fibers and are widely distributed through the atria and ventricles of the heart. The primary neurotransmitters of the sympathetic system are epinephrine and norepinephrine. Some of the specific activities of the heart that the sympathetic system increases are: automaticity, contractility, conduction rate, excitability, and dilation of the coronary blood vessels.

FIG. 1–6. EFFECTS OF THE SYMPATHETIC AND PARASYMPATHETIC SYSTEMS ON HEART RATE.

Sympathetic   Parasympathetic

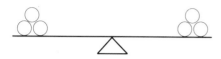

Balanced state = normal heart function (rate 60–100)

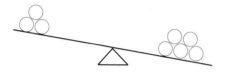

Too much parasympathetic = decreased heart function (Bradycardia—rate < 60)

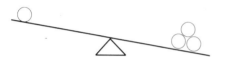

Not enough sympathetic = decreased heart function (Bradycardia—rate < 60)

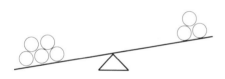

Too much sympathetic = increased heart function (Tachycardia—rate > 100)

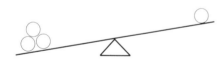

Not enough parasympathetic = increased heart function (Tachycardia—rate > 100)

AUTOMATICITY

One of the primary effects of epinephrine on the heart is to increase its automaticity which, in turn, increases its rate. A fast heart rate can be the result of increased sympathetic stimulation in the body, as well as suppression of the parasympathetic without any change in the sympathetic.

CONTRACTILITY

Not only will the heart beat faster, but its fibers will also shorten more during each contraction when the sympathetic system is stimulated. The end result of this extra shortening of the cardiac muscle fibers is that there is an increase in the force of contraction. As noted above, CO is a result of the heart rate and the force of contraction. When both elements are increased, the CO increases markedly.

CONDUCTION RATE

Although the determination of the rate of the cardiac cycle is primarily a function of the shortening of the diastolic or resting phase between the beats, in the presence of sympathetic stimulation, the rate at which the impulses are conducted from the SA node through the conduction system of the heart will also increase slightly. This increased conduction rate contributes both to an increase in the heart rate and an increase in the force of contraction.

EXCITABILITY

One effect of the epinephrine released from the sympathetic system on the cardiac tissues is to make it more sensitive to all types of stimuli. There is an increased sensitivity to outside stimuli (excitability), as well as an increase to internal stimuli (irritability). The net effect of this increased sensitivity is a tendency for premature ectopic beats.

DILATION OF THE CORONARY BLOOD VESSELS

Although epinephrine tends to constrict systemic arterioles to help in the control of bleeding when trauma occurs, it will cause an increase in the diameter of the coronary blood vessels at the same time. This increase in blood vessel size produces an increased blood flow to the cardiac muscle tissues to meet the increased demands for oxygen from the increased rate and force of contraction. Epinephrine also dilates other large blood vessels of the central circulatory system, increasing the blood supply to key organs such as the brain, liver, and pancreas. The net effect of the vascular changes is to increase the systemic blood pressure.

The parasympathetic system (also known as the cholinergic system, craniosacral system, or vegetative-homeostatic system) is responsible for reducing the activity of the heart in the absence of stressors. This system is important for maintaining the dynamic balance in the body that allows for normal growth, cell regeneration, digestion of food, and nourishment of the cells.

The main nervous fiber of the parasympathetic system is the vagus nerve (cranial nerve X). The primary neurotransmitter is acetylcholine. The vagus nerve is very long and is in contact through its branches with most of the internal organs, including the lungs, liver, kidneys, esophagus, stomach, intestines, rectum, and heart. The vagus nerve is known as the *inhibitory* nerve since it tends to slow the heart. Its effects are more localized and more discrete than the effects of the sympathetic system. In the heart, the parasympathetic system through the branches of the vagus nerve, is in contact primarily with the right atrium, in particular, the SA node and the AV node.

Stimulation anywhere along the vagus nerve (called vagal stimulation) has the potential to induce a reflex stimulation along the *whole* path of the vagus nerve.

In addition, sudden increases in blood pressure produces vagal stimulation. The effect on the heart of any type of vagal stimulation is a marked slowing of the rate. If the vagal stimulation is severe enough or for an extended period of time, the SA node may stop initiating impulses completely. If none of the backup pacemaker sites take over, then complete cardiac arrest is possible. Hearts that have been damaged through myocardial infarction or severe disease states are particularly sensitive to vagal stimulation.

The overall effect of the vagus nerve on the heart is to slow or reduce all those factors that the sympathetic system increased. This parasympathetic effect includes reducing automaticity, contractility, conduction rate, and irritability of the heart. The parasympathetic system also tends to constrict the coronary blood vessels, while dilating the systemic arteries to such organs as the stomach, intestines, and colon. Conversely, suppression of the parasympathetic system by medications or vagal suppression tends to increase the heart rate.

A variety of medications can be used to either increase or decrease both the sympathetic or parasympathetic systems. (see box, Medications That Affect the Autonomic Nervous System).

MEDICATIONS THAT AFFECT THE AUTONOMIC NERVOUS SYSTEM

Medications that Stimulate the Sympathetic System (Sympathetomimetics)

- Dobutamine hydrochloride (Dobutrex)*
- Dopamine hydrochloride (Intropin, Dopastat)*
- Epinephrine hydrochloride (Adrenalin)*
- Isoproterenol hydrochloride (Isuprel)*
- Norepinephrine [Levarterenol] (Levophed, Noradrenalin)*
- Ephedrine sulfate (Efedron)
- Metaproterenol sulfate (Alupent, Metaprel)
- Metaraminol bitartrate (Aramine)*
- Phenylephrine hydrochloride (Neo-synephrine)
- Ritodrine hydrochloride (Yutopar)

Medications that Suppress the Sympathetic System (Adrenergic Blocking Agents; Anti-adrenergics)

- Phentolamine mesylate (Regitine)*
- Metoprolol Tartrate (Lopressor, Betaloc)*
- Nadolol (Corgard)*
- Propanolol hydrochloride (Inderal)*
- Timolol maleate (Blocadren, Timoptic)
- Most narcotic agents and CNS depressant medications:
  Morphine sulfate
  Codeine
  Meperidine sulfate (Demerol)

(continued)

MEDICATIONS THAT AFFECT THE AUTONOMIC NERVOUS SYSTEM (*continued*)

Medications that Suppress the Sympathetic System (Adrenergic Blocking Agents; Anti-adrenergics)

Diazepam (Valium)
Chlordiazepoxide hydrochloride (Librium)

Medications that Stimulate the Parasympathetic System (Cholinergic Agents)

- Bethanechol chloride (Urecholine)
- Carbachol (Carbacel, Isopto)
- Metochlopramide hydrochloride (Reglan)
- Pilocarpine hydrochloride (Absorbocarpine, Pilocar)
- Edrophonium chloride (Tensilon)
- Neostigmine (Prostigmin)
- Pyridostigmine (Mestinon, Regonal)

Medications that Suppress the Parasympathetic System (Cholinergic Blocking Agents; Anticholinergic Agents)

- Atropine sulfate*
- Belladonna
- Benztropine mesylate (Cogentin)
- Glycopyrrolate (Robinul)
- Propantheline bromide (Pro-Banthine)
- Scopolamine hydrobromide
- Trihexyphenidyl hydrochloride (Artane)

* indicates medications used primarily for their cardiac and cardiovascular effects.

2

ECG BASICS

LEARNING OBJECTIVES

After studying this section, the learner will be able to:

1. Describe ECG paper and name the correct measurements of time and voltage as indicated by the ECG paper.
2. Identify the various parts of the ECG pattern.
3. Describe proper placement of ECG electrodes to achieve the best possible pattern.
4. Name the various leads that are used and describe the ECG patterns produced in each lead.
5. List the various types of artifact that can be produced on ECG tracings.

This chapter will provide basic information that forms building blocks to be used throughout the rest of the book. Spending extra time on this chapter will pay large dividends later in the analysis and interpretation of electrocardiogram (ECG) dysrhythmias.

ECG PATTERN

The ECG pattern is a result of the various electrical activities that take place in the heart during polarization, depolarization, and repolarization. The very small amount of electrical activity produced when the heart muscles depolarize and repolarize can be detected by sensitive monitoring equipment. A typical cardiac monitoring station consists of a bedside monitor, which is connected directly to the patient by wires; a central monitoring station, which is connected to the bedside monitor by a cable system of wires; and a recording machine, which is able to transfer the images produced on the monitor into a graphic representation. The monitor itself is a type of television set (also called an oscilloscope) that can convert the electrical activity in the heart into a displayed light pattern on the screen. Modern monitors are really computers that not only display the electrical activity in the heart on their screens but also process it in a number of ways.

ECG PAPER

The actual "hard" copy of the electrical activity in the heart (called the ECG tracing, ECG pattern, or just ECG) is made by the recording machine on a special type of heat-sensitive paper. The paper on which the tracing is recorded is called ECG paper. ECG paper is a type of graph paper composed of small square blocks and large square blocks (Fig. 2-1). The small blocks are 1 millimeter by 1 millimeter (1 mm^2 square). The large blocks are marked by a darker line and are 5 millimeters by 5 millimeters (5 mm^2 square) and contain 25 small blocks.

FIG. 2–1. ECG PAPER.

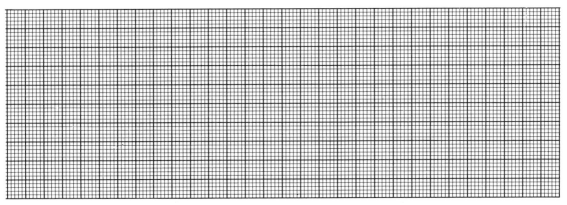

On standard ECG paper, each small block is 1 millimeter by 1 millimeter. The large blocks are 5 millimeters by 5 millimeters. (actual size)

Most standard ECG paper comes in rolls or packs. This paper is 50 mm high (50 small blocks or 10 large blocks) or about 2 inches high, and an undetermined length across. While it is unusual to find ECG paper that is higher than 50 mm, to save space, many types of portable monitoring systems and bed-side defibrillators use paper that is less than 50 mm high. Even if the paper is only 30 mm high, the size of the individual squares remains the same. ECG paper also comes in different colors depending on the manufacturer. Some of the common colors are grey, light green, and pink. The actual tracings produced on the paper are usually black or dark blue in color, which contrast with the background color of the paper.

Throughout the world, ECG paper is the same. The standard speed at which ECG paper is rolled out of the recording machine is 25 mm/sec (about 1 inch/sec). With some types of monitoring equipment, this speed can be increased to

50 mm/sec or slowed to 12.5 mm/sec. Any changes in the speed of the paper should be noted because it will change the basic pattern. Because it is difficult to handle very long rolls of ECG paper once they are out of the machine, the tracings produced on the paper are usually limited to shorter sections of ECG paper, from 6 to 12 inches long, that are called ECG strips.

The ECG paper measures the two elements of time and voltage. The horizontal plane of the paper measures time. Each small block on the horizontal plane or scale is equal to 0.04 second of time. Because the large blocks are five times the size of the small blocks, the large blocks are equal to $0.04 \times 5 = 0.20$ second. These are important measurements to learn because they will be used in all analyses of every ECG strip in this book (Fig. 2-2).

FIG. 2–2. TIME AND VOLTAGE MEASUREMENTS ON ECG PAPER.

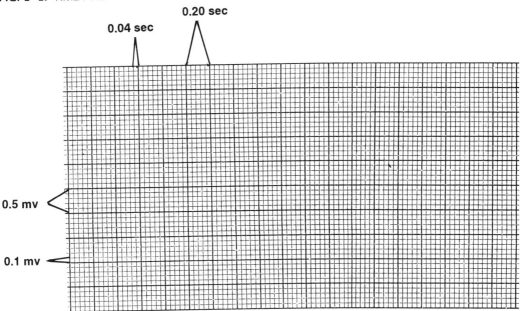

(strip two times normal size)

The vertical plane or scale of the ECG paper measures voltage. On single lead ECG strips, as are found in this book, this measurement is not as important as the time measurement since the size of the ECG pattern can be adjusted through a "gain" control on the monitor. In single lead ECG tracings, the size of the pattern is usually adjusted so that all the wave forms can be seen clearly. On standardized (to 1 millivolt or 10 mm) ECG tracing such as the 12 lead ECG that is used for diagnostic purposes, the measurement of the voltage of the complexes is more important. In general, it is the direction and magnitude of the electrical activity in the heart that determines the size of the pattern on the ECG paper. A strong electrical activity, such as the depolarization of the ventricles, will produce a very tall or large wave form. A weaker electrical activity, such as the depolarization of the atria, will produce a smaller wave form. No electrical activity at all will produce a straight line on the ECG paper.

Each small block on a standardized ECG in the vertical plane represents 0.1 millivolt (mv), which is an extremely small amount of electrical energy. A large block in the vertical plane represents 0.5 mv (0.1 mv × 5 = 0.5 mv). On a standardized 12 lead ECG, a standardization artifact (mark) of 1 mv (10 small blocks) is inserted during each lead change to help in the determination of the actual size of the patterns being produced (see Fig. 2-2).

ELECTRODES

Some method of detecting the small amounts of electrical energy produced in the heart and transferring that information to the ECG monitoring equipment is required to produce an ECG pattern. The most sensitive method of detecting cardiac electrical activity would be to insert wires directly into the myocardial tissue that would then be connected to the monitoring equipment.

Most external electrodes used today consist of a piece of some type of adhesive tape that has on its "sticky" side a small conductive jell pad. The reverse side of the tape has a small metal connector button that is in contact with the jelled pad and can be connected to the cable from the monitor (Fig. 2-3). The jelled pad is a good conductor of electrical activity and will easily pick up, through the skin of the chest wall or other locations in the body, the electrical activity produced by the heart.

Sometimes electrodes are referred to as leads. This is an inaccurate use of the term "lead." An electrode is a device that is in contact with the skin for the purpose of detecting and relaying information about the electrical activity in the heart to the monitoring equipment, whereas a lead is a particular arrangement of electrodes that produce a particular pattern on the ECG paper. Any time an electrode is moved from one location on the body to another, even if it is only a short distance, the monitoring lead will change to some degree. It is extremely important to notify whoever is watching the monitors that an electrode has been moved.

Without electrodes, there is no ECG pattern on the monitor. Certain actions can be taken to improve the contact of the electrode with the skin. These actions include the following:

1. Remove extra hair in the area where the electrode is to be placed. Hair not only interferes with the ability of the electrode to stick to the skin but also will keep the jelled pad away from the skin.
2. Cleanse the skin well. Oils on the skin, as well as dirt or perspiration, will prevent the electrode from sticking and will prevent good contact with the skin.
3. Abrade the skin. This action is an additional step in the cleansing of the skin. Many electrode manufacturers place a small piece of very fine sandpaper on one side of the electrode. Rubbing this sandpaper lightly on the skin will improve the conduction through the skin. Some caution should be taken in using this method. The jelled pads tend to be irritating and abrading the skin may increase the irritation. Abrading of the skin probably should only be used with individuals who have a tough outer layer of skin.

FIG. 2–3. ELECTRODE CARE.

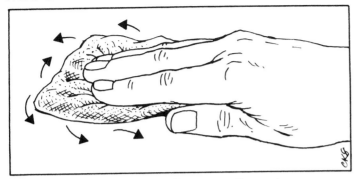

I   Clean skin well removing oils, sweat, dirt, and excess
hair. Clean an area slightly larger than the electrode.

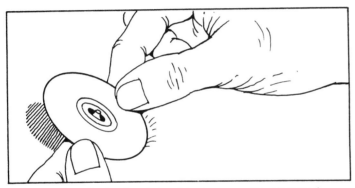

II   Place the electrode sticky side down on the cleansed
area, starting in on corner. Avoid touching the sticky side.

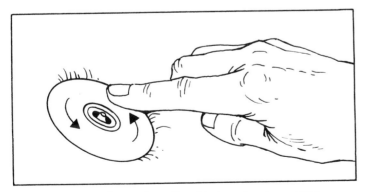

III   Smooth the electrode on the skin in a circular motion.
Make sure the saline pad is in good contact with the skin.
Connect the monitor wire to the center of the electrode.

4. Press the electrode on firmly. A firm, even pressure around the outer edge of the electrode will help it to adhere securely to the skin and optimize the contact area of the jelled pad.

5. Add a small amount of contact medium to the jelled pad. On occasion, the pads become dry even before they are used. Addition of a small dab of a saline-based contact medium, such as used with Doppler probe stethoscopes, will increase the conduction of the electrical impulses from the heart through the skin to the electrode. Given the option, it would probably be better to apply fresh pads that have fresh jell than to add jell to dry pads (see Fig. 2-3).

COMPONENTS OF THE ECG PATTERN

The ECG pattern is composed of components or parts that have very specific definitions to those who work with ECG patterns. The main components are: the baseline, the wave, the segment, the interval, and the complex.

THE BASELINE OR ISOELECTRIC LINE

The baseline (Fig. 2-4) is defined as the part of the ECG pattern that appears as a straight line and is between the wave forms of the ECG pattern. The baseline indicates that the electrical charges are balanced on each side of the line so it does not deflect in either direction.

FIG. 2–4. BASELINE (ISOELECTRIC LINE) ON THE ECG.

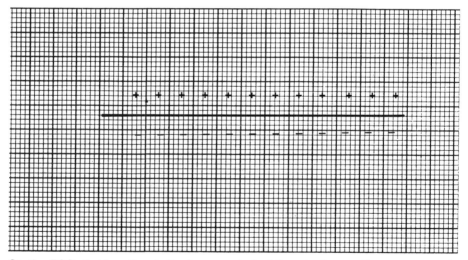

On the ECG, the baseline indicates a period of time in the cardiac cycle when the electrical charges are balanced against each other. The baseline is between wave forms and ECG patterns.

THE WAVE

A wave (Fig. 2-5) is defined as a positive (upward) or a negative (downward) deflection that generally begins at the baseline and ends at the baseline. A wave is an electrical representation of the depolarization of one of the large groups of cardiac muscle tissue in the heart, such as the atria or the ventricles. Waves can also represent repolarization of the chambers of the heart. Waves are named individually depending on their location.

FIG. 2–5. WAVE FORMS ON THE ECG.

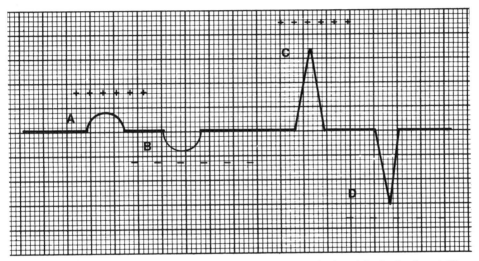

On the ECG, waves represent large changes in the electrical activity in the heart. They can be upright (positive) in their deflection as waves A and C, or downward (negative) in deflection, as waves B and D. They can also either be rounded (waves A and B) or peaked (waves C and D).

THE SEGMENT

The segment (Fig. 2-6) is defined as the length of baseline between two waves. It is usually named by the wave before it and the wave after it. For example, the ST segment is the section of baseline between the S wave and the T wave.

THE INTERVAL

In ECG terminology, an interval (Fig. 2-7) is either the length of a wave or the length of a wave with its following segment. It is named by the wave that begins it and the wave that ends it. For example, the PR interval is the distance covered by the P wave plus the interval that follows the P wave up to the point where the QRS complex begins.

FIG. 2–6. SEGMENT ON THE ECG.

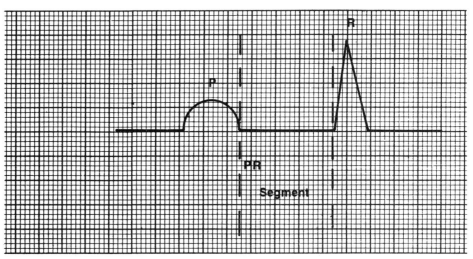

On the ECG, a segment is the short section of baseline between two waves. It is named by the wave before and the wave that ends it. In this example, the PR segment starts at the end of the P wave and ends at the beginning of the R wave.

FIG. 2–7. INTERVAL ON THE ECG.

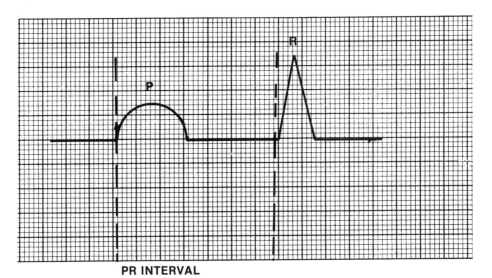

PR INTERVAL

On the ECG, an interval is the width of a wave plus the segment that follows it. It is named by the wave that begins it and the wave that terminates the segment. Occasionally, a wave will be so wide that there is no segment following it. In that case, the wave becomes the interval.

THE COMPLEX

The complex (Fig. 2-8) is a group of waves that follows one after the other without any segments or intervals between them. There is only one complex called the QRS complex. This complex is usually composed of three waves: the Q wave, the R wave, and the S wave.

FIG. 2–8. WAVE COMPLEX ON THE ECG.

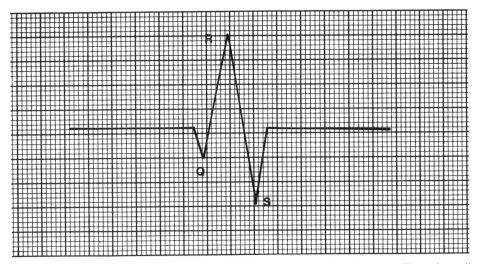

In general, a complex on the ECG is a group of waves together in a row. There is really only one complex that is considered on the ECG; that is the QRS complex. Even though all three wave forms may not be present, it is still referred to as the QRS complex.

THE LAW OF WAVE FORMATION ON THE ECG

As discussed above, the various phases of cardiac activity produce a measurable electric current, which can be detected and reproduced as the ECG pattern. The direction of the various wave forms is due to the placement of the positive and negative electrodes in relationship to the electrical flow in the heart. The usual flow of electrical activity in the heart is from the SA node in the superior right atrium downward toward the apex of the left ventricle. In the body, this current flow is from the right arm toward the left leg of the patient. The law of wave formation states that if the current flow in the heart is generally toward the positive electrode, the major wave form patterns produced on the ECG will be upright (or positive). Conversely, if the current flow in the heart is generally away from the positive (toward the negative) electrode, the primary wave forms produced will be downward (or negative) (Fig. 2-9).

FIG. 2–9. CURRENT FLOW IN THE HEART.

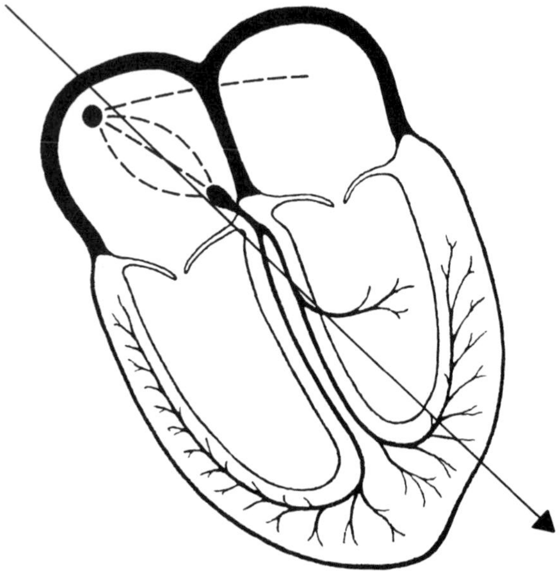

The normal current flow in the heart is along the conduction pathways from the sinoatrial node to the ventricles. This produces a normal direction (vector) of current flow from the upper right chest toward the left foot.

LEADS USED TO PRODUCE THE ECG PATTERN

As defined earlier in this chapter, a monitoring lead is a particular arrangement of the positive and negative electrodes that will produce a particular pattern on the ECG paper. To have a monitoring lead, a minimum of two electrodes, one positive and one negative, is required. Many monitoring systems may have as many as five electrodes, but only two of the five electrodes are being used at any given time in the formation of the ECG pattern on the monitor. Of the remaining three electrodes, one serves as a "ground" to help decrease the amount of electrical interference while the other two are inactive. The monitoring equipment can be made to switch between electrodes to produce different ECG patterns that will give different electrical views of the heart. In a 12 lead ECG, the chest or V leads require all the other leads to make the negative.

There are many different leads that can be used in assessing the electrical activity in a patient's heart. Although not absolutely essential for basic dysrhythmia analysis and interpretation, a knowledge of the locations of the electrode placement for the basic 12 lead ECG is useful in understanding how a diagnosis can be made from this test.

The 12 lead ECG actually "looks" at the heart electrically from two different planes in 12 different positions. Each one of these 12 positions will produce a different ECG pattern, depending on the relationship of the positive and negative electrodes to the flow of electrical activity in the heart.

The first 6 leads of the 12 lead ECG are called the *limb leads* and are named lead I, lead II, lead III, lead AVR, lead AVL, and lead AVF (Fig. 2-10). The electrodes on the limb leads are placed on the arms and legs and look at the heart along the right and left frontal (vertical) planes from the top to the bottom right and left. The positive and negative electrodes are moved in relationship to each other, depending on which lead is being assessed at the time.

FIG. 2–10. LOCATION AND NAMES OF THE LIMB LEADS.

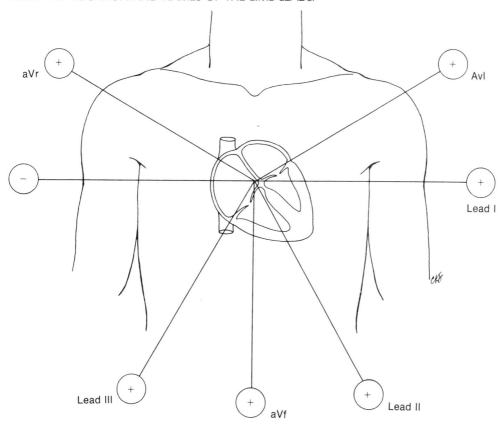

The second 6 leads in the 12 lead ECG are the *chest leads* and are placed on the chest of the patient in a semicircle around the heart. These leads are also called the "V leads" because of the way they are designated or named. The names of the chest leads are V_1, V_2, V_3, V_4, V_5, and V_6 (Fig. 2-11). The V leads look across the heart in the horizontal plane from the six positions indicated. With the 12 lead ECG, each one of the V positions is a positive electrode, while the center of the heart (AV node) acts as the negative electrode because it combines the RA, LA, and LL information.

Three other leads sometimes used for diagnostic purposes are the X, Y, and Z leads. The electrode placement for the X lead is the positive electrode at the left axilla and the negative electrode at the right axilla. The electrode placement for the Y lead is the positive electrode on the anterior lower chest in the midline and the negative electrode on the neck in the midline. The electrode placement for the Z lead is the positive electrode on the anterior chest, fifth intercostal space to the left of the sternum, and the negative electrode on the back to the left of the spine at the level of the heart (Fig. 2-12).

Although any of these leads may be used for monitoring purposes, the two primary leads in use in most hospitals today for continuous cardiac monitoring are lead II and lead MCL_1.

FIG. 2–11. LOCATION AND NAMES OF THE CHEST LEADS.

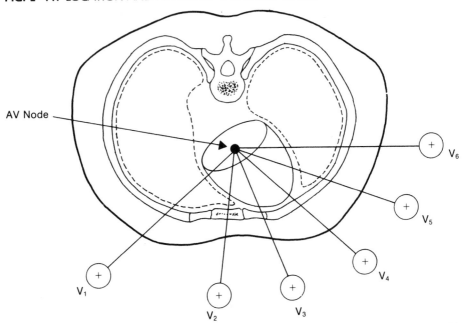

The chest leads look at the heart electrically in a cross section. Each lead is a positive electrode with the center of the heart acting as the negative electrode.

Lead II, which produces a pattern essentially identical to limb lead II, was the earliest and most commonly used lead for monitoring. The electrode placement in lead II is the positive electrode on the lower extreme left side of the left chest and the negative electrode on the second intercostal space in the midline of the upper right chest. In this particular configuration, the electrical current in the heart flows from the negative electrode directly toward the positive electrode. In accordance with the law of ECG wave formation, in lead II, most wave forms of the ECG pattern are upright. The ECG pattern produced in lead II is the "classical ECG pattern" demonstrated in most ECG books (Fig. 2-13).

The monitoring lead MCL_1 has gained much popularity during recent years and is now the most common long-term monitoring lead used by hospitals. The MCL_1 lead most closely approximates the ECG pattern produced by the chest lead V_1. The electrode placement is a positive electrode at the fourth intercostal space just to the right of the sternum and the negative electrode at the second intercostal space midline on the upper left chest or the outer third of the left clavicle preferably on the back.

The designation MCL_1 stands for modified chest lead left chest with the positive electrode in the V_1 position. The modification of the chest lead occurs because of the actual placement of a negative electrode on the left side of the chest rather than having the center of the heart function as the negative as in the V leads.

FIG. 2–12. ELECTRODE PLACEMENT FOR THE X, Y, AND Z LEADS.

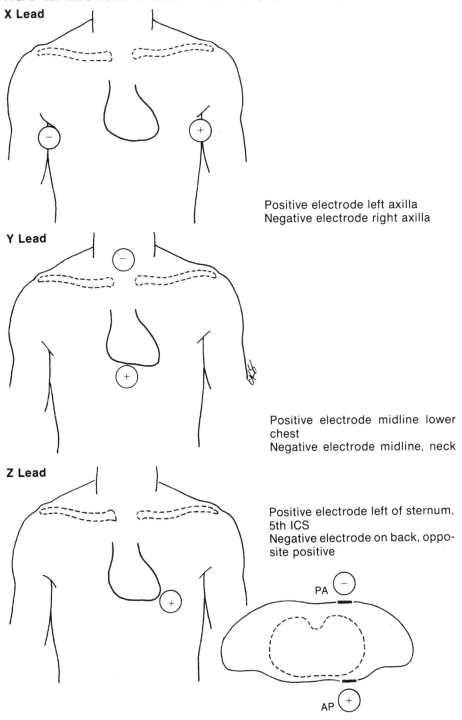

X Lead

Positive electrode left axilla
Negative electrode right axilla

Y Lead

Positive electrode midline lower chest
Negative electrode midline, neck

Z Lead

Positive electrode left of sternum, 5th ICS
Negative electrode on back, opposite positive

PA

AP

FIG. 2–13. LEAD II: ELECTRODE PLACEMENT
AND PATTERN PRODUCED.

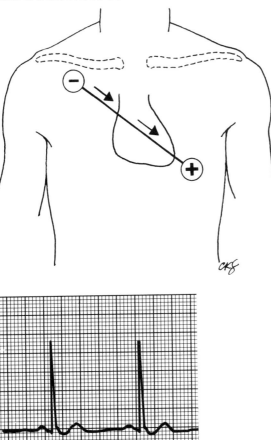

The current flow in the heart is to-
wards the positive electrode in a
Lead II. The pattern produced on
the ECG will have all major wave
forms upright positive.

Since the current flow of the heart is generally away from the positive electrode
in the MCL_1 lead, the ECG wave forms produced in this lead tend to be downward
or negative (Fig. 2-14).

Because the MCL_1 lead is so often used, all of the ECG patterns in this book
are from the MCL_1 lead unless indicated otherwise. The major advantage the
MCL_1 has over the lead II is better visualization of ventricular activity on the
ECG, a fact that will become more evident later in the book. The one advantage
that lead II may have over lead MCL_1 is the determination of atrial activity on
the ECG. The wave forms produced by the atria in the MCL_1 lead can take several
configurations; it may be difficult to distinguish normal sinus P wave forms from
abnormal ones.

FIG. 2–14. LEAD MCL$_1$: ELECTRODE POSITION AND PATTERN PRODUCED.

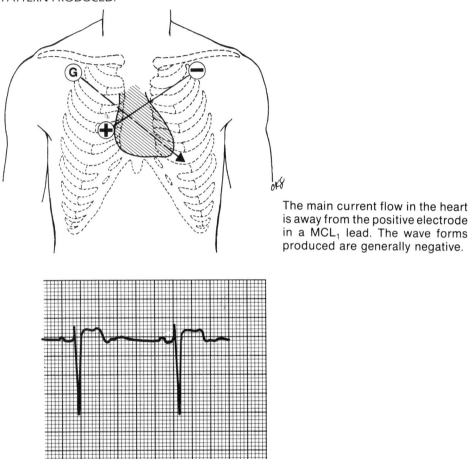

The main current flow in the heart is away from the positive electrode in a MCL$_1$ lead. The wave forms produced are generally negative.

ECG WAVE FORMS AND MEASUREMENTS

The pattern produced by the electrical activity in the heart that is then recorded by the ECG monitoring equipment is composed of a series of waves, intervals, and segments. In a normal ECG pattern, these waves, intervals, and segments follow a regular sequence and have normal ranges for their durations (Fig. 2-15).

P WAVE

The P wave is the first upward deflection of a normal ECG pattern in a lead II or lead MCL$_1$. The P wave represents discharge of the SA node and atrial depolarization. The normal P wave should be upright (positive), rounded, and less than

FIG. 2–15. NORMAL ECG PATTERN (LEAD MCL$_1$).

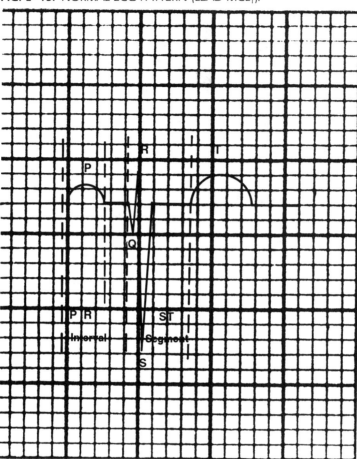

0.12 second in duration in lead II. In a lead MCL$_1$, normal P waves may have some alternative appearances, but they should all be the same no matter what the shape.

QRS COMPLEX

The QRS complex is a series of wave forms that usually follow shortly after the P wave. The Q wave is the first downward (negative) deflection after the P wave. The R wave is the first upward (positive) deflection after the Q wave. The S wave is the first downward (negative) deflection after the R wave. Often, the Q wave is not present. Although all the individual wave forms may not be present, this wave form is commonly called the *QRS complex*. The QRS complex represents the ventricular muscle depolarization. The normal QRS complex should measure between 0.06 and 0.10 second in duration. Any delay in the conduction through the ventricles will produce a wider-than-normal QRS complex.

PR INTERVAL

The PR interval includes the P wave and the short section of baseline called PR segment that follows the P wave. The PR interval extends from the beginning of the P wave to the beginning of the QRS complex. This determination may be a little misleading because, if the Q wave is present, the interval (strictly speaking) is the PQ interval even though it is still called the PR interval. The PR interval represents atrial depolarization (the P wave), the delay of the impulse in the AV node (PR segment), and conduction through the bundle branches to the Purkinje fibers. The normal PR interval has a normal range of 0.12–0.20 second in duration.

T WAVE

The T wave is the first upward deflection after the QRS complex in a normal ECG pattern. The T wave represents the electrical activity in the ventricles during repolarization. T waves are not as important in single lead ECG patterns as they are in the 12 lead ECG. In the single lead ECG, the T wave shape can be changed by electrode placement and often normal T waves appear inverted (negative) or even flattened.

ST SEGMENT

The ST segment is a short section of baseline that begins at the end of the S wave and ends at the beginning of the T wave. The ST segment represents the early phase of repolarization of the ventricles. The ST segment on the single lead ECG pattern is not as significant as it is on the 12 lead ECG. The ST segment may be elevated or depressed (Fig. 2-16).

FIG. 2–16. EXAMPLES OF ELEVATED AND DEPRESSED ST SEGMENTS.

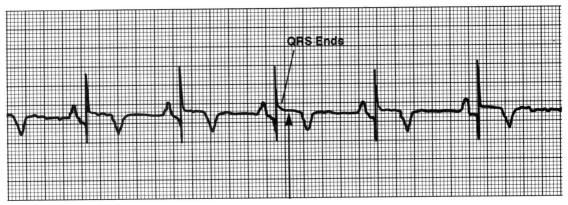

QRS Ends

A

Elevated ST Segment

(continued)

FIG. 2–16. EXAMPLES OF ELEVATED AND DEPRESSED ST SEGMENTS (continued).

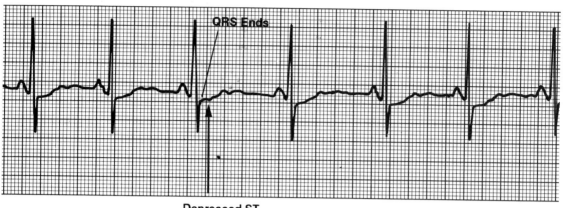

**Depressed ST
Segment**

B

THE ECG PATTERN AND THE REFRACTORY PERIODS

As discussed earlier, as the heart proceeds through its various stages of polarization, depolarization, and repolarization, it has various refractory periods. These refractory periods can be compared to the various phases of the ECG pattern (Fig. 2-17).

DIMINISHED REFRACTORY PERIOD

On the normal ECG pattern, the diminished refractory period (DRP) extends from near the end of the T wave (the end of ventricular repolarization) across the baseline (repolarization), through the P wave (atrial depolarization) and PR segment (delay of the impulse in the AV node), and travels through the ventricular conduction system). The DRP ends at the beginning of the QRS complex. The DRP is the phase of the cardiac cycle when the myocardium is particularly sensitive to any type of strong external stimulus.

ABSOLUTE REFRACTORY PERIOD

On the normal ECG pattern, the absolute refractory period extends from the beginning of the QRS complex (ventricular depolarization) across the ST segment (early phase of ventricular repolarization) to the beginning of the T wave (still early ventricular repolarization). The absolute refractory period is the phase of the cardiac cycle during which the ventricular myocardium will not respond to any stimulus, no matter how strong it is.

FIG. 2–17. ECG PATTERN WITH REFRACTORY PERIODS.
DRP = DIMINISHED REFRACTORY PERIOD; ARP = ABSOLUTE
REFRACTORY PERIOD; AND RRP = RELATIVE REFRACTORY
PERIOD.

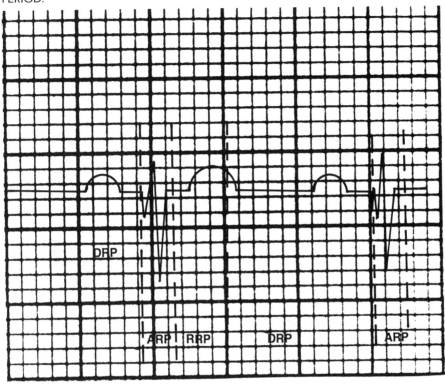

RELATIVE REFRACTORY PERIOD

On the normal ECG pattern, the relative refractory period (RRP) begins near the beginning of the T wave (early ventricular repolarization) and includes most of the T wave (middle and late ventricular repolarization). The RRP ends at the point where the DRP begins. The RRP's beginning and ending points are variable from individual to individual. The RRP is considered the "dangerous" part of the cardiac cycle because a strong stimulus that strikes during this part of the cycle is likely to produce partial or abnormal depolarization of the ventricles, leading to dysrhythmias, which can be fatal to the patient unless immediate corrective action is taken.

ARTIFACT

Artifact is any type of electrical activity on the ECG that is noncardiac in origin, that is, not produced by inherent cardiac electrical activity. Artifact can be divided into two main groups.

The first group of artifact includes those types of noncardiac electrical activities on the ECG that are intentional and useful. In this group are the standardization artifact and artificial pacemaker artifact (often called a spike), which indicates when an artificial pacemaker discharges (Fig. 2-18).

The second group of artifact is composed of those noncardiac electrical activities that interfere with the ECG pattern, making analysis and interpretation of the pattern difficult. In non-ECG terminology, this type of artifact is sometimes referred to as "garbage," "junk," or "interference." There are four main types of artifact in this group although it is possible to have combinations of two or more of these types in the same ECG pattern.

FIG. 2–18. EXAMPLES OF STANDARDIZATION AND PACEMAKER ARTIFACT.

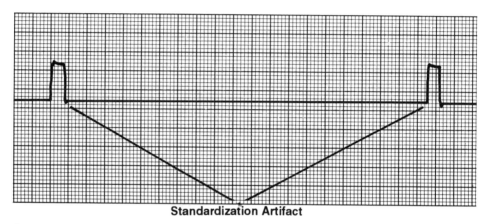

Standardization Artifact

A

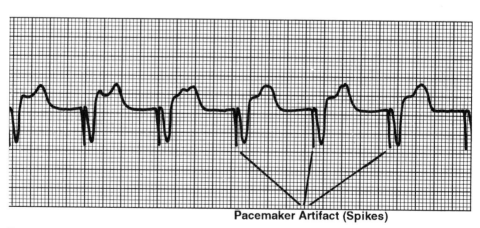

Pacemaker Artifact (Spikes)

B

ARTIFACT PRODUCED BY LOOSE ELECTRODES, BROKEN CABLES, OR BROKEN WIRES

This pattern (Fig. 2-19) has a wandering baseline that is often interspersed with wide, unusual wavelike fluctuations. This type of artifact is simple to eliminate by either replacing the electrodes, the broken wires, or both.

ARTIFACT PRODUCED BY PATIENT MUSCULAR TREMORS

This type of artifact (see Fig. 2-19) includes such involuntary patient activities as tensed muscles, shivering, tremors from Parkinson's disease, or seizure activity. This ECG pattern has a very jagged, irregular baseline, which will interfere not only with the visualization of the P waves but also the QRS complexes. Correction of this pattern requires controlling the underlying condition of the patient.

FIG. 2–19. ARTIFACT ON ECG PATTERNS.

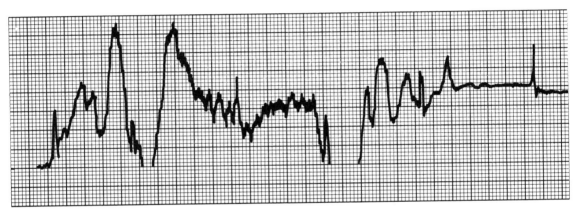

A Loose Electrodes

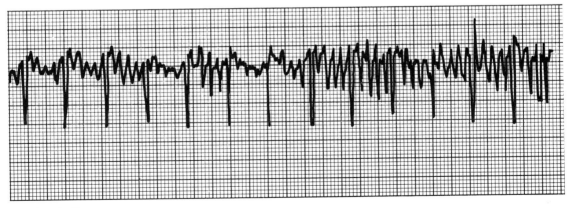

B Muscle Tremors

(continued)

FIG. 2–19. ARTIFACT ON ECG PATTERNS (continued).

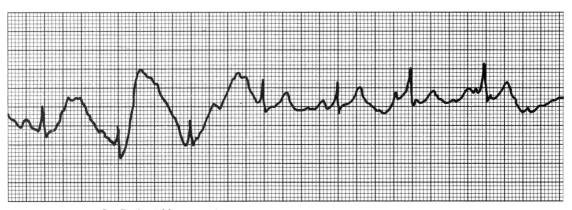

C Patient Movements

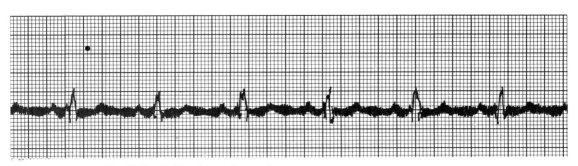

D 60-Cycle Electrical Current

ARTIFACT PRODUCED BY PATIENT MOVEMENTS

This artifact (see Fig. 2-19) may appear similar to the involuntary muscle tremor artifact at times but is caused by voluntary movement on the part of the patient. These movements would include such activities as brushing teeth, brushing hair, turning in bed, changing positions (*e.g.*, sitting up), or even taking a deep breath.

ARTIFACT PRODUCED BY 60-CYCLE INTERFERENCE

All the electrical equipment used in the hospital, ranging from light bulbs to ventilators and intravenous pumps, operate on alternating electric current. At the electric generating plant, the electric current is produced by rotating a group of wires quickly through a magnetic field. As this group of wires is rotated, the polarity of the electric current is switched quickly back and forth (actually 60 times in 1 second) between the positive and negative poles, thus, the term *alternating current.* This switching of the direction of the current is normally so fast that it cannot be detected by the human eye.

Occasionally, there will be a leakage of a small amount of current in a piece of equipment so the electric current does not all stay in the particular circuit of that equipment. All equipment used in modern hospitals is supposed to be grounded so that this stray electric current is carried off harmlessly to a place where it will not create any danger.

This stray electric current can be detected by the cardiac monitor and appears as a wide, dark baseline on the ECG. A closer look at this baseline with a magnifying glass will actually show 60 regular, even, small spikelike deflections in a 1-second interval. Electrical equipment that contains electric motors, such as intravenous pumps, ventilators, beds, and so on will produce this type of artifact most often.

If this type of artifact is present on an ECG tracing, it is important to identify the equipment that is producing it and have it evaluated by the biomedical department of the hospital. There may be nothing wrong with the equipment, in which case the electric outlet that the offending equipment is plugged into may have to be changed. It is often a trial-and-error procedure to discover which piece of equipment is causing the artifact and then find an outlet to plug it into so that the artifact is eliminated. All modern monitoring equipment has built-in electronic filters that detect artifact and, to some degree, eliminate it from the ECG pattern.

CHAPTER

3

ECG ANALYSIS

LEARNING OBJECTIVES

After studying this section, the learner will be able to:

1. Describe analysis as the primary means of ECG rhythm strip interpretation.
2. List the elements that go into analyzing any ECG rhythm strip to make an interpretation.
3. Describe the questions to ask about each of the elements in ECG rhythm strip interpretation.
4. Identify the various forms that a QRS complex can assume.

Various methods can be used in the analysis and interpretation of electrocardiogram (ECG) rhythms. Strip analysis is a method that breaks the ECG strip into its key elements, compares these elements to what the findings should be for a normal rhythm, and then accounts for anything that is abnormal in the strip in the interpretation. This method requires that the learner know what the norms are for a normal rhythm, as well as what the abnormals are for any given dysrhythmia. These norms are sometimes referred to as the *rules* or *criteria* for dysrhythmias. (This book will use the term *criteria* when referring to the rules for the various dysrhythmias.) It is also important in the analysis to relate the abnormal findings back to the actual electrical activity in the heart's conduction system, which is producing the dysrhythmia. Not only will understanding the pathophysiology of the dysrhythmia help in the interpretation, but it will also aid in the understanding of the treatment method for that particular rhythm problem.

There are a number of analysis methods for ECG dysrhythmia interpretation. While all of these methods share some common elements, the order of these elements and their names will vary from author to author. The analysis method used throughout this book was developed from years of teaching beginning students ECG dysrhythmia interpretation; it has met with much success. The method follows the conduction system through the heart and asks specific questions about the particular areas reflected on the ECG rhythm strip. Where the answers to the questions vary from the normal findings, the learner must account for the abnormals in the interpretation of the strip.

ANALYSIS SCHEMA FOR ECG RHYTHM STRIPS

Whenever the learner looks at a rhythm strip, these are the questions he or she should ask to make an interpretation.

RHYTHM

What is the rhythm of the strip? Rhythm refers to the *regularity* of the pattern. It asks: Is the rhythm regular or irregular? To determine whether the rhythm is regular or irregular, the learner must be able to measure and compare the P to P intervals and the R to R intervals. While the majority of the rhythm determinations depend upon the R to R (QRS complexes), there are several dysrhythmias where the P to P interval (atrial activity) is significant.

The R to R interval (and/or P to P interval) needs to be measured across the entire 6-second rhythm strip to make a determination about the regularity of the pattern (Fig. 3-1). If all of the intervals are equal, then the pattern on that strip is regular, which is normal. If the intervals are not all equal, then the pattern is irregular. One difficulty with irregular ECG patterns is that they can take several forms, which the learner must distinguish.

FIG. 3–1. MEASURING THE R TO R INTERVAL (A) AND THE P TO P INTERVAL (B).

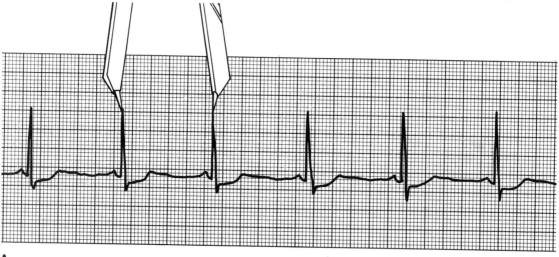

A

If the R to R intervals are all equal, as they are on this strip, the pattern is considered regular. Make sure to measure across the whole strip.

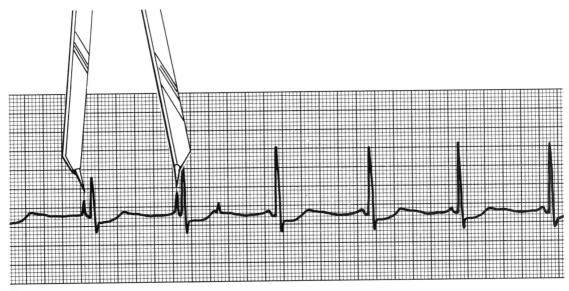

B

The P to P intervals are also regular on this strip, which is the most common finding since the sinoatrial node is a very regular pacemaker. Make sure to measure P to P intervals across the whole strip.

The forms of irregular patterns are as follows:

Slightly irregular. Is the difference between the R to R intervals (or P to P intervals) three small blocks or less (0.12 second)? Slightly irregular patterns are usually considered normal, particularly when the rates are slow (below 60). From experience, it has been observed that in most rhythms, the faster the rate, the more regular the rhythm becomes (Fig. 3-2).

Basically regular. In this pattern of irregularity, the underlying or predominant pattern is regular, but it is interrupted by *ectopic beats*. Ectopic beats are wave forms or complexes that arise from some part of the heart other than the sinoatrial (SA) node. Ectopic beats are recognized by the abnormal shapes they produce on the ECG strip because they are not following the normal conduction system of the heart. There are two basic types of ectopic beats that cause irregular rhythms: premature and escape.

Premature ectopic beats. These beats are caused by irritable areas in the heart (either the atrium, atrioventricular [AV] junction, or ventricles), that "fire" or discharge before the next regular beat from the SA node. They are recognized by wave forms or complexes that come early in the cardiac cycle, that is, before the next scheduled sinus beat should arrive (Fig. 3-3). These beats are usually just called *premature.*

FIG. 3–2. SLIGHTLY IRREGULAR PATTERN.

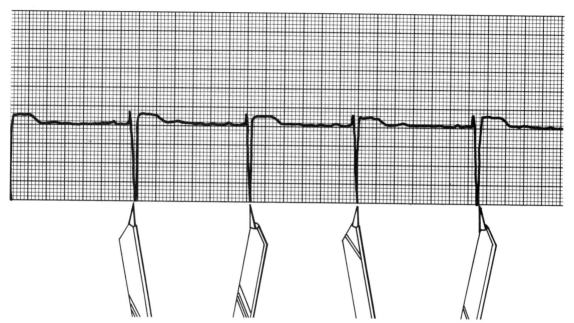

In slightly irregular patterns, there is a variation of three small blocks or less in between the R to R intervals (or in this example, the S to S interval) from the previous or following interval.

FIG. 3–3. PREMATURE ECTOPIC BEATS.

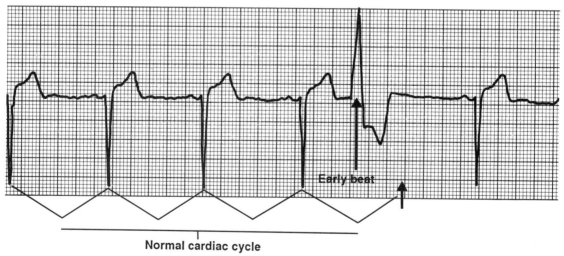

Early beat

Normal cardiac cycle

A

Premature ectopic beats can have either a normal QRS complex that is the same configuration as the rest of the strip (**B**) or the QRS can be a different configuration (**A**). In either case, it comes early in the cardiac cycle.

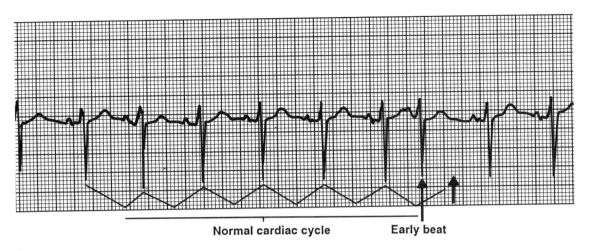

Normal cardiac cycle   **Early beat**

B

Escape ectopic beats. These abnormal wave forms or complexes arise from the same areas as the premature beats (atria, AV junction, or ventricles), except that they are a function of the safety or backup mechanisms built into the heart to protect it from complete arrest. These escape beats are often a result of the failure of the SA node to fire on time. These beats are recognized by their abnormal shapes, as well as the fact that they come late in the cardiac cycle, that is, after the next scheduled sinus beat should have arrived (Fig. 3-4). These ectopic escape beats are preceded by a long pause or interval. These beats are usually called *escape beats.*

FIG. 3–4. ESCAPE ECTOPIC BEATS.

Normal cardiac cycle   **Late beat**

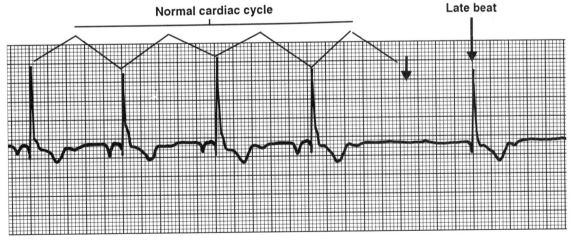

A

Late ectopic beats (escape beats) can have either a normal QRS complex (**A**) or the QRS can be different in configuration (**B**). In either case, it comes late in the cardiac cycle.

(*continued*)

FIG. 3–4. ESCAPE ECTOPIC BEATS (continued).

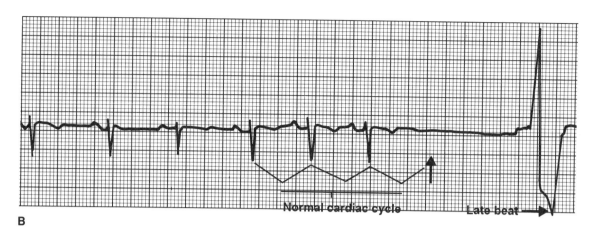

B

Regularly irregular. In this pattern of irregularity, there is a pattern of normal beats and ectopic beats grouped together that repeat over and over. It is an irregular pattern that repeats itself. The ectopic beats can be from any area of the heart and can result in a number of grouping patterns, many of which have special names that will be discussed in later chapters (Fig. 3-5).

Irregularly irregular. In this pattern of irregularity (also called totally irregular), there is no pattern and all of the R to R intervals (and/or P to P intervals) are all different from one another, with an interval greater than three small blocks (0.12 second; Fig. 3-6).

FIG. 3–5. REGULARLY IRREGULAR PATTERNS (PATTERNS OF GROUPED BEATS).

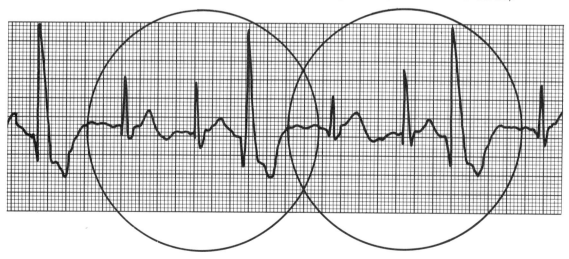

A

In strip **A,** there is a pattern of two normal beats and one ectopic beat that is repeated over and over. In strip **B,** there is a pattern of one normal beat and one ectopic beat that is repeated. The ectopics may or may not be in the same configuration as the nonectopic beats.

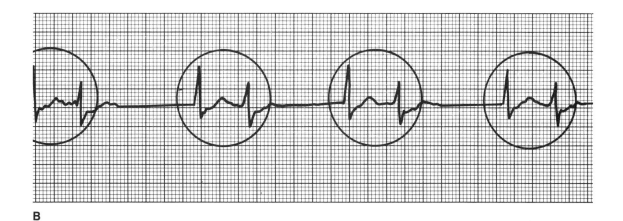

B

FIG. 3–6. IRREGULARLY IRREGULAR (TOTALLY IRREGULAR).

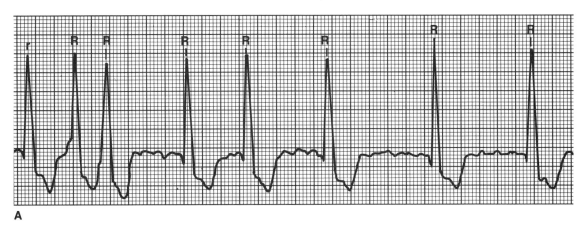

A

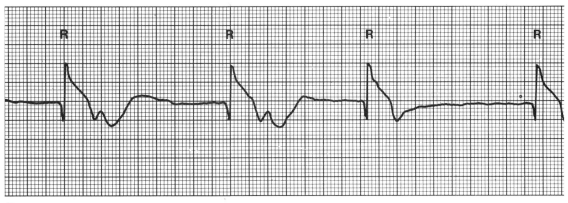

B

In this pattern of irregularity, all of the R to R intervals are different and there is no repeat of a pattern. The QRS complexes can be in a normal configuration (**A**) or be abnormally shaped (**B**). The rhythm may be fast, normal, or slow.

RATE

What is the rate of the heart beat? Since there are two areas in the heart that can, at times, function independently of each other (the atria and the ventricles), there is, at times, a need to determine the rates of these two areas separately. To determine the rate of the atria, the P waves must be considered. To determine the rate of the ventricles, the QRS complexes are essential. There are several methods to determine rate. It is important to decide whether the pattern is regular or irregular before attempting to determine the rate, because the methods used for regular patterns will not work on most irregular patterns.

Rate Determination for Regular Patterns

- Determine the R to R interval (or P to P) and count the number of small blocks within one interval. Since the pattern is regular, the intervals will all be the same. After determining the number of small blocks, divide that number into 1500. (The number 1500 is used because there are 1500 small blocks in a 1-minute strip of ECG paper.) This method is extremely accurate in determining rate (Fig. 3-7).

FIG. 3–7. DETERMINING RATE BY COUNTING SMALL BLOCKS.

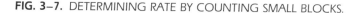
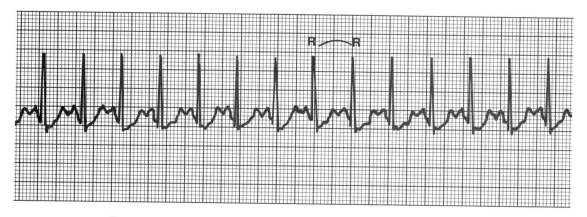

The pattern is regular (all the R to R intervals are equal). Count the number of small blocks between two R waves. There are 11 small blocks between two R waves on this strip. Then divide 1500 by the number of small blocks. (eg, 1500 ÷ 11 = 136). The rate of this strip is 136 beats/min.

- Determine the R to R interval (or P to P) and count the number of large blocks within one interval. After deciding the number of large blocks, divide that number into 300. (The number 300 is used because there are 300 large blocks in a 1-minute strip.) An alternate to this method is to memorize what the rates are as they fall on the dark lines of the ECG paper. The dark lines are measured off in rates of 50, 60, 75, 100, 150, and 300. This method is less accurate than

FIG. 3–8. DETERMINING RATE BY COUNTING LARGE BLOCKS.

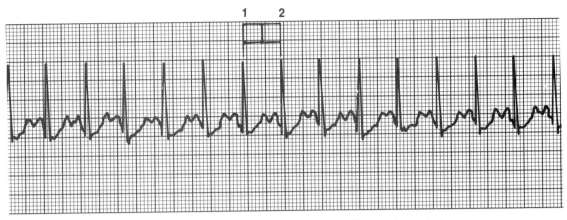

Using the same strip as is used in Fig. 3–7, count the number of large blocks between two R waves. There are two large blocks between the R to R intervals. Divide 300 by the number of large blocks (300 ÷ 2 = 150). The approximate rate using this method of rate determination is 150 beats/min. It is quicker but less accurate than using the number of small blocks.

using the small blocks but, with less math involved, somewhat faster (Figs. 3-8 and 3-9C).
- Use a rate ruler or some other measurement instrument to determine the rate. These measurement instruments all use the small block/1500 system but have worked the math out for the rate determination ahead of time. (Fig. 3-9).

Rate Determination for Irregular Patterns

- Since there is no regular and consistent R to R interval (or P to P interval) in irregular patterns, all of the methods discussed above are inaccurate in determining the rate. The simplest method is to count the number of cardiac cycles (R to R/P to P intervals) in a 6-second strip and multiply by 10. To determine a 6-second strip, the markers at the top of the ECG paper must be identified. Almost all ECG paper in use today has some type of marker system (slashes, short lines, or dots), which is at 3-second intervals along the top of the paper (Fig. 3-10). The multiplication factor of 10 is used because there are 6 × 10 (60) seconds in a minute. This method of rate determination will also work with regular patterns but is less accurate. Ectopic beats are usually counted in the rate determination of irregular patterns, although there is some controversy about this practice.
- Run a minute strip. This method works both for irregular and regular patterns and is extremely accurate. The idea is to let the ECG machine run off a strip for 1 full minute (20 three-second markers) and then count the number of cardiac cycles on that strip. The major problems with this method are that it is extremely time-consuming and also uses a great deal of expensive ECG paper.

FIG. 3–9. DETERMINING RATE USING A RATE RULER OR MEMORIZATION OF RATE INTERVALS.

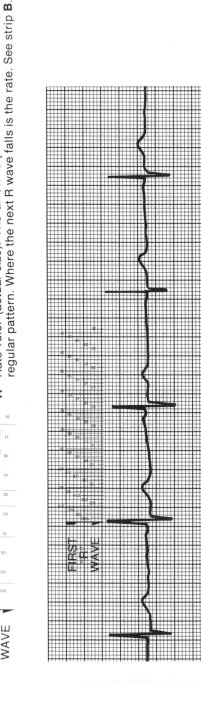

A Rate ruler (actual size). The arrow is placed on one R wave of a regular pattern. Where the next R wave falls is the rate. See strip **B**.

FIRST "R" WAVE

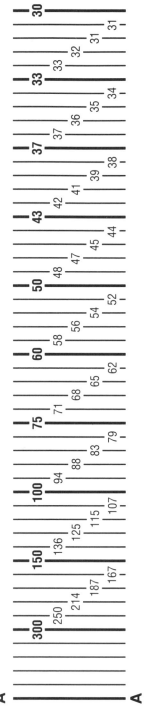

B Measuring with a rate ruler. Rate = 49.

C Rate scale: This device is similar to a rate ruler and is based on the small block/1500 method of rate determination. The dark and light lines correspond with the dark and light lines on the ECG paper and can be used to determine rates of regular patterns. The R to R are compared to the scale and the rate determined. The dark lines are relatively easy to memorize (300, 150, 100, 75, 60, 50).

FIG. 3–10. THREE-SECOND MARKERS ON ECG PAPER.

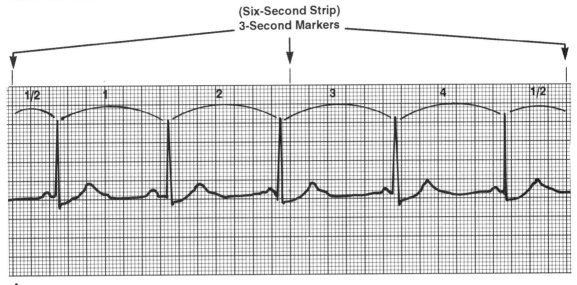

A
5 complete R to R intervals in the 6-second strip. Approximate rate is 5 × 10 = 50

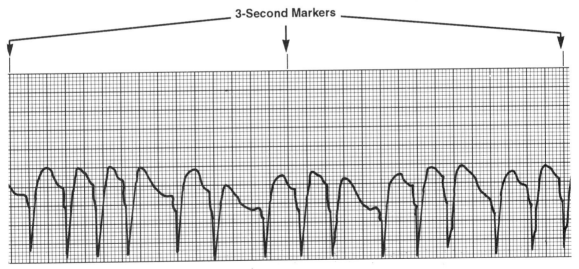

B
14.5 R to R interval in the 6-second strip. Approximate rate is 14.5 × 10 = 145

(*continued*)

FIG. 3–10. THREE-SECOND MARKERS ON ECG PAPER (continued).

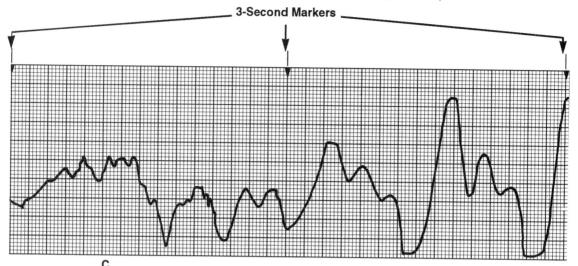

3-Second Markers

C
It is difficult to determine rate on this strip since the QRS complexes are not distinct.

THE NORMAL RATE

One other factor to consider in rate determination is the normal rate. For an adult, the normal heart rate is between 60 and 100 beats per minute. Any rates above or below these ranges may be abnormal and must be accounted for in the interpretation. Also, the other normal condition for the rate is that the atrial rate (P waves) should be the same rate as the ventricles (QRS complexes). If these two rates are different, the separate rates should be noted in the rate part of the analysis and then accounted for in the interpretation of the pattern.

ATRIAL CONDUCTION

In considering the atrial conduction, the P waves are the most significant factor to examine and analyze. Some questions that must be considered in analyzing the P waves include the following:

- Are there P waves present? The normal is to have P waves in the cardiac cycle representing atrial depolarization on the ECG strip.
- Is there a P wave for each QRS complex? The normal is to have one P precede each QRS complex.
- Is the P wave before or after the QRS complex? In certain abnormal rhythms, the P wave will follow the QRS.
- What is the shape of the P wave? Normal P waves in a lead II are upright, rounded, and less than 0.12 second in duration. In the lead MCL$_1$, the P waves may take on some abnormal shapes as compared with the lead II yet to be considered normal. The key in looking at P waves in MCL$_1$ is to observe if they are the same shape for the whole rhythm strip, because the unusual shape is more a function of lead placement than abnormal atrial activity (Fig. 3-11).

FIG. 3–11. POSSIBLE NORMAL CONFIGURATIONS
FOR P WAVES.

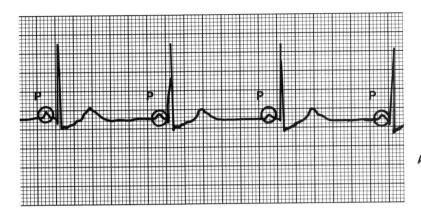

A Lead II: Normal P waves are upright and rounded. One P wave for each QRS.

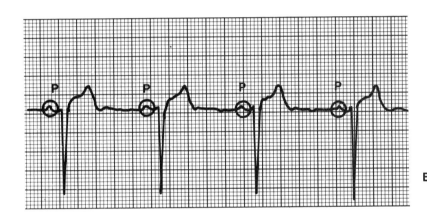

B Lead MCL₁. P waves are often upright and rounded as in Lead II.

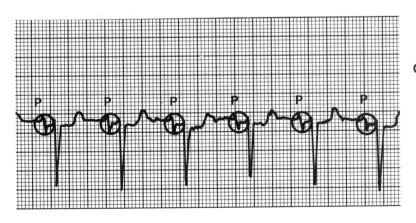

C Lead MCL₁. P waves sometimes take on atypical forms as in this strip where they are diphasic (they have both a positive and negative deflection). These P waves are considered normal since they are all the same and there is one P for each QRS.

- Do all the P waves look alike? This question is appropriate for both lead II and lead MCL$_1$. If there are P waves that look different from the majority of the other P waves on the strip, then that is an indication that there is an abnormal atrial activity taking place.
- If there are ectopic beats, are there any abnormal-shaped P waves in relationship to these beats? This question is particularly important for premature ectopic beats, which can arise from several areas in the heart and can be determined by the associated P waves.
- Are there more P waves than QRS complexes? If there are, then an abnormal condition exists in the heart's functioning. The rate for the P waves needs to be established, and a determination of whether the P waves are being conducted to the ventricles needs to be made. The conduction is the next step in the analysis.
- Are there any buried (also called lost or hidden) P waves in the pattern? It is important to remember that the SA node is a very reliable and regular pacemaker for the heart. The result of this regularity is that P waves are produced at very regular and consistent intervals most of the time. When measuring the P to P intervals across a rhythm strip, note any places where P waves should, but cannot, be seen; they may be hidden. The principle that governs this factor is that on the ECG strip, higher voltage electrical activities in the heart will cover up or hide lower voltage electrical activities. In practice, this principle translates into the fact that if the ventricles and the atria depolarize at the same time, the ECG paper will record the QRS complexes but not the P waves. This phenomenon also occurs to some degree with T waves and P waves, although the P waves that occur at the same time as the T waves may distort the T wave in some manner (such as making it more peaked or notched) (Fig. 3-12).
- If there are no visible P waves, what does the area on the ECG look like where the P waves are supposed to be? The baseline before the QRS complex can take on various forms that will help in the determination of the type of atrial activity taking place. These forms include an uneven, undulating baseline, a sawtooth pattern, or just a straight line. (These forms will be discussed in more detail in Chapter 5.) It is important to note them in the atrial conduction portion of the analysis.

**PITFALLS IN
P WAVE INTERPRETATION**

Beginning learners should be aware of several problems inherent in P wave recognition. On the one hand, P waves are sometimes difficult to identify and easy to overlook. On the other hand, many types of artifacts look like P waves and are easy to misinterpret as P waves when they are not. Practicing analyzing ECG strips and identifying P waves will eventually sharpen the learner's ability to make accurate determinations and analyses of P waves.

FIG. 3–12. T WAVE DISTORTION DUE TO SIMULTANEOUS P WAVES.

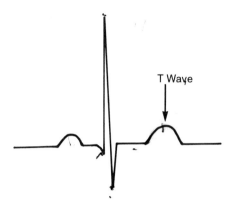

T Wave

A Normal sinus pattern on ECG with normal T wave.

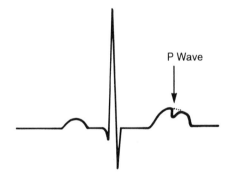

P Wave

B P wave that falls on a T wave may cause distortion of the T wave.

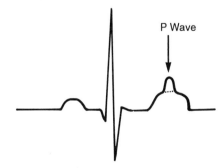

P Wave

C P waves that fall on the T wave may cause the T wave to be "taller."

AV CONDUCTION

The part of the ECG to consider for the AV conduction is the PR interval. The PR interval reflects atrial depolarization and the delay of the impulse in the AV node before it travels to the ventricular muscle tissue. Abnormalities of the PR interval reflect pathology of the conduction system from the SA node to the Purkinje fibers, including the AV node. Questions that should be asked about the PR interval include the following:

- Is the PR interval normal? The normal PR interval is 0.12–0.20 second in duration. If it is either shorter or longer than this range, it reflects a problem with the AV conduction.
- Are all the PR intervals the same? In a normal pattern, all of the PR intervals measure the same duration across the whole strip.
- If the PR intervals are different, is there a pattern to them or are they associated with any ectopic beats? Certain types of repetitive patterns of PR intervals that change can be the key to interpretation of certain specific conduction problems. Abnormally long PR intervals indicate some type of block in the AV conduction that either slows the impulses for too long a time or completely prevents them from going to the ventricular muscle tissues. In association with ectopic beats, the PR interval may vary from the normal due to the unusual area of impulse formation in the atria, which results in changes in conduction times for the impulse. The PR interval will vary in association with ectopic beats because the impulse is not following the normal conduction pathways in the heart.
- If there is no PR interval, where is the P wave? This question refers the learner back to the atrial conduction part of the analysis. If there is no P wave or if the P wave comes after the QRS complex, then there is no means to measure the PR interval. Also, in certain patterns of atrial conduction such as the uneven, undulating baseline or the sawtooth pattern, the PR interval is not measured because there is no conclusive means of determining which impulse is being conducted to the ventricles to stimulate their depolarization.

PITFALLS IN AV CONDUCTION DETERMINATION

There is really only one major difficulty in determining AV conduction times. The questions most often asked are "Where does the P wave start?" and "Where does the QRS complex start?" Since the PR interval begins at the beginning of the P wave and ends at the beginning of the QRS complex, these questions become extremely important. In some complexes and waves, the beginning of the form is clearly seen as a sharp-angled departure from the baseline. In other patterns, the beginning of the P wave in particular, but sometimes the QRS complex, is a slurred upstroke from the baseline, with no clear, sharp angle. In these situations, accurate measurements become a matter of practice. Often, there will be a variation in the measurement from interpreter to interpreter within an acceptable range.

VENTRICULAR CONDUCTION

The part of the ECG to consider for determination of the ventricular muscle depolarization is the QRS complex. The QRS complex represents depolarization of the ventricular muscle tissues. Ventricular depolarization determination is very important because the ventricles of the heart actually produce circulation through the vascular system. This circulation causes the oxygenation of the blood and supplies the tissues and organs of the body with nutrients and oxygen for survival. Questions to ask in the analysis of the ventricular conduction include the following:

- Are the QRS complexes normal? A normal QRS complex measures 0.06–0.10 second. Any deviation from the normal myocardial depolarization will produce a QRS complex of 0.12 second or greater.
- Are all the QRS complexes of the same duration? QRS complexes that vary in duration, even if they are all within the normal range, indicate some type of conduction problem in the ventricles. A more commonly seen situation is the mixture of longer-than-normal QRS complexes with normal QRS complexes.
- Do all the QRS complexes look the same? Even if the complexes all measure the same duration, if they are changing shape (or morphology) on the ECG strip, there is a conduction abnormality present in the ventricles.
- If there are ectopic beats (either premature or escape beats), are the QRS complexes of these beats abnormal in configuration or duration? QRS complexes that are abnormal in shape and duration that are also ectopic may indicate a ventricular focus for that beat. Since ventricular premature beats are the most common type of ectopic beat after a person has suffered myocardial injury or damage, it is important to be able to recognize these ectopics and treat them effectively. Ventricular ectopic beats and rhythms will be discussed in more detail in later chapters.
- If there are no visible or recognizable QRS complexes, what does the area of the ECG strip where the QRS complexes are supposed to be look like? In the absence of QRS complexes, the baseline of the ECG may assume a variety of configurations, ranging from a straight line to very irregular and chaotic wave forms. Since no circulation is produced when there are no QRS complexes, accurate analysis and interpretation of these patterns will determine appropriate treatment, which may save a person's life. It is important to note these patterns in the ventricular conduction portion of the ECG analysis.

PITFALLS IN VENTRICULAR CONDUCTION ANALYSIS

QRS complexes are usually the largest wave forms on the ECG strip, but there is sometimes a question concerning what QRS complexes should look like. In general usage, any pattern or group of wave forms produced by ventricular depolarization is called a QRS complex even if all three wave forms (Q wave, R wave, and S wave) are not present. Some examples of the forms that the QRS complex can take are provided in Figure 3–13.

FIG. 3-13. VARIOUS FORMS OF QRS COMPLEXES.

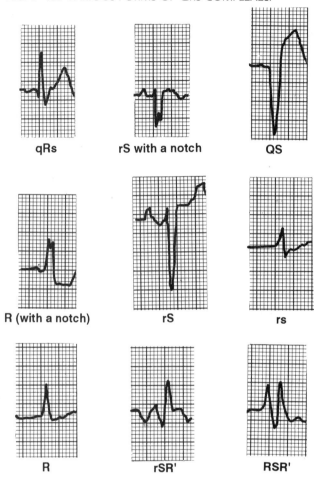

(Note: All of these are called QRS complexes, even though they may only have one wave form. Upper case letters are used when the wave is 5 mm or more; lower case letters are used when the wave is less than 5 mm.

PRACTICE ECG STRIPS FOR CHAPTER 3

Directions. On the following practice ECG strips, identify the P waves and QRS complexes. Analyze the strips for rhythm, rate (both atrial and ventricular), and atrial conduction; measure the PR interval, and the width of the QRS complexes. Note if any of the findings are abnormal. (See Appendix II for interpretations.)

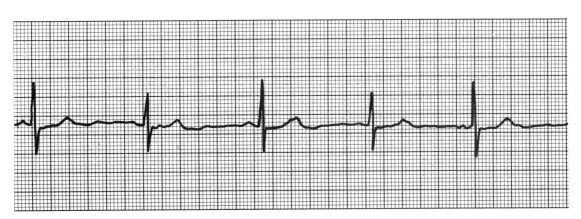

3–1

RHYTHM: _____ SINUS _____

RATE: _____ 60 _____

ATRIAL CONDUCTION: _____ YES _____

AV CONDUCTION: _____ YES _____

VENTRICULAR CONDUCTION: _____ YES _____

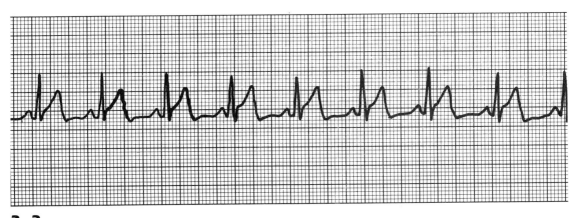

3–2

RHYTHM: _____ SINUS _____

RATE: _____ 100 _____

ATRIAL CONDUCTION: _____ YES _____
_____ YES _____

AV CONDUCTION: _____ YES _____

VENTRICULAR CONDUCTION: _____ YES _____

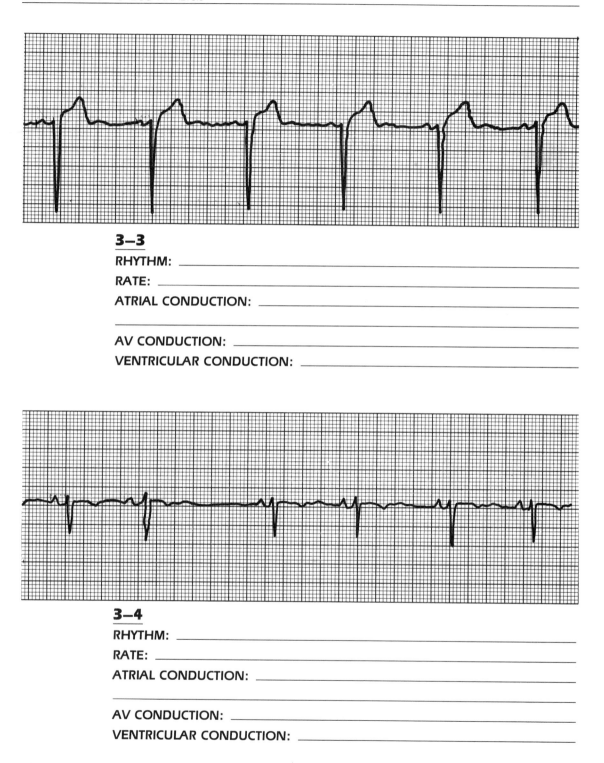

3—3

RHYTHM: _____

RATE: _____

ATRIAL CONDUCTION: _____

_____

AV CONDUCTION: _____

VENTRICULAR CONDUCTION: _____

3—4

RHYTHM: _____

RATE: _____

ATRIAL CONDUCTION: _____

_____

AV CONDUCTION: _____

VENTRICULAR CONDUCTION: _____

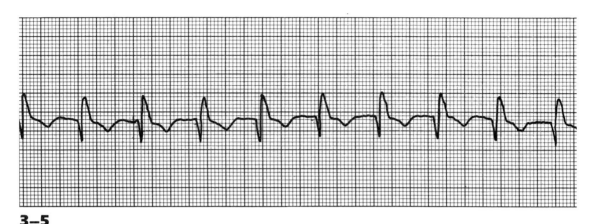

3–5

RHYTHM: _____

RATE: _____

ATRIAL CONDUCTION: _____
_____

AV CONDUCTION: _____

VENTRICULAR CONDUCTION: _____

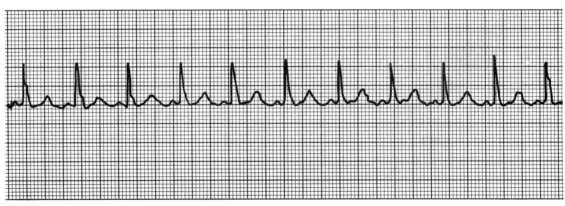

3–6

RHYTHM: _____

RATE: _____

ATRIAL CONDUCTION: _____
_____

AV CONDUCTION: _____

VENTRICULAR CONDUCTION: _____

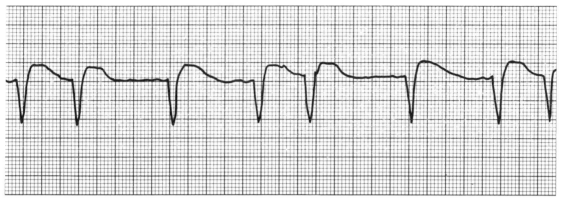

3–7

RHYTHM: _____

RATE: _____

ATRIAL CONDUCTION: _____

_____

AV CONDUCTION: _____

VENTRICULAR CONDUCTION: _____

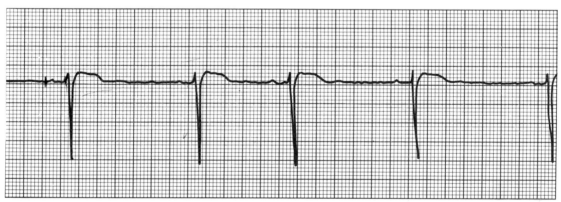

3–8

RHYTHM: _____

RATE: _____

ATRIAL CONDUCTION: _____

_____

AV CONDUCTION: _____

VENTRICULAR CONDUCTION: _____

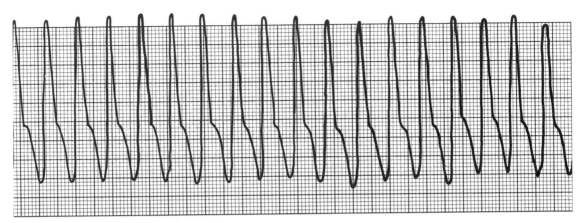

3–9

RHYTHM: _____

RATE: _____

ATRIAL CONDUCTION: _____

_____

AV CONDUCTION: _____

VENTRICULAR CONDUCTION: _____

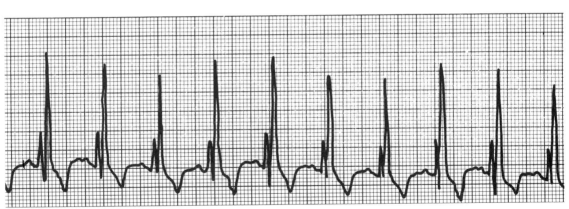

3–10

RHYTHM: _____

RATE: _____

ATRIAL CONDUCTION: _____

_____

AV CONDUCTION: _____

VENTRICULAR CONDUCTION: _____

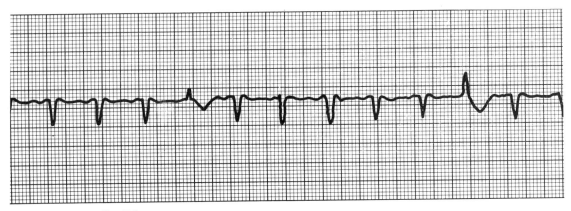

3–11

RHYTHM: _____

RATE: _____

ATRIAL CONDUCTION: _____
_____

AV CONDUCTION: _____

VENTRICULAR CONDUCTION: _____

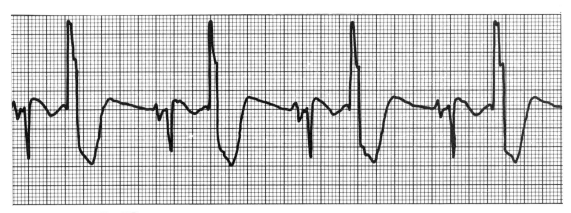

3–12

RHYTHM: _____

RATE: _____

ATRIAL CONDUCTION: _____
_____

AV CONDUCTION: _____

VENTRICULAR CONDUCTION: _____

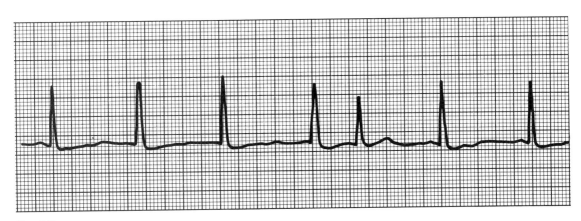

3–13

RHYTHM: _____

RATE: _____

ATRIAL CONDUCTION: _____

_____

AV CONDUCTION: _____

VENTRICULAR CONDUCTION: _____

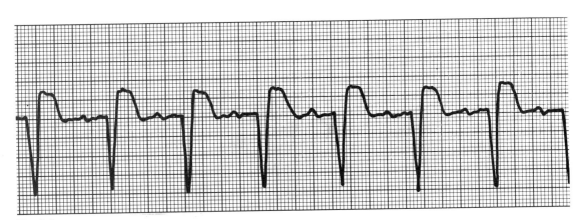

3–14

RHYTHM: _____

RATE: _____

ATRIAL CONDUCTION: _____

_____

AV CONDUCTION: _____

VENTRICULAR CONDUCTION: _____

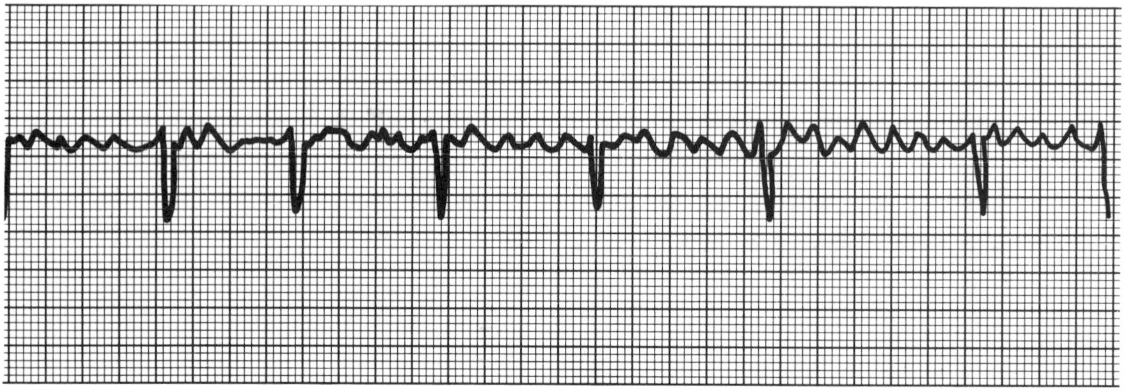

3–15

RHYTHM: _____

RATE: _____

ATRIAL CONDUCTION: _____

_____

AV CONDUCTION: _____

VENTRICULAR CONDUCTION: _____

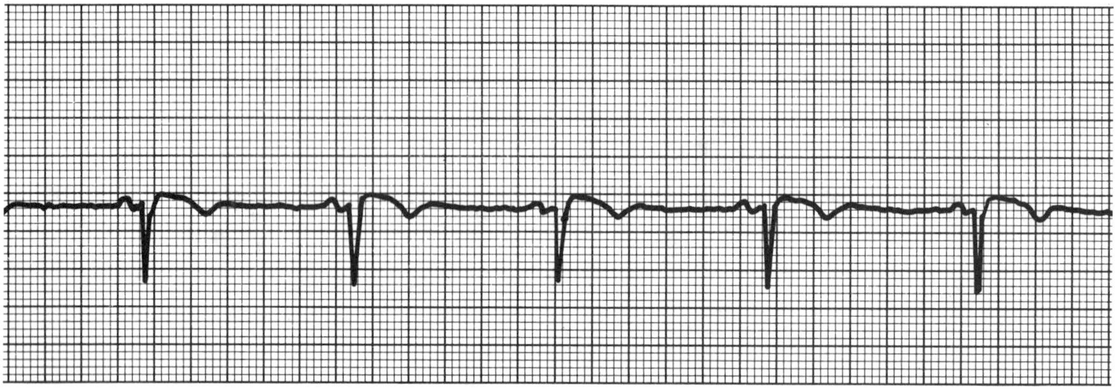

3–16

RHYTHM: _____

RATE: _____

ATRIAL CONDUCTION: _____

_____

AV CONDUCTION: _____

VENTRICULAR CONDUCTION: _____

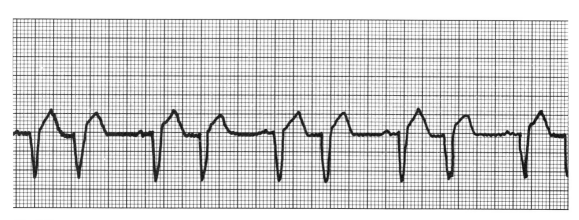

3–17

RHYTHM: _____

RATE: _____

ATRIAL CONDUCTION: _____

_____

AV CONDUCTION: _____

VENTRICULAR CONDUCTION: _____

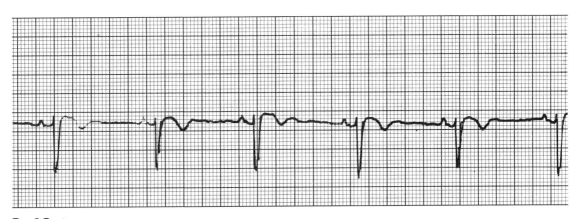

3–18

RHYTHM: _____

RATE: _____

ATRIAL CONDUCTION: _____

_____

AV CONDUCTION: _____

VENTRICULAR CONDUCTION: _____

4

NORMAL SINUS RHYTHM AND DYSRHYTHMIAS ASSOCIATED WITH THE SINUS NODE

LEARNING OBJECTIVES

After studying this section, the learner will be able to:

1. Name the criteria for normal sinus rhythm.
2. Identify the criteria for dysrhythmias that arise from the sinoatrial node.
3. Discuss the common causes for the various dysrhythmias that are associated with the sinoatrial node.
4. Identify the dysrhythmias that most severely compromise cardiac output and describe the symptoms commonly seen with these dysrhythmias.
5. Describe the treatment and care modalities for each of the various dysrhythmias.

The normal and usual location for the origin of the impulses that depolarize the heart is the sinus node in the right atrium. In healthy hearts and even some hearts that are not very healthy, the sinus node is an extremely reliable and regular pacemaker. The sinus node produces impulses at a consistent rate when it is allowed to depolarize without interference from factors outside of the heart. The sinus node is also affected by a variety of factors from outside the heart. These factors include the sympathetic and parasympathetic systems; hormones such as epinephrine, norepinephrine, and thyroid; and a variety of medications such as digoxin, calcium blockers, and beta blockers. All of these factors affect either the rate or regularity of the impulse production in the sinus node. Many of the dysrhythmias associated with the sinus node are related to these factors or to serious cardiac disease.

One key element in the rhythms and dysrhythmias that originate from the sinus node is the P wave and its variation from the "normal" shape. Another key element is that the QRS complex in sinus nodal dysrhythmias is usually normal in shape and duration because the impulses follow the normal conduction pathways through the ventricles. Other conduction system abnormalities can occur in conjunction with sinus node dysrhythmias, and may tend to complicate the analysis and interpretation.

NORMAL SINUS RHYTHM

Normal sinus rhythm (also called NSR, regular sinus rhythm, RSR, sinus rhythm, SR) is the strict and accurate term to use for a pattern that originates in the sinoatrial (SA) node and follows the normal conduction pathways through the rest of the heart, producing normal depolarization of the atria and the ventricles at normal rates and intervals. Although the other names of normal sinus rhythm are used, it would be more accurate to call it sinus rhythm (Fig. 4-1) any time there is any deviation from the normal criteria in a cardiac pattern.

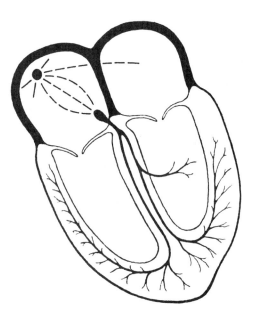

FIG. 4–1. SINUS NODE DISCHARGES IMPULSES AT A REGULAR AND NOR-MAL RATE IN NORMAL SINUS RHYTHM. THE IMPULSES FOLLOW THE NORMAL CONDUCTION PATHWAYS THROUGH THE REST OF THE HEART.

An important factor to remember about normal sinus rhythm is that it produces maximal cardiac output because all of the parts of the heart are functioning the way they are supposed to function. All dysrhythmias alter the cardiac output to some degree. There are a few dysrhythmias that will actually increase cardiac output, but the vast majority of the dysrhythmias decrease cardiac output. The greater the reduction in cardiac output, the more likely the patient is to have symptoms and the more serious the classification of the dysrhythmia.

It is extremely important that the learner memorize the criteria for each of the dysrhythmias. It is even more important that the learner know the criteria for normal sinus rhythm because this is the yardstick against which all patterns are compared to determine normalcy of the pattern that they are analyzing. Any deviations from the "normal" of normal sinus rhythm must be accounted for in the interpretation of the strip.

While it will seem to be a great deal of material to master at first, by relating the criteria back to the conduction system of the heart and the activity that is taking place in the heart, it will make the information easier to understand and more logical. One of the major difficulties with electrocardiogram (ECG) analysis and interpretation is that there is an exception to almost every criterion that is stated. The criteria will be presented first; if these are understood, then the exceptions will be easier to understand (Fig. 4-2).

FIG. 4–2. EXAMPLE OF NORMAL SINUS RHYTHM.

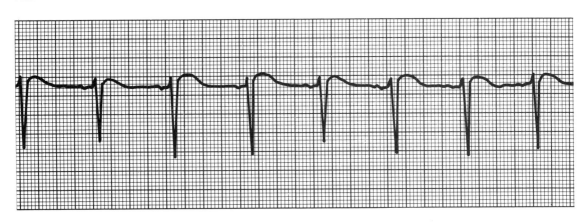

CRITERIA FOR NORMAL SINUS RHYTHM

Rhythm: Regular.

Rate: 60–100 beats/min.

Atrial Conduction: One P wave before each QRS; normal shape; consistent in shape.

AV Conduction: PRI = 0.12–0.20 second; same across the strip; may vary with the rate.

Ventricular Conduction: QRS = 0.06–0.10 second; uniform in shape.

SINUS BRADYCARDIA

Sinus bradycardia (SB) (Fig. 4-3) is a dysrhythmia that originates in the sinus node and follows the normal conduction pathways through the heart, producing normal depolarization and a normal ECG pattern. Therefore, the criteria are identical to that for normal sinus rhythm except for one factor: the rate (in the adult) is less than 60 beats/min (brady = slow).

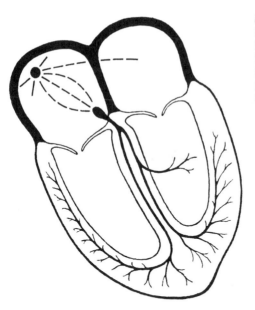

FIG. 4–3. SINUS NODE DISCHARGES IMPULSES AT REGULAR TO SLIGHTLY IRREGULAR INTERVALS BUT AT A RATE SLOWER THAN NORMAL IN SINUS BRADYCARDIA. IMPULSES FOLLOW THE NORMAL PATHWAYS THROUGH THE REST OF THE CONDUCTION SYSTEM.

CAUSES

Sinus bradycardia may be a normal variation of a normal heart rhythm in some individuals, such as athletes or individuals who exercise regularly and vigorously. These individuals have developed their heart muscle (*i.e.*, increased the muscle tone of the heart) to such a degree that at rest the heart can maintain a normal cardiac output even at a slower rate. Medications that suppress the myocardium can cause sinus bradycardia. These medications include: digoxin, beta blockers, calcium blockers, and certain types of antihypertensives. Central nervous system depressant medications also tend to slow the heart rate indirectly through the autonomic nervous system. These medications include: morphine sulfate and other narcotic medications, sedatives, and tranquilizers.

Sinus bradycardia can also be a result of direct pathologic damage to the heart tissue either from acute cardiac events such as an myocardial infarction (MI) or from long-standing cardiac disease such as sclerotic coronary arteries or high blood pressure. Finally, sinus bradycardia can result from stimulation of the vagus nerve (cranial nerve X). Some of the common causes of vagal stimulation include vomiting, deep bronchial sectioning of patients, Valsalva's maneuver, carotid massage, and gagging. Hypoxia can also cause sinus bradycardia.

SYMPTOMS

If the rate of the bradycardia is not very slow, most individuals tolerate it without any major symptoms. In general, symptoms associated with all dysrhythmias are due to lower-than-normal cardiac output. Low cardiac output causes a decreased blood flow to the brain, heart, and other organs, producing a set of symptoms that are similar for many of the dysrhythmias that lower cardiac output markedly.

These symptoms can be grouped into two major categories: (1) neurologic signs and symptoms, including dizziness, weakness, syncope, disorientation, and seizures; and (2) cardiac signs and symptoms, including chest pain, chest pressure, chest tightness, shortness of breath, diaphoresis, pallor of the skin, coolness of the skin, low blood pressure, and weak peripheral pulses.

TREATMENT

The main goal of treatment for sinus bradycardia is to increase the heart rate. One point to remember in the treatment of any dysrhythmia is that the patient's clinical condition must be thoroughly assessed before any treatment is given. If the patient is tolerating the bradycardia (*i.e.*, blood pressure is normal, patient is oriented and awake, skin is warm and dry), then he or she probably does not need treatment. If the patient is developing symptoms with the dysrhythmia, then he or she probably requires treatment.

Some methods of treating sinus bradycardia include the following:

- Eliminate the cause of the bradycardia. If a patient has been receiving digoxin and the blood level is in the toxic range, holding the medication brings the level down. The same treatment can be used if the blood levels of the calcium blockers or beta blockers are elevated. If the cause is related to vagal stimulation or hypoxia, correcting these conditions returns the heart to a normal rate.

- Suppress the parasympathetic system and allow the sympathetic system to take over. The primary group of medications used to produce this effect is the anticholinergics. The principal medication in this group is atropine sulfate (0.5–1.0 mg IV push). It can be repeated every 15 minutes, as needed, up to 2 mg total dose or until the rate returns to normal or some other action is taken. As a rule, atropine sulfate is the medication of choice for *any* slow rhythm, regardless of the cause. Atropine works to speed up the SA node if it is discharging at a too slow rate or even to cause the SA node to start producing impulses if it has stopped completely. Atropine has few lethal side effects, and it also has a short half-life so that the body can recover from its effects quickly.

- Directly stimulate the SA node with medications that stimulate the sympathetic nervous system. The most common medication used for this purpose is epinephrine (0.5–1 mg IV push). Other medications that can be used for sinus bradycardia are dopamine (although its effects are dose-dependent), norepinephrine, and metaraminol bitartrate. This latter group also has vasoconstrictive actions and will increase the cardiac output and raise the blood pressure. These medications have the advantage of raising the ventricular rate even if there is no sinus node activity, which is not the problem in sinus bradycardia.

- Use a pacemaker. The pacemaker may be either a temporary pacemaker or a permanent implanted pacemaker. The temporary external pacemaker is often used when there has been cardiac damage, as from an MI, which may produce a temporary bradycardia. In these situations, the bradycardia will often correct itself within 48–72 hours after the damage. If it is not corrected by that time and the patient is symptomatic with the dysrhythmia, a permanent pacemaker may be required (Fig. 4-4).

FIG. 4–4. EXAMPLE OF SINUS BRADYCARDIA.

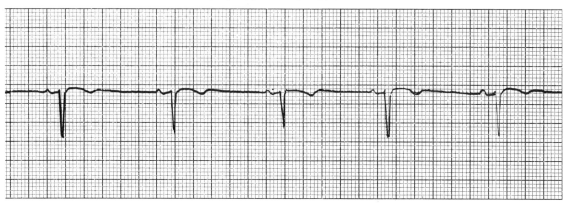

CRITERIA FOR SINUS BRADYCARDIA

Rhythm: Regular to slightly irregular.

Rate: Less than 60 beats/min.

Atrial Conduction: One P wave before each QRS; normal shape; consistent.

AV Conduction: PRI 0.12–0.2 second; consistent across the whole strip.

Ventricular Conduction: QRS 0.06–0.10 second; uniform in shape.

SINUS TACHYCARDIA

Sinus tachycardia (also called ST, sinus tach) (Fig. 4-5) is a dysrhythmia that originates in the sinus node and follows the normal conduction pathways through the heart, producing normal depolarization and a normal ECG pattern. Therefore, the criteria are identical to those for normal sinus rhythm except for the rate. The rate in the adult will be faster than 100 beats/min (tachy = fast).

CAUSES

Sinus tachycardia is one of the most common of all the dysrhythmias because an accelerated heart rate is one of the body's adaptive mechanisms to a variety of conditions and illnesses. Some of the most common physiologic factors that can produce a sinus tachycardia include fever, anxiety, fear, injury to any part of the body, physical activity, pain, sexual stimulation, anemia, lung disease, hypoxia, hemorrhage, and hypotension.

Sinus tachycardia can also be produced by medications that either affect the heart directly (atropine, quinidine sulfate, epinephrine, and dopamine) or by central nervous system stimulant medications that cause an indirect stimulation on the heart (amphetamines, cocaine, caffeine, and nicotine). Hormones such as

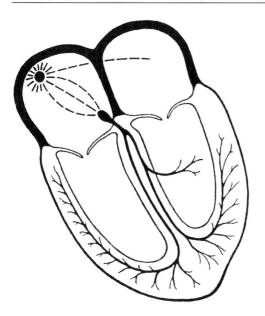

FIG. 4–5. SINUS NODE DISCHARGES IMPULSES AT REGULAR INTERVALS BUT AT A FASTER RATE THAN NORMAL IN SINUS TACHYCARDIA. IMPULSES FOLLOW THE NORMAL CONDUCTION PATHWAYS THROUGH THE REST OF THE HEART.

thyroid will also cause an increase in the heart rate, as well as the general metabolism of the body.

The third common cause of sinus tachycardia is from damage to the heart tissue itself, from either acute injury such as an MI, trauma or infection, or chronic cardiac problems such as coronary heart disease, congestive heart failure, or cor pulmonale.

SYMPTOMS

Sinus tachycardia actually increases the cardiac output, up to a point. This means that there are many times a patient is in sinus tachycardia but has no symptoms. Usually symptoms do not develop until the rate exceeds 160 beats/min. The major difficulty for patients who have sinus tachycardia is that, with high rates over an extended period of time (days to weeks), the heart does not have a chance to rest and recover properly, leading to weakness in the muscle tissue and ineffective contractions. The end result of this episode is either heart failure or another more serious dysrhythmia.

The patient symptoms observed with sinus tachycardia are similar to those seen with sinus bradycardia. They include (1) neurologic signs and symptoms such as dizziness, weakness, syncope, disorientation, and seizures, and (2) cardiovascular signs and symptoms such as chest pain, chest pressure, chest tightness, shortness of breath, diaphoresis, pallor of the skin, low blood pressure, weak pulses, occasional palpitations, or "fluttering" feeling in the chest.

TREATMENT

The main goal of treatment is to slow the heart rate down to a level where optimal cardiac output is obtained with minimal strain on the cardiac muscle tissues. In general, the goal is to reduce the heart rate to less than 100 beats/min. As in all dysrhythmia treatments, the clinical condition of the patient must be considered. If the patient is asymptomatic and shows no signs of developing congestive heart failure secondary to the fast rate, then he or she may require no treatment. If the patient is symptomatic or is showing signs of excessive heart strain from the fast rate in the form of heart failure, then treatment is required. Sinus tachycardia can be treated by the following:

- Eliminate the cause of the tachycardia. If the tachycardia is a result of a high fever, reducing the fever will bring the heart rate down. If the tachycardia is a result of fear, anxiety, or pain, relief from these factors helps to reduce the rate to normal. The same principle works for sinus tachycardia that is a result of stimulating medications. Elimination of these from the body reduces the heart rate.
- Use central nervous system depressant medications. This group of medications include the minor tranquilizers and antianxiety agents such as diazepam (Valium), chlordiazepoxide (Librium), oxazepam (Serax), alprazolam (Xanax), as well as narcotic medications such as morphine sulfate and meperidine hydrochloride (Demerol).
- Use specific cardiac medications to slow the heart rate. These medications tend to be more effective in their use when the sinus tachycardia is a result of cardiac damage secondary to an MI, congestive heart failure, or other type of cardiac injury. These medications include digoxin, the beta-blockers such as propranolol (Inderal), and the calcium channel blockers, particularly verapamil (Calan) (Fig. 4-6).

FIG. 4–6. EXAMPLE OF SINUS TACHYCARDIA.

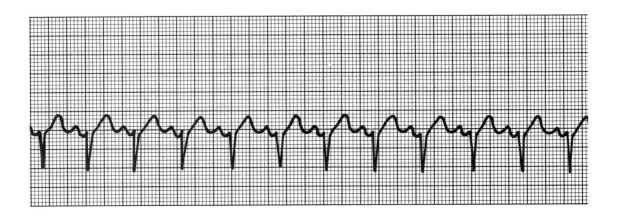

CRITERIA FOR SINUS TACHYCARDIA

Rhythm: Regular.

Rate: Above 100 beats/min.

Atrial Conduction: One P wave before each QRS; normal shape; consistent.

AV Conduction: PRI 0.12–0.20 second; same across the whole strip.

Ventricular Conduction: QRS 0.06–0.10 second; uniform in shape.

SINUS DYSRHYTHMIA

Sinus dysrhythmia (also called sinus arrhythmia, SA, respiratory pattern) (Fig. 4-7) is a dysrhythmia that is caused by irregular impulse formation in the SA node. After the impulses leave the SA node, they follow the normal conduction system through the rest of the heart, producing normal depolarization and a normal ECG pattern. The general criteria are identical to those for a normal sinus rhythm except for the rhythm. The rhythm will be totally irregular but will correspond to the respiratory cycle. Usually the rate will increase with inhalation and decrease with exhalation.

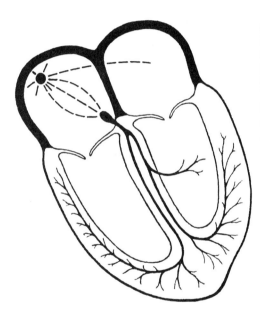

FIG. 4–7. SINUS NODE DISCHARGES IMPULSES AT IRREGULAR INTERVALS BUT GENERALLY AT NORMAL RATES IN SINUS DYSRHYTHMIA. THE IRREGULARITY IS OFTEN IN RESPONSE TO CHANGES IN INTRATHORACIC PRESSURE. THE IMPULSES FOLLOW THE NORMAL CONDUCTION PATHWAYS THROUGH THE REST OF THE HEART.

CAUSES

Most commonly, sinus dysrhythmia is associated with the normal changes in pressure in the chest cavity during inspiration and expiration. There are many other structures in the chest cavity other than the lungs and heart. The structures most affected by the changes in pressure during the breathing process are the great blood vessels, in particular, the vena cava, which is a relatively thin-walled vessel. As the individual breathes in, a negative pressure is created in the chest cavity, which allows air to rush in from the outside. This negative pressure also tends to expand the vena cava, thus allowing for an increase in blood return to the right side of the heart (increased preload). The heart responds to the increased blood supply by increasing its rate. When the individual breathes out, a positive pressure is created in the chest that tends to constrict the vena cava, thereby reducing the blood returning to the right side of the heart (decreased preload). The heart responds to the decrease in blood volume by slowing down its rate. The overall effect of this process on the ECG is a rhythm that gradually speeds up, then gradually slows down. On a long enough ECG strip, this process becomes evident. On a short 6-second strip, the interpreter usually only sees the speeding up phase or the slowing down phase. Overall, the rhythm may appear irregular.

A sinus dysrhythmia pattern may be a normal variation in all individuals but is particularly common in children and young adults. It tends to produce only minimal compromise in cardiac output. Patients who are on positive pressure ventilators often display a type of sinus dysrhythmia pattern due to the major alterations in intrathoracic pressure produced by the ventilator.

Sinus dysrhythmia that is a result of cardiac damage from an MI, rheumatic heart disease, cardiac ischemia, or coronary heart disease tends to be more serious in nature and has the potential to lead to other dysrhythmias. Sinus dysrhythmia may also be caused by digoxin toxicity. Aggressive treatment in these latter situations is sometimes required.

SYMPTOMS

Since there is a minimal decrease or no decrease in cardiac output from this dysrhythmia, there usually are no symptoms associated with the dysrhythmia itself. Unless the patient is on a monitor or telemetry, the only real way of detecting this dysrhythmia is to note an irregular pulse when taken for 1 full minute.

TREATMENT

If there is no decrease in cardiac output and no symptoms associated with the dysrhythmia, it does not require treatment. There is no specific treatment for sinus dysrhythmia. In some instances, the basic sinus dysrhythmia may also be present when there is a sinus tachycardia, called *sinus tachy-dysrhythmia,* or when there is an underlying sinus bradycardia, called *sinus brady-dysrhythmia.* If there are symptoms associated with the tachycardia or the bradycardia, the treatment would be the same as for those specific dysrhythmias (see above). A very slow sinus brady-dysrhythmia can be a manifestation of a serious dysrhythmia, namely, sick sinus syndrome. A pacemaker is the usual treatment for sick sinus syndrome (Fig. 4-8).

CRITERIA FOR SINUS DYSRHYTHMIA

Rhythm: Irregular with evidence of increases or decreases in rate. The difference between the time for the two fastest beats and the two slowest beats should be greater than 0.12 second.

Rate: Usually in the normal range (60–100 beats/min) but it can be faster or slower.

Atrial Conduction: One P wave before each QRS; normal in shape; consistent.

FIG. 4–8. EXAMPLE OF SINUS DYSRHYTHMIA.

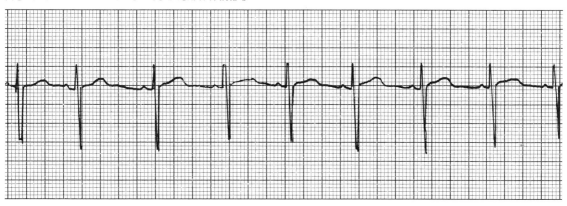

AV Conduction: PRI 0.12–0.20 second; same across the whole strip.

Ventricular Conduction: QRS 0.06–0.10 second; uniform in shape.

SINUS EXIT BLOCK

Sinus exit block (also called sinus block, SA block, blocked sinus beats) (Fig. 4-9) refers to a dysrhythmia that occurs when impulses from the sinus node are blocked immediately after they are initiated by the sinus node. The sinus node

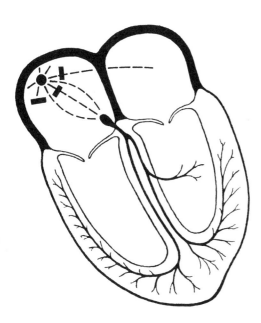

FIG. 4–9. SINUS NODE DISCHARGES IMPULSES AT REGULAR INTERVALS AND AT A NORMAL RATE, BUT THEY ARE BLOCKED HIGH IN THE ATRIAL CONDUCTION SYSTEM; THEREFORE, NO P WAVE AND NO QRS COMPLEX ARE INSCRIBED ON THE ECG PAPER.

continues to produce impulses but none of them are conducted to the atrial muscle tissue or any other part of the conduction system of the heart (sometimes called atrial asystole).

If no backup pacemaker areas of the heart take over, there is a long pause during which there is no P wave, no PR interval, and no QRS complex (*i.e.,* no ECG pattern). Since the sinus node continues to discharge impulses at its normal rate and rhythm, when the block is relieved and the impulses can travel to the rest of the heart, the pattern produced is "in cycle" and has the same rate as the pattern before the pause. To determine if a beat is "in cycle," measure the distance between three normal beats prior to the missed beat or pause. If the beat immediately after the pause falls where a beat would normally be expected to fall, then it is in cycle. If it does not fall there, then the beat is "out of cycle" and it is another type of dysrhythmia (Fig. 4-10). If the pause is longer than one beat, an alternate method of measuring the cycle can be used. This method involves measuring the distance between two normal beats and reproducing that interval across the pause until the next beat is encountered. If this beat is where it would be expected to be, then it is in cycle. If the beat is either before or after the expected location, then it is out of cycle.

CAUSES

Sinus blocked beats are often associated with conditions that may cause sinus bradycardia. These conditions include vagal stimulation, cardiac depressant medications, and central nervous system depressant medications. More commonly, sinus blocks are caused by serious cardiac diseases such as MI, congestive failure, arterial sclerotic heart disease, and occlusion of the sinus nodal artery. Congenital heart defects such as atrial-septal defects may also produce sinus blocked beats.

SYMPTOMS

If the block is transient and infrequent, there may be no symptoms associated with its presence. If the episodes of blocked beats are more frequent, often there will be complaints of palpitations or "skipped beats" in the chest due to the long filling period of the ventricles during the missed beat. If the pauses from the blocked beats are excessively long (3 or more seconds), there will most likely be complaints of some dizziness, weakness, or even transient syncope with chest pressure or pain. Sinus blocked beats usually do not last for more than 3 seconds and tend to be transient in nature. In the presence of a recent MI, the patient must be monitored closely for episodes of asystole.

TREATMENT

If the patient is asymptomatic and the block is infrequent and transient, no treatment may be required. If the block is caused by cardiac medication therapy, then removal of those medications from the patient's treatment or reduction in dosage is required. In the event that the sinus block is severe, producing symptoms and asystole, it is treated more aggressively. Atropine sulfate IV is the usual first-line treatment to attempt to stimulate the SA node. It also improves conduction through the blocked conduction pathways in the atria. The atropine may be used alone or in conjunction with medications such as isoproterenol (IV drip) or epinephrine (IV push) or other cardiac stimulant medications. If the sinus block does not respond to any of the medication treatments, a pacemaker may need to be inserted. A temporary pacemaker is used if the sinus block is secondary to an acute MI, because these blocks have the potential to be transient after the myocardial healing process begins and the swelling from the injured area is reduced. If the sinus block seems to be a permanent condition, or serious and frequent enough to cause symptoms, a permanent pacemaker may be used.

FIG. 4–10. EXAMPLE OF SINOATRIAL BLOCK.

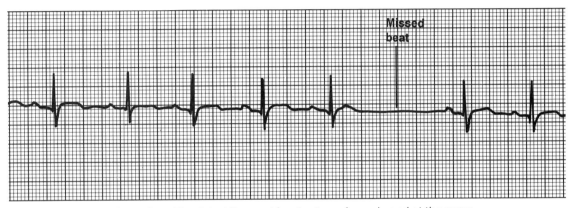

In sinus block there is a missed beat, but the next beat returns in cycle and at the same rate as the rhythm prior to the missed beat.

CRITERIA FOR SINUS BLOCK

Rhythm: Overall irregular pattern with a pause of one or more missed beats that return in cycle at the same rate as the rhythm before the pause. The rhythm may be regular before and after the pause.

Rate: Basic rate may be normal (60–100 beats/min), faster than normal or slower than normal. The overall rate will usually be slower due to the missed beats.

Atrial Conduction: One P wave before each QRS; normal shape; consistent.

AV Conduction: PRI 0.12–0.20 second; same across the whole strip.

Ventricular Conduction: QRS 0.06–0.10 second; uniform in shape.

SINUS ARREST

Sinus arrest (also called SA arrest, sinus pause, pause) (Fig. 4-11) is a dysrhythmia that occurs when the sinus node fails to discharge an impulse for one or more cycles. The sinus node is "arrested," that is, stops producing impulses. Sinus

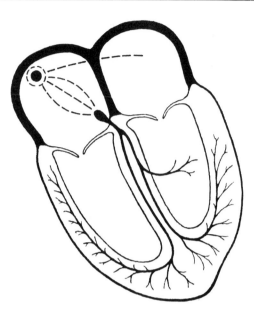

FIG. 4–11. THE SINUS NODE STOPS DISCHARGING IMPULSES FOR ONE OR MORE CYCLES IN SINUS ARREST. DURING THE ARREST PERIOD, THE SINUS NODE RESETS ITSELF SO THAT WHEN IT DOES START DISCHARGING IMPULSES AGAIN, THE RETURNING BEAT IS OUT OF CYCLE AND THE RATE IS OFTEN DIFFERENT FROM THE RATE BEFORE THE PAUSE.

arrest is a more serious condition than sinus blocked beats because the underlying pathology has affected the sinus node itself, not just the conduction system in the atria. When the sinus node fails to initiate an impulse and if the backup pacemakers do not take over the pacing functions of the heart, there is a long pause during which there is no P wave, no PR interval, and no QRS complex. Because the sinus node is not discharging any impulses during this time span, when it does start producing impulses, the ECG pattern will be out of cycle and at a different rate than the pattern before the pause. (See the previous section for an explanation of how to measure cardiac cycle.)

CAUSES

Although the factors that produce sinus block have the potential to produce sinus arrest, sinus arrest is more often caused by severe cardiac disease states. These disease states include infectious inflammatory diseases of the heart (rheumatic heart disease, endocarditis, pericarditis, and myocarditis); coronary heart disease; MI; autoimmune disorders; cardiomyopathy; surgical injuries to the atria; and metastatic diseases of the heart. A small group of individuals may be classified as having idiopathic sinus arrest where no specific physiologic factor can be found.

SYMPTOMS

The symptoms are similar to those for sinus block except that patients with sinus arrest tend to have more severe symptoms. These symptoms result from the fact that sinus arrest often produces longer (3–9 seconds) and more frequent pauses. The symptoms are the ones usually seen when there has been a significant decrease in cardiac output. Neurologically, the patient is dizzy, lightheaded, and weak, and may have episodes of transient syncope. These episodes of transient syncope are called *transient syncope attacks*, *Stokes-Adams Syndrome*, or *syncope*. Cardiac symptoms include chest pressure or pain, shortness of breath, diaphoresis, low blood pressure, cool skin, and weak, irregular pulses.

TREATMENT

Since the potential for sinus arrest to develop into asystole is greater than that for sinus block, the treatment is usually more aggressive. If the dysrhythmia is medication-induced, removal of the medication or a reduction in its dosage would be required. If the sinus arrest is caused by cardiac disease, a permanent demand pacemaker is often inserted. The same medications used to treat sinus block and sinus bradycardia are used in sinus arrest (atropine sulfate, epinephrine, and isoproterenol) for short-term management, to maintain an adequate tissue perfusion until a pacemaker can be inserted. In some patients, sinus arrest may be a temporary and transient condition that produces minimal decrease in cardiac output and no symptoms. In these patients, the key to treatment is to monitor them closely until the condition resolves itself (Fig. 4-12).

FIG. 4–12. EXAMPLE OF SINOATRIAL ARREST.

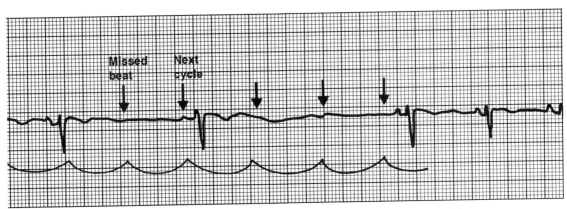

In sinoatrial arrest, there is a missed beat and the next beat returns out of cycle. The rate after the missed beat is different from the rate of the pattern before the missed beat.

CRITERIA FOR SINUS BLOCK

Rhythm: Overall irregular pattern with a pause of one or more missed beats with return out of cycle and often at a different rate than the pattern before the pause. The rhythm may be regular or irregular before or after the pause.

Rate: The basic rhythm may be normal (60–100 beats/min), faster than normal, or slower than normal. The overall rate, which includes the pauses, is bradycardic due to the pause.

Atrial Conduction: One P wave before each QRS; normal shape; consistent.

AV Conduction: PRI 0.12–0.20 second; same for whole strip.

Ventricular Conduction: QRS 0.06–0.10 second; uniform in shape.

PRACTICE ECG STRIPS FOR CHAPTER 4

Directions. On the following practice ECG strips, analyze each strip according to its rhythm, rate, atrial conduction, AV conduction, and ventricular conduction. Arrive at an interpretation of the strip based upon the analysis and criteria for dysrhythmias originating in the SA node as learned in this chapter. (See Appendix II for interpretations.)

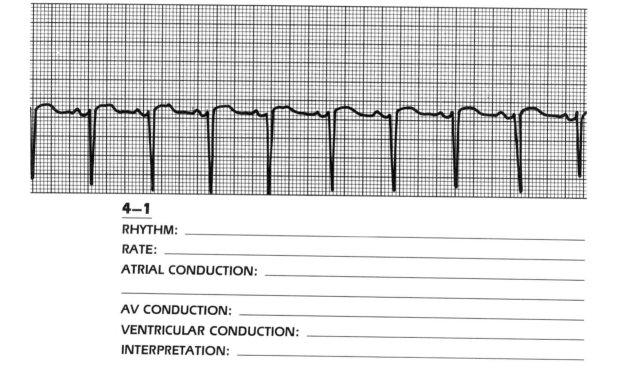

4–1

RHYTHM: _____

RATE: _____

ATRIAL CONDUCTION: _____

_____

AV CONDUCTION: _____

VENTRICULAR CONDUCTION: _____

INTERPRETATION: _____

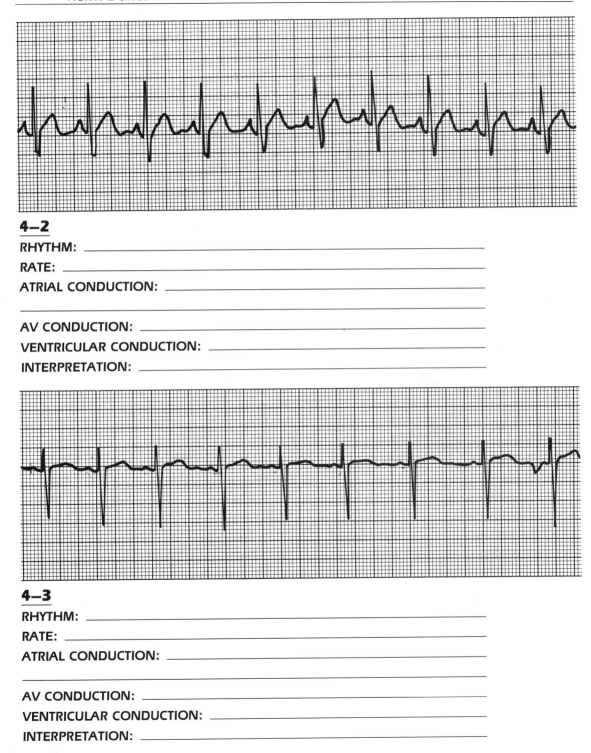

4–2

RHYTHM: _____

RATE: _____

ATRIAL CONDUCTION: _____

_____

AV CONDUCTION: _____

VENTRICULAR CONDUCTION: _____

INTERPRETATION: _____

4–3

RHYTHM: _____

RATE: _____

ATRIAL CONDUCTION: _____

_____

AV CONDUCTION: _____

VENTRICULAR CONDUCTION: _____

INTERPRETATION: _____

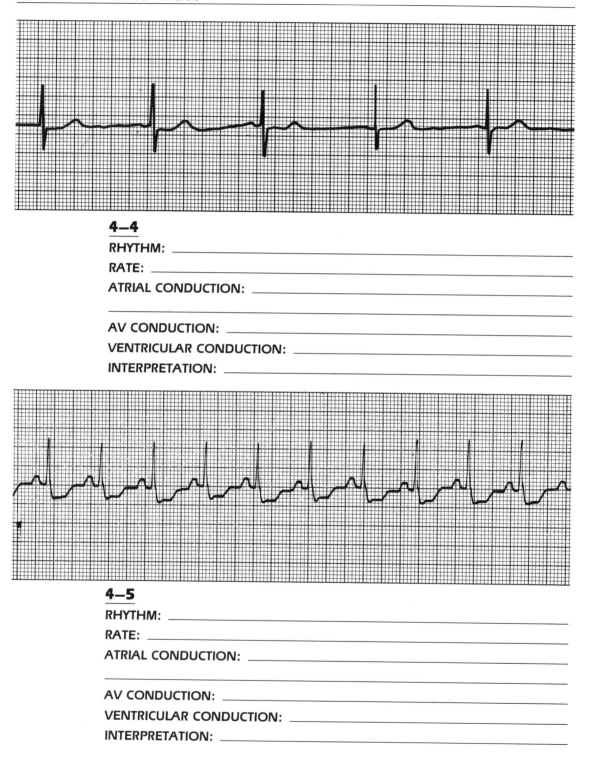

4–4

RHYTHM: _____

RATE: _____

ATRIAL CONDUCTION: _____

_____

AV CONDUCTION: _____

VENTRICULAR CONDUCTION: _____

INTERPRETATION: _____

4–5

RHYTHM: _____

RATE: _____

ATRIAL CONDUCTION: _____

_____

AV CONDUCTION: _____

VENTRICULAR CONDUCTION: _____

INTERPRETATION: _____

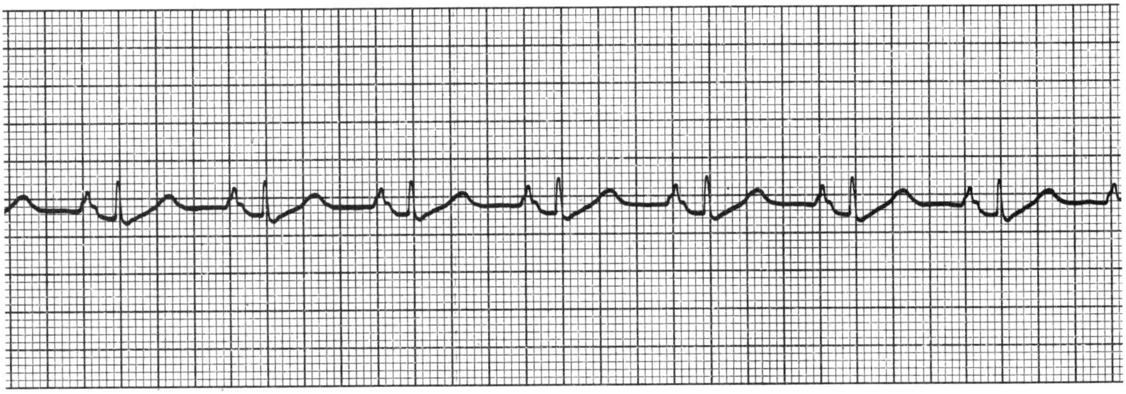

4–6

RHYTHM: _____

RATE: _____

ATRIAL CONDUCTION: _____

_____

AV CONDUCTION: _____

VENTRICULAR CONDUCTION: _____

INTERPRETATION: _____

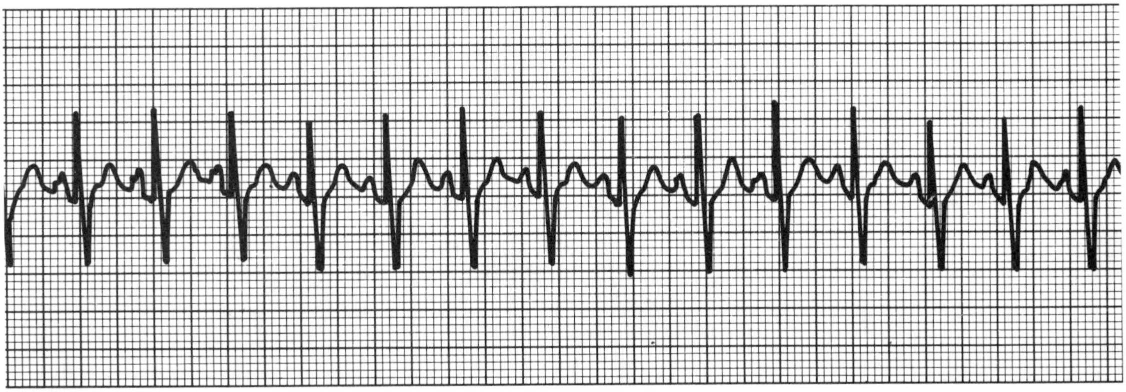

4–7

RHYTHM: _____

RATE: _____

ATRIAL CONDUCTION: _____

_____

AV CONDUCTION: _____

VENTRICULAR CONDUCTION: _____

INTERPRETATION: _____

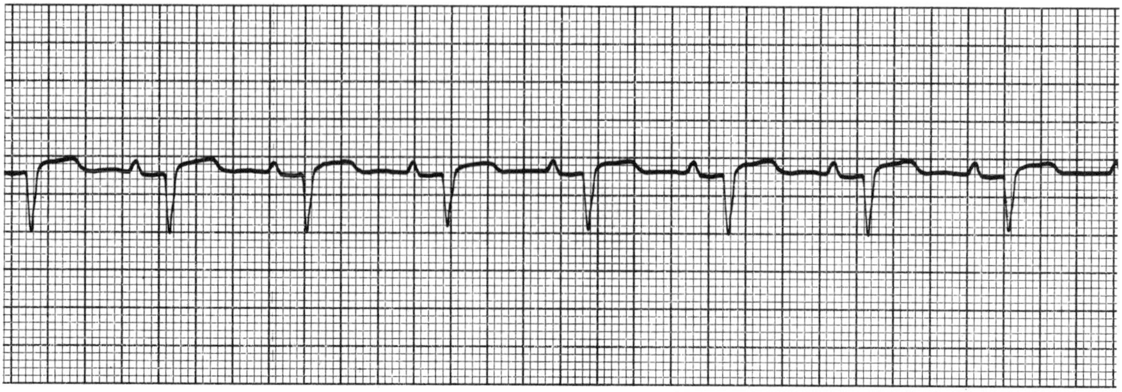

4–8

RHYTHM: _____

RATE: _____

ATRIAL CONDUCTION: _____

_____

AV CONDUCTION: _____

VENTRICULAR CONDUCTION: _____

INTERPRETATION: _____

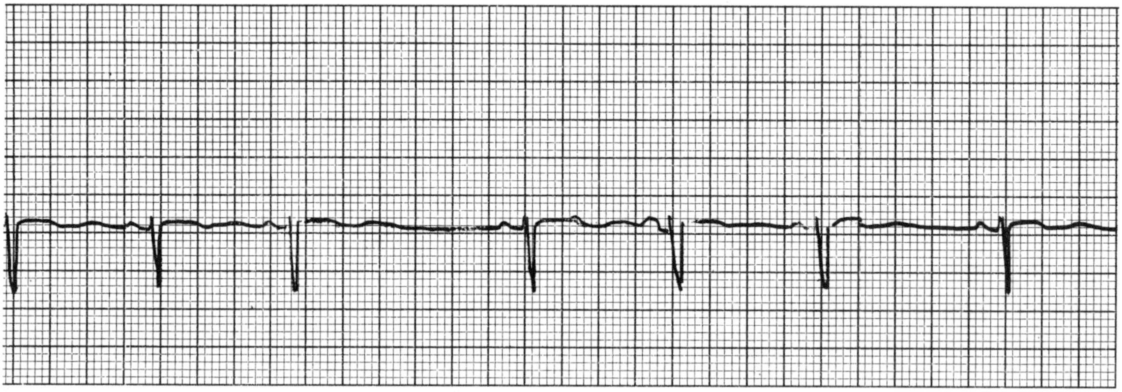

4–9

RHYTHM: _____

RATE: _____

ATRIAL CONDUCTION: _____

_____

AV CONDUCTION: _____

VENTRICULAR CONDUCTION: _____

INTERPRETATION: _____

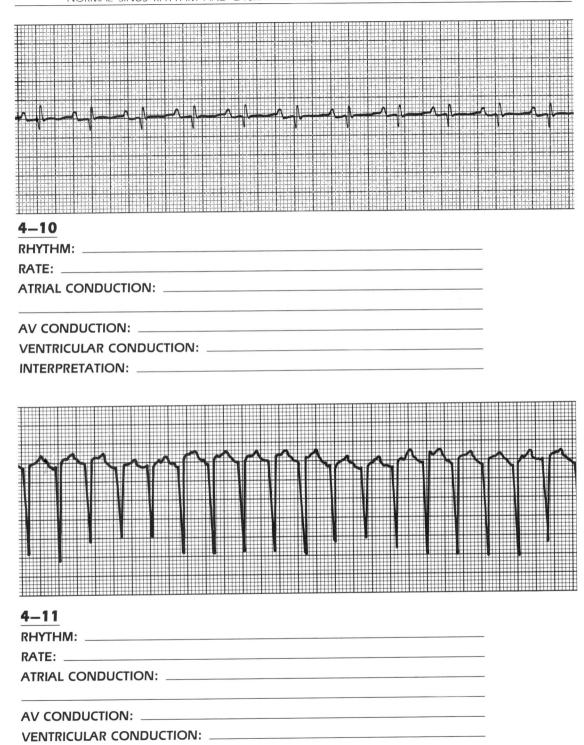

4—10

RHYTHM: _____

RATE: _____

ATRIAL CONDUCTION: _____

_____

AV CONDUCTION: _____

VENTRICULAR CONDUCTION: _____

INTERPRETATION: _____

4—11

RHYTHM: _____

RATE: _____

ATRIAL CONDUCTION: _____

_____

AV CONDUCTION: _____

VENTRICULAR CONDUCTION: _____

INTERPRETATION: _____

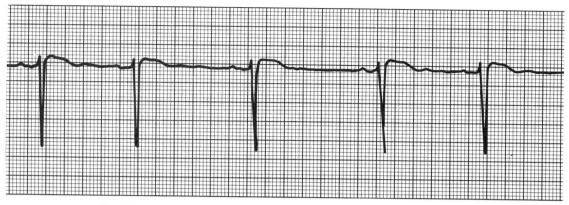

4–12

RHYTHM: _____

RATE: _____

ATRIAL CONDUCTION: _____
_____

AV CONDUCTION: _____

VENTRICULAR CONDUCTION: _____

INTERPRETATION: _____

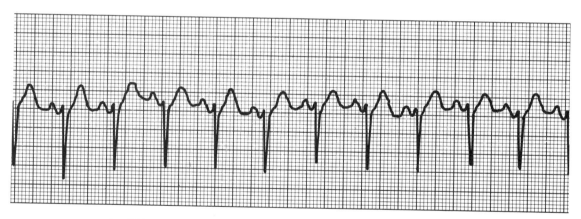

4–13

RHYTHM: _____

RATE: _____

ATRIAL CONDUCTION: _____
_____

AV CONDUCTION: _____

VENTRICULAR CONDUCTION: _____

INTERPRETATION: _____

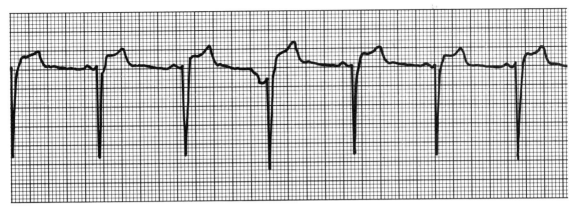

4—14

RHYTHM: _____

RATE: _____

ATRIAL CONDUCTION: _____

_____

AV CONDUCTION: _____

VENTRICULAR CONDUCTION: _____

INTERPRETATION: _____

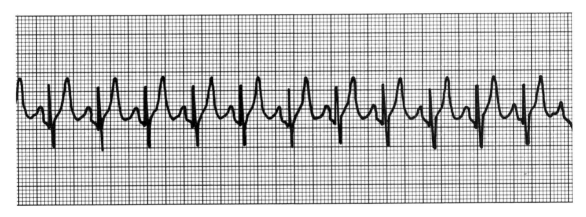

4—15

RHYTHM: _____

RATE: _____

ATRIAL CONDUCTION: _____

_____

AV CONDUCTION: _____

VENTRICULAR CONDUCTION: _____

INTERPRETATION: _____

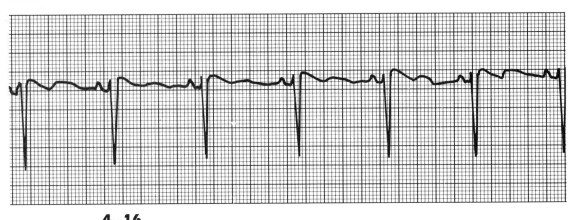

4–16

RHYTHM: _____

RATE: _____

ATRIAL CONDUCTION: _____

_____

AV CONDUCTION: _____

VENTRICULAR CONDUCTION: _____

INTERPRETATION: _____

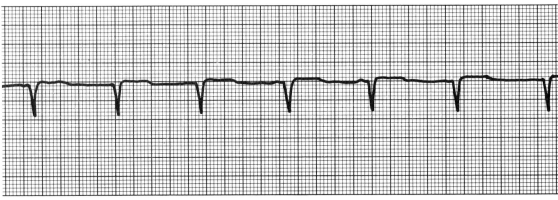

4–17

RHYTHM: _____

RATE: _____

ATRIAL CONDUCTION: _____

_____

AV CONDUCTION: _____

VENTRICULAR CONDUCTION: _____

INTERPRETATION: _____

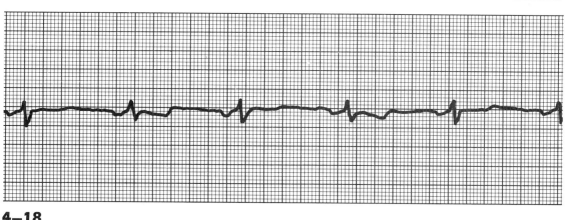

4—18

RHYTHM: _____

RATE: _____

ATRIAL CONDUCTION: _____
_____

AV CONDUCTION: _____

VENTRICULAR CONDUCTION: _____

INTERPRETATION: _____

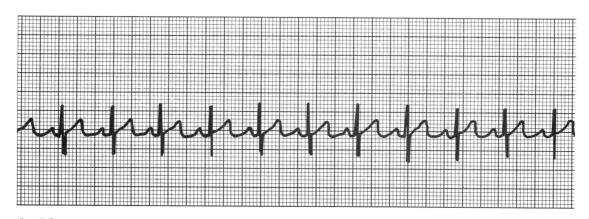

4—19

RHYTHM: _____

RATE: _____

ATRIAL CONDUCTION: _____
_____

AV CONDUCTION: _____

VENTRICULAR CONDUCTION: _____

INTERPRETATION: _____

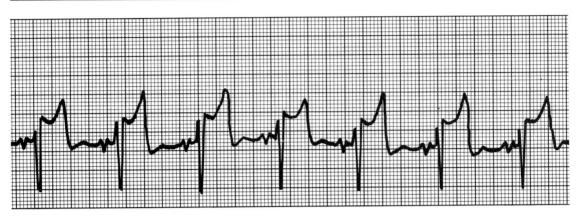

4–20

RHYTHM: _____

RATE: _____

ATRIAL CONDUCTION: _____

_____

AV CONDUCTION: _____

VENTRICULAR CONDUCTION: _____

INTERPRETATION: _____

CHAPTER

5

DYSRHYTHMIAS ASSOCIATED WITH THE ATRIA

LEARNING OBJECTIVES

After studying this section, the learner will be able to:

1. Describe the abnormal P wave configurations produced by atrial impulse initiation.
2. Discuss the common causes of atrial dysrhythmias.
3. Identify the atrial dysrhythmias that most severely compromise cardiac output.
4. List the most frequent symptoms associated with atrial dysrhythmias.
5. List the treatments for each of the atrial dysrhythmias discussed in the chapter.

The normal originating point for the depolarizing currents in the heart is the sinoatrial (SA) node. If the SA node should fail, the atria are the next place in the conduction system from which impulses can originate and act as a backup pacemaker. Also, the atria become irritable very easily and can quickly take over the pacemaker function of the heart. Since the conduction system of the atria and the cardiac muscle fibers themselves are very similar in structure to those of the SA node, the inherent rates for atrial pacemaker sites tend to be near the same rate as the inherent rate of the SA node.

The conduction patterns initiated by the atria are sometimes called "rougher" than those patterns initiated by the SA node. This rougher atrial pattern becomes evident on the electrocardiogram (ECG) strip in the form of abnormal-shaped P waves. In lead II, P waves are normally rounded, upright, and less than 0.11 second duration. Lead II is the best lead to look for normal P waves. In lead MCL_1, the P waves often appear different due to electrode placement. The key feature on the ECG in the determination of atrial dysrhythmias is the abnormal-shaped P wave (Fig. 5-1).

FIG. 5–1. VARIOUS SHAPES AND FORMS P WAVES CAN TAKE IN ATRIAL DYSRHYTHMIAS.

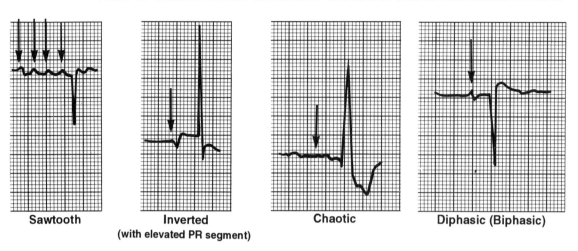

| Sawtooth | Inverted (with elevated PR segment) | Chaotic | Diphasic (Biphasic) |

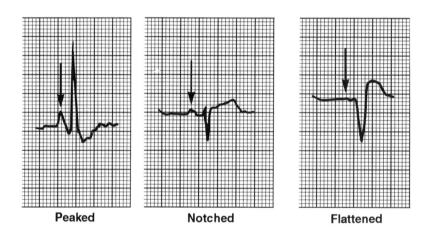

| Peaked | Notched | Flattened |

WANDERING PACEMAKER

Wandering pacemaker (also called WP, wandering atrial pacemaker, WAP) is a dysrhythmia that occurs when the pacemaker site switches location from beat to beat or during longer runs of beats from different pacemaker locations. The usual locations for a wandering pacemaker include the sinus node, any place in the atria, and the atrioventricular (AV) junction. Strictly speaking, any type of ectopic beat (premature or escape) could be considered a wandering pacemaker location. What distinguishes a wandering pacemaker as a dysrhythmia from ectopic beats is that the basic rhythm in the wandering pacemaker pattern remains regular or nearly regular as the pacemaker site changes, without any long pauses before or after QRS complexes (Fig. 5-2).

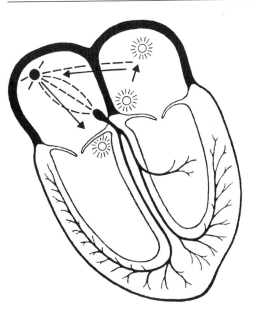

FIG. 5–2. IN WANDERING PACEMAKER, THE PACEMAKER SITE SWITCHES PERIODICALLY FROM ONE AREA OF THE ATRIA TO ANOTHER, OR TO THE SINOATRIAL NODE OR EVEN THE ATRIOVENTRICULAR JUNCTION. THE IMPULSES FOLLOW THE NORMAL CONDUCTION PATHWAYS THROUGH THE VENTRICLES.

The means of differentiating one pacemaker site from another is through close observation of the P wave. P waves that originate from the sinus node will have the normal P wave shape of being upright, rounded, and less than 0.11 second in lead II. P waves that originate from the atria have a different shape or morphology than the normal P waves. These atrial P waves may appear peaked, flattened, notched, diphasic, inverted, or in some way different from the sinus node initiated P waves.

P waves that originate from the AV junction also are different from the sinus node P waves. While the junctional dysrhythmias will be discussed in detail in Chapter 6, junctional P waves are characteristically inverted and frequently hidden in the QRS complex, therefore, there appears to be no P wave before the QRS complex.

Wandering pacemaker is considered to be an atrial rhythm even though some of the impulses may originate from the AV junction. After the impulses pass through the AV node, they follow the normal conduction pathways through the ventricles, resulting in normal QRS complexes. The PR interval will be in the normal range unless there is some other conduction defect present. If measured very closely, the PR intervals will often change slightly as the pacemaker site changes, because the conduction times through the atria will change, depending on the location of the pacemaker site. There will be no PR interval if the P wave is hidden, or comes after the QRS complex, as is found with junctional pacemaker site.

CAUSES

Wandering pacemaker may be a normal variation without a specific cause in some individuals. It is often found in individuals who have a history of recent cardiac disease such as a myocardial infarction (MI) or acute congestive heart failure, but can also be found in individuals with long-term cardiac disease such as coronary heart disease, angina, and cardiac ischemia from any cause. Wandering pacemaker can also be caused by high levels of cardiac medications, with digoxin as the most common one.

SYMPTOMS

Most patients who have wandering pacemaker have no symptoms with the dysrhythmia. It causes little reduction in cardiac output and is not evident unless the patient's ECG is being monitored. Wandering pacemaker is usually a transient dysrhythmia that terminates on its own.

TREATMENT

Since the wandering pacemaker dysrhythmia causes no symptoms, there is no specific treatment. If it has been caused by excessive cardiac medications, the stopping or reducing of these medications eliminate the dysrhythmia. In patients with a recent acute MI, wandering pacemaker may be the harbinger of other types of atrial dysrhythmias. These patients should be monitored closely for changes in their ECG patterns (Fig. 5-3).

FIG. 5–3. *EXAMPLE OF WANDERING PACEMAKER.*

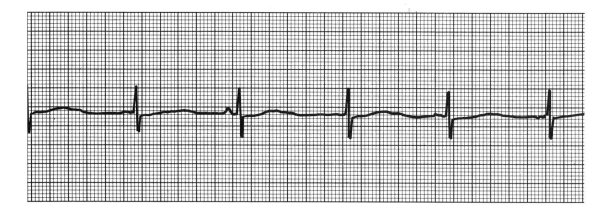

CRITERIA FOR WANDERING PACEMAKER

Rhythm: Regular to slightly irregular. The R to R interval will change slightly as the pacemaker site changes.

Rate: Usually 60–100 beats/min but may be slower or faster depending on the underlying rhythm.

Atrial Conduction: P waves will change shape as the pacemaker site changes. One P wave before each QRS except when the pacemaker site is junctional. Then the P wave may be hidden or after the QRS complex. The P to P interval will be slightly irregular as the pacemaker site changes. There must be at least three different-shaped P waves in the strip.

AV Conduction: PRI 0.12–0.20 second; the PRI may change slightly as the pacemaker site changes. No PRI when P waves are hidden or after the QRS complex.

Ventricular Conduction: QRS 0.16–0.10 second; uniform shape.

PREMATURE ATRIAL CONTRACTIONS

Premature atrial contractions are also called PACs, atrial premature contractions, APCs, premature atrial beats, and PABs (Fig. 5-4). They are produced when a single irritable area in the atria discharges an impulse before the next regular SA node impulse is due to discharge. This early discharge interrupts the regularity of the underlying rhythm with premature ectopic beats. Since these impulses arise from the atria, the ectopic beat has an abnormal-shaped P wave before the QRS complex. The QRS complex itself should be normal because the depolarization of the ventricles takes place in the normal way.

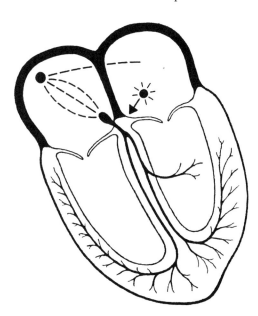

FIG. 5–4. A SINGLE IRRITABLE AREA IN THE ATRIA DISCHARGES EARLY IN THE CARDIAC CYCLE AT IRREGULAR IN-TERVALS PRODUCING PREMATURE EC-TOPIC BEATS. AFTER PASSING THROUGH THE ATRIO-VENTRICULAR NODE, THE IM-PULSES FOLLOW THE NORMAL PATHWAYS THROUGH THE VENTRICLES.

   Premature atrial contractions are probably one of the most common premature beats. It is important to remember that it is just a single beat that interrupts another rhythm. Interpretation of PAC must also include the interpretation of the underlying rhythm. It is possible to have PACs that occur in patterns with the underlying rhythm to produce a regularly irregular type rhythm. The names of these patterns will be discussed later in the book.

CAUSES

Most people, even those with no history of cardiac disease, will have PACs from time to time. Premature atrial contractions are most frequently caused by some common factors found in most people's lives. These factors include feelings of fear and anxiety, exercise, consumption of caffeine-containing beverages, use of tobacco, consumption of alcoholic beverages, or use of a wide variety of nervous system stimulant medications ranging from therapeutic medications (such as aminophylline) to street drugs (such as amphetamines and cocaine).

Premature atrial contractions are also caused by cardiac diseases such as MIs, congestive failure, and coronary heart disease. In individuals who have a history of cardiac disease, frequent PACs may precede a change in the person's basic cardiac rhythm. These individuals must be monitored closely.

SYMPTOMS

Although most individuals have no symptoms associated with the presence of PACs, there is a small group who complain of palpitations or feeling skipped beats in their chest, particularly if the PACs are frequent. Since the ventricles are contracting normally, cardiac output is only slightly reduced with PACs and the premature beats usually can be palpated in the peripheral vascular system, that is, they perfuse.

TREATMENT

Premature atrial contractions are usually not treated unless they are frequent or follow an MI. If the cause is an increased intake of caffeine, alcohol, or tobacco, reducing the intake of these substances should eliminate the dysrhythmia. Mild sedation with the minor tranquilizers will often help the individual who has PACs caused by anxiety. Some cardiac medications used in the treatment of PACs are quinidine sulfate in conjunction with digoxin, procainamide, and the calcium channel blockers (Fig. 5-5).

FIG. 5–5. EXAMPLE OF PREMATURE ATRIAL CONTRACTION.

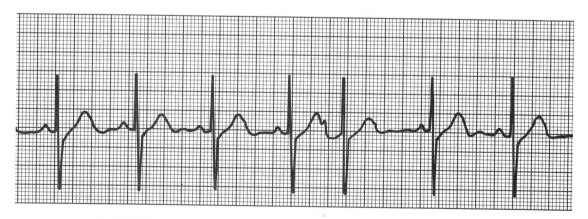

CRITERIA FOR PREMATURE ATRIAL CONTRACTIONS

Rhythm: Basically regular rhythm that is interrupted by single premature ectopic beats. If the underlying rhythm is irregular as in sinus dysrhythmia, the interpretation is made based on the P waves. The premature ectopic beat is followed by an incomplete compensatory pause (Fig. 5-6).

Rate: The rate of the basic or underlying rhythm determines the overall rate of the pattern. Premature atrial contractions are counted in the total rate.

Atrial Conduction: The P wave of the premature ectopic beat will be different from the P waves of the basic rhythm. There will be one P wave before each QRS complex. The P waves for the basic rhythm should be consistent.

AV Conduction: PRI 0.12–0.20 second. The PRI for the PAC may be slightly different from the PRI for the basic rhythm. If it is, record both the basic rhythm PRI and the PAC PRI.

Ventricular Conduction: QRS 0.06–0.10 second; the QRS for the PAC should be the same shape and duration as the QRS in the basic rhythm. (Note: Not all premature P waves have QRS complexes after them and some premature P waves conduct aberrantly.)

INCOMPLETE COMPENSATORY PAUSE
VERSUS COMPLETE COMPENSATORY PAUSE

After a premature beat of any type, there is often a pause during which the SA node of the heart "resets" itself for the next beat. To measure the pause when there is a regular underlying rhythm, measure the interval covered by three normal beats. Compare that interval to the interval produced by the premature beat by placing the point of one of the legs of the calipers on the normal beat just before the premature beat. If the normal beat following the premature beat occurs *before* the point where the second leg of the caliper is located, then it is an *incomplete compensatory pause*. If the following normal beat occurs at the point where the second leg of the calipers is located, then it is a *complete* (full) *compensatory pause* (sometimes just called a compensatory pause) (Fig. 5-6A, B).

FIG. 5–6. (A) INCOMPLETE COMPENSATORY PAUSES MOST OFTEN FOLLOW PACS ALTHOUGH THIS IS NOT AN ABSOLUTE ELEMENT IN DETERMINING A PAC.

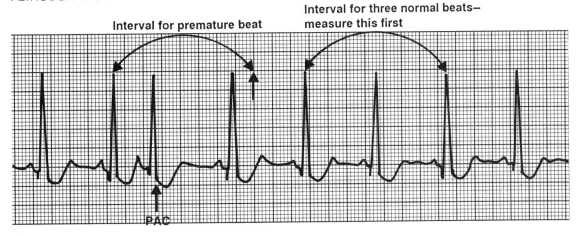

A

(continued)

FIG. 5–6. (continued) **(B)** COMPLETE COMPENSATORY PAUSES MOST OFTEN FOLLOW PRE-MATURE VENTRICULAR CONTRACTIONS, ALTHOUGH THIS IS NOT A 100% RELIABLE RULE. INDIVIDUAL PATTERNS MAY VARY AS TO COMPENSATORY PAUSES.

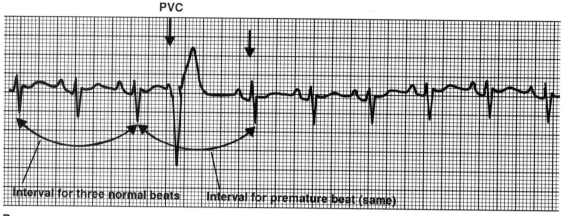

B

ATRIAL TACHYCARDIA

Atrial tachycardia (also called AT, paroxysmal atrial tachycardia, and PAT) (Fig. 5-7) is a rapid dysrhythmia that originates in the atria. It is usually faster than sinus tachycardia and is caused by a single area anywhere in the atria that has become extremely irritable and takes over the pacemaker functions in the heart.

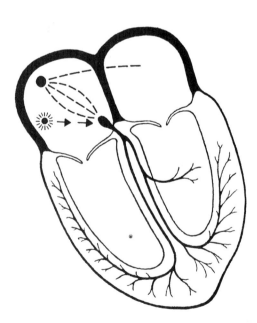

FIG. 5–7. ONE AREA IN THE ATRIA BECOMES VERY IRRITABLE AND INITIATES IMPULSES RAPIDLY ONE AFTER ANOTHER, TAKING OVER THE PACEMAKER FUNCTION FROM THE SINOATRIAL NODE. ALL IMPULSES ARE CONDUCTED THROUGH THE ATRIO-VENTRICULAR NODE TO THE VENTRICLES THROUGH THE NORMAL CONDUCTION PATHWAYS.

It can be thought of as a whole series of PACs occurring one after another. Because of the rapid rate of this dysrhythmia, the ventricles of the heart are unable to fill sufficiently and there can be a decrease in cardiac output.

Paroxysmal atrial tachycardia has the same mechanisms of production as atrial tachycardia except that it starts suddenly and often ends suddenly (paroxysmal = sudden onset). Paroxysmal atrial tachycardia is sometimes faster than atrial tachycardia and can compromise cardiac output even more.

CAUSES

The same factors that can cause PACs are also capable of producing AT. In addition, atrial tachycardia can occur without any specific cause. It is occasionally seen in women between 18 and 35 years of age who have no history of cardiac disease and no other reason to have the dysrhythmia.

SYMPTOMS

Depending on the rate of the dysrhythmia and the degree of compromise of cardiac output, many signs and symptoms are possible. These include the neurologic signs and symptoms of weakness, dizziness, and syncope, and the cardiac symptoms of chest pain or pressure, shortness of breath, chest palpitations (described as a fluttering or pounding), weak rapid pulses, and low blood pressure. One distinguishing sign in atrial tachycardia is a blood pressure that is lower than normal with a small pulse pressure. It is not unusual to obtain blood pressures in 86/80 range. The closeness of the diastolic pressure to the systolic pressure is due to the short time of diastolic filling caused by the rapid rate. Many patients can tolerate this type of pressure as long as their activity is restricted to bed rest.

TREATMENT

As with all dysrhythmias, the patient's clinical status must be considered before treatment is initiated. Atrial tachycardia is always treated but the aggressiveness of the treatment depends directly upon how well the dysrhythmia is being tolerated. The treatments can be divided into five approaches, which can be used independently or in combination.

Stimulation of the vagus nerve. These treatments rely on the fact that when the vagus nerve is stimulated, the parasympathetic system will cause the heart rate to slow. Some of the common methods used to stimulate the vagus nerve, either directly or indirectly, include the following: (1) carotid massage (indirect); (2) stimulating the gag reflex; (3) stimulating the anal sphincter; (4) pressure on the eyes; and (5) Valsalva's maneuver (indirect).

Medications that increase the blood pressure rapidly. These medications, when administered intravenous (IV) push, cause a sudden rapid rise in the systemic blood pressure. The body's response to a rapid rise in blood pressure through the parasympathetic system is to slow the heart rate. These medications are not used as often as they once were but still are very effective treatment of atrial tachycardia. The dosages of the medications are individualized to the patient, based on size, weight, and clinical condition. Monitoring blood pressure and heart rate during administration is essential. These medications include the following: metaraminol bitartrate (Aramine); oxymetazoline hydrochloride (Neo-Synephrine); and edrophonium chloride (Tensilon).

Medications that directly slow or block the impulse production. This group of medications has become the primary mode of medication treatment for atrial tachycardia. The calcium channel blocker verapamil hydrochloride (Calan, Isoptin) administered IV push is highly effective in stopping atrial tachycardia. Its tendency to lower the blood pressure rapidly and significantly requires very close monitoring of the blood pressure during IV administration.

The cardiac glycoside, digoxin (Lanoxin) is also effective in the termination of atrial tachycardia. This medication, even when administered IV push, tends to be slower acting than the medications listed above, but it is appropriate for patients who are tolerating the dysrhythmia.

Calming measures and sedation. In patients who are tolerating the atrial tachycardia well, who do not have any underlying cardiac disease, and who do not need immediate conversion to sinus rhythm, placing them in a calm, quiet environment may be enough to produce a slowing and eventual cardioversion of the atrial tachycardia. Sedative medications such as diazepam (Valium) and oxazepam (Serax) may also aid in the conversion of the atrial tachycardia to a slower rhythm.

Electrical cardioversion. This mode of treatment is indicated when the patient is extremely symptomatic with the dysrhythmia or when the other modes of treatment have not worked. An electrical current is passed through the heart from the cardioversion machine, stopping all intrinsic electrical activity in the heart. When the electrical activity of the heart resumes, it is hoped that the SA node will take over the pacemaker function and produce a normal sinus rhythm (Fig. 5-8).

FIG. 5–8. EXAMPLE OF ATRIAL TACHYCARDIA.

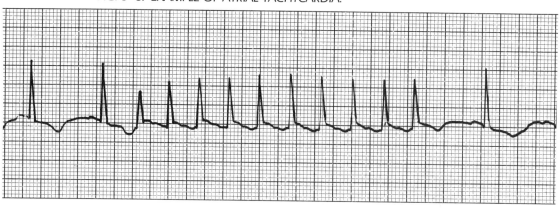

CRITERIA FOR ATRIAL TACHYCARDIA

Rhythm: Regular to slightly irregular. Paroxysmal atrial tachycardia shows a sudden onset from the basic rhythm.

Rate: Usual rate 150–250 beats/min.

Atrial Conduction: P waves will have shapes that are different from the P waves of the patient's sinus rhythm. If unable to identify normal sinus P waves, look for the abnormal-shaped P waves characteristic of atrial rhythms. Due to very rapid rates, P waves may be hidden in preceding T waves or QRS complexes.

AV Conduction: PR interval should be in the normal range of 0.12–0.20 second. It may be difficult to measure due to the rapid rate and hidden P waves.

Ventricular Conduction: QRS complex should be normal 0.06–0.10 second in duration and be consistent.

ATRIAL FLUTTER

Atrial flutter (Fig. 5-9) is a dysrhythmia that is produced when the atria become extremely irritable and contract at a rate that exceeds the rate at which the ventricles are capable of contracting. Physiologically, the atria are capable of contractions up to the rate of 400 times per minute. The ventricles can rarely exceed 250 contractions per minute because of their larger muscle mass and long conduction system. The rapid "fluttering" type beats produced in the atria originate in a single irritable area anywhere in the atria.

The AV node plays an important part in preventing damage to the ventricles from an excessively fast rate by acting as a filter or gatekeeper to prevent too many impulses from reaching the ventricles from the fluttering atria. The AV

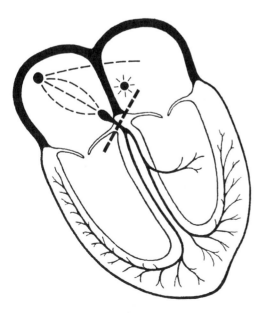

FIG. 5–9. A SINGLE AREA IN THE ATRIA BECOMES EXTREMELY IRRITABLE AND INITIATES IMPULSES AT A RATE FASTER THAN THE VENTRICLES ARE ABLE TO CONTRACT. THE ATRIO-VENTRICULAR NODE BEGINS TO BLOCK SOME OF THE IMPULSES FROM GETTING TO THE VENTRICLES. THE IMPULSES THAT DO TRAVEL THROUGH THE ATRIO-VENTRICULAR NODE FOLLOW THE NORMAL CONDUCTION PATHWAYS THROUGH THE VENTRICLES.

node selectively blocks impulses from the atria when the rate is excessive. The AV node may block one out of two atrial impulses (2 : 1 ratio); two out of three atrial impulses (3 : 1 ratio); three out of four atrial impulses (4 : 1 ratio); or it may vary the ratio from impulse to impulse (variable ratio). In any of these ratios, there will always be more flutter waves than QRS complexes.

CAUSES

Since the fluttering of the atria is caused by an irritable area in the atria, the same factors that can cause PACs will also produce atrial flutter. Atrial flutter is considered a more serious dysrhythmia because it is usually caused by more serious cardiac disease. Three to five percent of post MI patients will develop atrial flutter. It is also caused by long-term coronary heart disease, hypertension, chronic obstructive pulmonary disease, rheumatic heart disease, and pericarditis.

SYMPTOMS

Many patients report no or very minor symptoms with atrial flutter, including a rapid fluttering feeling, palpitations in the chest, or the feeling of "skipped beats." A small group of patients report the symptoms of dizziness, weakness, and chest pressure or pain with shortness of breath and some activity intolerance, particularly when the ventricular rate is rapid. Changes in blood pressure readings are usually minor.

TREATMENT

One of two approaches may be taken when treating atrial flutter.

First, if the dysrhythmia is a recent development and associated with a recent acute episode of cardiac disease such as an MI, the goal of the treatment would most likely be to attempt to convert the dysrhythmia back to a sinus rhythm. This course of treatment would be followed whether or not the patient was symptomatic with the dysrhythmia. Medications such as digoxin (Lanoxin), verapamil hydrochloride (Calan, Isoptin), quinidine sulfate, or even propranolol (Inderal) may be given either IV or PO to convert the atrial flutter to sinus rhythm. If these medications do not produce the required change in rhythm, then DC electrocardioversion may be used.

Second, if the dysrhythmia is long-term and caused by long-standing cardiac disease such as coronary heart disease, the goal of treatment would most likely be to keep the ventricular rate below 100 beats/min. Cardioversion in these individuals is either impossible or very short-lived. The same medications are used to slow the ventricular rate as are used to cardiovert the dysrhythmia, including digoxin and verapamil. They are usually administered PO and titrated to keep the rate below 100 beats/min. The patient needs to be cardiac monitored during treatment to prevent excessive slowing of the ventricular rate or even potential complete heart block (Fig. 5-10).

CRITERIA FOR ATRIAL FLUTTER

Rhythm: The atria and ventricles have two separate rhythms that should be analyzed separately.

FIG. 5–10. EXAMPLE OF ATRIAL FLUTTER.

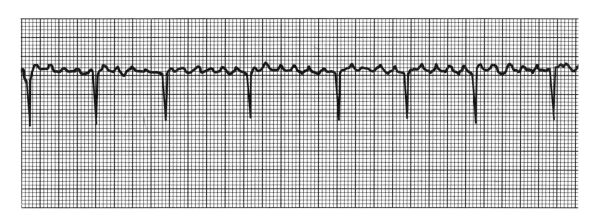

Atrial Rhythm: The P to P (flutter wave) interval should be regular.
Ventricular Rhythm: The R to R interval may be regular to irregular depending on whether the ratio of P to QRS is fixed or variable.

Rate: There are also two separate rates with this dysrhythmia that require separate analysis.
Atrial Rate: The most common rate at which the atria flutter is 300 beats/min, particularly when the dysrhythmia has not been treated. It will usually range between 250 and 300 beats/min.
Ventricular Rate: The rate at which the ventricles will contract is totally dependent on the ratio of blocked to conducted beats established by the AV node. For example, if the atria are contracting at 300 beats/min and the AV node has established a 4 : 1 ratio, the resultant ventricular rate will be 75 beats/min. As a rule of thumb, if the dysrhythmia has never been treated, the ratio will be 2 : 1 (ventricular rate of 150 beats/min). After treatment is well established, the ratio will usually be 4 : 1. During the period when the cardiac medication is reaching a therapeutic level, the ratio will be variable (2 : 1, 3 : 1, 4 : 1), with a variety of possible ventricular rates. Since keeping the ventricular rate below 100 beats/min is an important goal of treatment, it is usually noted in the interpretation if the dysrhythmia is *controlled* (less than 100 beats/min) or *uncontrolled* (more than 100 beats/min).

Atrial Conduction: P waves in atrial flutter assume a characteristic "sawtooth" pattern. They are peaked, at regular intervals, and uniform in shape and size; there are more of them than there are QRS complexes. These P waves of atrial flutter are sometimes called *F waves* or *flutter waves*. Occasionally, the atrial flutter P waves appear rounded, depending on lead placement.

AV Conduction: PR interval is not measured in atrial flutter because it is impossible to determine which of the flutter waves is being conducted through the AV node to produce the QRS complex.

Ventricular Conduction: QRS complexes should be normal 0.06–0.10 second in duration and consistent. Occasionally, the QRS complex is distorted in shape because of P waves that "push into" the complex on the ECG pattern.

ATRIAL FIBRILLATION

Atrial fibrillation (also called atrial fib) (Fig. 5-11) is a dysrhythmia of the atria that exists when the atria have become so irritable that multiple areas in the atria begin initiating depolarizing impulses. Unlike atrial tachycardia and atrial flutter, which have a single irritable atrial focus that results in a unified atrial contraction, atrial fibrillation results in small areas of the atria contracting independently of each other. The end result of this type of contraction is a "quivering" of the atria and loss of any atrial filling. The rate of these multiple impulses may range between 350 to 500 per minute.

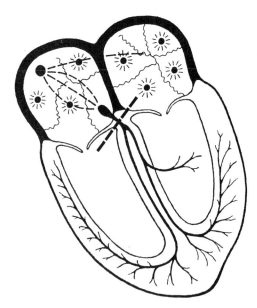

FIG. 5–11. THE ATRIA ARE SO IRRITABLE THAT MULTIPLE AREAS BEGIN TO INITIATE IMPULSES. THE ATRIO-VENTRICULAR NODE BLOCKS MANY OF THESE IMPULSES FROM TRAVELING TO THE VENTRICLES. THE IMPULSES THAT DO GET THROUGH FOLLOW THE NORMAL CONDUCTION PATHWAYS THROUGH THE VENTRICLES.

Because any or all of these atrial impulses have the potential to be conducted through the conduction system of the heart to the ventricles and produce a ventricular contraction, the AV node again becomes an important gatekeeper. As in atrial flutter, the AV node blocks a large number of these impulses, permitting only enough to pass through to allow for adequate cardiac output. Since there is no regularity at all to the pattern of these fibrillating impulses, the AV node allows them to pass through at totally random intervals, producing a totally irregular ventricular pattern.

CAUSES

Although many factors may cause atrial fibrillation, including those factors that cause PACs, atrial tachycardia, and atrial flutter, atrial fibrillation is usually associated with more serious cardiac disease. Most commonly it is caused by MIs, long-standing coronary heart disease, atrial-septal defects, and chronic obstructive lung disease.

SYMPTOMS

Because all atrial contraction is lost with atrial fibrillation, the cardiac output is reduced 10% to 15%. While most individuals who have healthy hearts have at least this much reserve capacity and would not miss the atrial "kick," the majority of patients with this dysrhythmia will show symptoms associated with the loss of output because of the underlying cardiac disease and decreased reserve capacity. The usual low cardiac output symptoms of dizziness, weakness, syncope, chest pressure or pain, shortness of breath, and low blood pressure may occur individually or in combination.

Additional complications of atrial fibrillation that may also produce symptoms include pulmonary emboli and congestive heart failure. Pulmonary emboli result when blood in the quivering atria of the patient with atrial fibrillation becomes static and begins to form clots. When these clots become large enough, they separate and travel through the right ventricle into the pulmonary artery and the lungs. The primary symptoms of pulmonary emboli include chest pain (pleuritic in nature), shortness of breath, and blood-tinged sputum. Congestive heart failure results from the long-term reduction in cardiac output. One of the effects of this reduction is poor profusion of the kidneys, resulting in decreased urinary output and increased pressures on the right and left sides of the vascular system. Symptoms associated with congestive heart failure include peripheral edema, distended neck veins, and lung congestion.

TREATMENT

Although atrial fibrillation is a more serious dysrhythmia than atrial flutter, the treatment modalities are almost identical. If the dysrhythmia is of recent origin in a patient with an MI or other acute cardiac disease and if the patient is symptomatic, the treatment will most likely involve the attempt to convert the atrial fibrillation to sinus rhythm. The same medications or electrocardioversion used for atrial flutter would also be used with atrial fibrillation. When the patient is asymptomatic and the cause of the dysrhythmia is long-term cardiac disease, the most likely goal of treatment will be to keep the ventricular rhythm below 100 beats/min. The same medications, including digoxin, verapamil, and quinidine, or a combination of these, would be used to control the rate (Fig. 5-12).

FIG. 5–12. EXAMPLE OF ATRIAL FIBRILLATION.

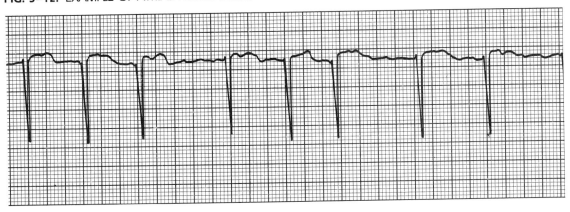

CRITERIA FOR ATRIAL FIBRILLATION

Rhythm: Totally irregular R to R intervals. If the rate is extremely fast, the R to R intervals tend to become more regular but usually display some periods of irregularity. Ashman's pattern of R to R intervals may occur in atrial fibrillation, often at slower rates (below 70 beats/min). This pattern is marked by long R to R intervals followed by short R to R intervals. It is caused by a conduction phenomenon in the ventricles, so it may be seen in other types of dysrhythmias (Fig. 5-13).

FIG. 5–13. *EXAMPLE OF ATRIAL FIBRILLATION WITH ASHMAN'S PATTERN*

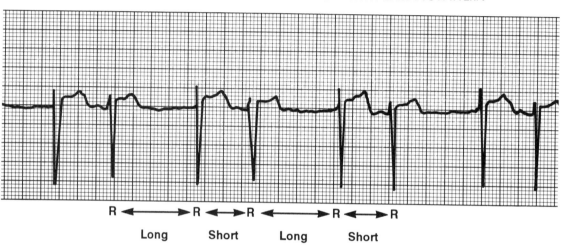

In an Ashman's Pattern, a long R to R interval is followed by a short R to R interval. This pattern is produced by conduction qualities of the ventricles and is not associated exclusively with atrial fibrillation.

Rate: There are two separate rates in this dysrhythmia.
Atrial Rate: Very fast but usually unable to determine because there are no distinct P waves.
Ventricular Rate: Untreated atrial fibrillation is usually very fast and can range from 100 to 250 beats/min. After it has been treated, it will slow to below 100 beats/min. Because an important goal of treatment is to keep the rate below 100 beats/min, it is important to note whether the dysrhythmia is controlled (less than 100 beats/min) or uncontrolled (more than 100 beats/min).

Atrial Conduction: P waves in atrial fibrillation are not distinct. The baseline where the P waves should be appears as a jagged, uneven, disorganized series of bumps. These P waves of atrial fibrillation are sometimes referred to as *f waves*, *fib waves*, or an *undulating baseline*. These fibrillation wave patterns can range from large, fairly distinct wave forms to very small, flat, indistinguishable forms, which may be referred to as *straight line atrial fibrillation*.

AV Conduction: PR interval is not measured in atrial fibrillation since there are no distinct P waves.

Ventricular Conduction: QRS complexes should be normal 0.06–0.10 second in duration and consistent. Occasionally, some QRS complexes are distorted due to the effect of the abnormal f waves on the QRS complex.

VARIATIONS ON THE ATRIAL FIBRILLATION PATTERN

ATRIAL FIBRILLATION/FLUTTER

Atrial fibrillation/flutter is also called atrial fib/flutter, atrial flutter/fib, and coarse atrial fibrillation) (Fig. 5-14). It is a pattern that seems to combine both dysrhythmias into one strip. For part of the strip, the P waves have the characteristic sawtooth flutter pattern, and then they will degenerate into the indistinct pattern of P waves for atrial fibrillation. These two patterns alternate with each other. The R to R interval remains irregular, with normal QRS complexes.

FIG. 5–14. EXAMPLE OF ATRIAL FIBRILLATION/FLUTTER.

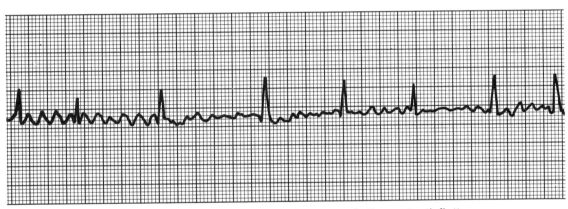

The pattern of the P waves alternates between those that appear in the sawtooth flutter pattern and those that have the chaotic atrial fibrillation pattern. R to R intervals are irregular.

ATRIAL FIBRILLATION WITH COMPLETE AV BLOCK

Atrial fibrillation with block (also called atrial fib with junctional escape rhythm) (Fig. 5-15) occurs when the AV node no longer conducts *any* of the irregular impulses produced by the fibrillating atria to the ventricles. This block can be caused by cardiac disease but is most often the result of the medication treatment of atrial fibrillation. All of the medications used to slow the rate have the potential to produce AV block. For there to be any ventricular contractions, a backup pacemaker must take over. The most usual area of backup pacemaker location is the AV junction. Atrial fibrillation with block will still have the typical irregular P wave formation, but the R to R intervals will be regular with a slower rate (AV junction has an inherent rate of 40–60 beats/min). QRS complexes should be normal in duration and shape.

FIG. 5–15. EXAMPLE OF ATRIAL FIBRILLATION WITH BLOCK.

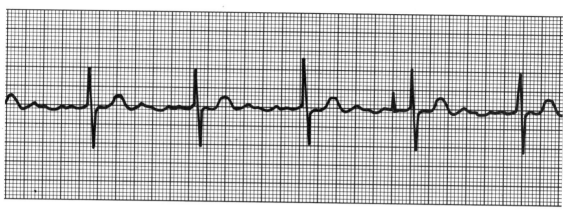

Although the P waves are in the chaotic, irregular atrial fibrillation pattern, the R to R intervals remain regular because a regular backup pacemaker site (atrio-ventricular junction) has taken over. The rate is frequently slower than a nonblocked atrial fibrillation because the backup rhythm is often an accelerated junction rhythm (especially in block caused by digoxin toxicity).

CHAOTIC ATRIAL RHYTHM

Chaotic atrial rhythm is also called multifocal atrial tachycardia, chaotic atrial tachycardia, and PACs with block (Fig. 5-16). Chaotic atrial rhythm is one of several "catch-all" categories in dysrhythmia analysis and interpretation; it is used when certain patterns occur that do not seem to fit anywhere else. The main feature of chaotic atrial rhythm is that there are irregular shaped P waves

FIG. 5–16. EXAMPLE OF CHAOTIC ATRIAL RHYTHMS.

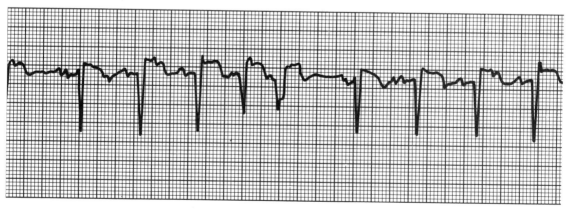

The P waves in chaotic atrial rhythms are irregular in interval and different shapes. The R to R intervals are also irregular but the QRS complexes remain normal in duration and shape.

(indicating multiple areas of impulse production in the atria) occurring at irregular intervals and at a fairly rapid rate (100–200 per minute). The P wave configuration at times degenerates into the fibrillation pattern of f waves. Sometimes there are more P waves than QRS complexes, although, in some instances, the conduction can be 1 to 1. The QRS complexes are normal in duration and shape but the R to R intervals are totally irregular. The ventricular rate may vary between 100 and 150 beats/min. (At rates between 60 and 100 beats/min with 1 : 1 conduction, the rhythm is wandering atrial pacemaker.)

PRACTICE ECG STRIPS FOR CHAPTER 5

Directions. On the following practice ECG strips, analyze each strip according to its rhythm, rate, atrial conduction, AV conduction, and ventricular conduction. Arrive at an interpretation of the strip based on the analysis and criteria for the dysrhythmias originating in the atria as learned in this chapter. (See Appendix II for interpretations.)

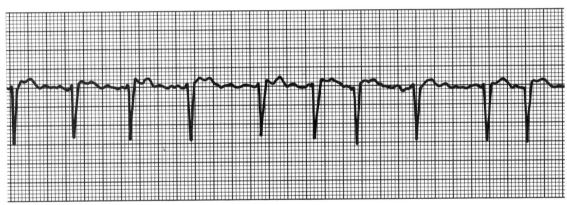

5–1

RHYTHM: _____

RATE: _____

ATRIAL CONDUCTION: _____

_____

AV CONDUCTION: _____

VENTRICULAR CONDUCTION: _____

INTERPRETATION: _____

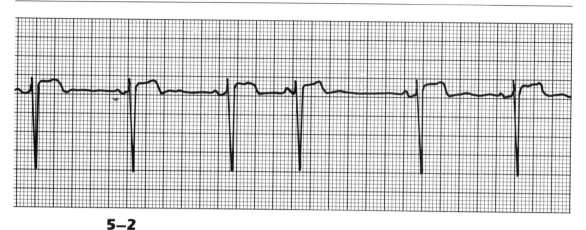

5–2
RHYTHM: _____

RATE: _____

ATRIAL CONDUCTION: _____

_____

AV CONDUCTION: _____

VENTRICULAR CONDUCTION: _____

INTERPRETATION: _____

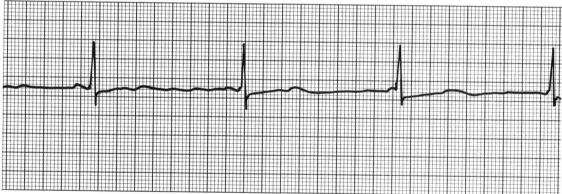

5–3
RHYTHM: _____

RATE: _____

ATRIAL CONDUCTION: _____

_____

AV CONDUCTION: _____

VENTRICULAR CONDUCTION: _____

INTERPRETATION: _____

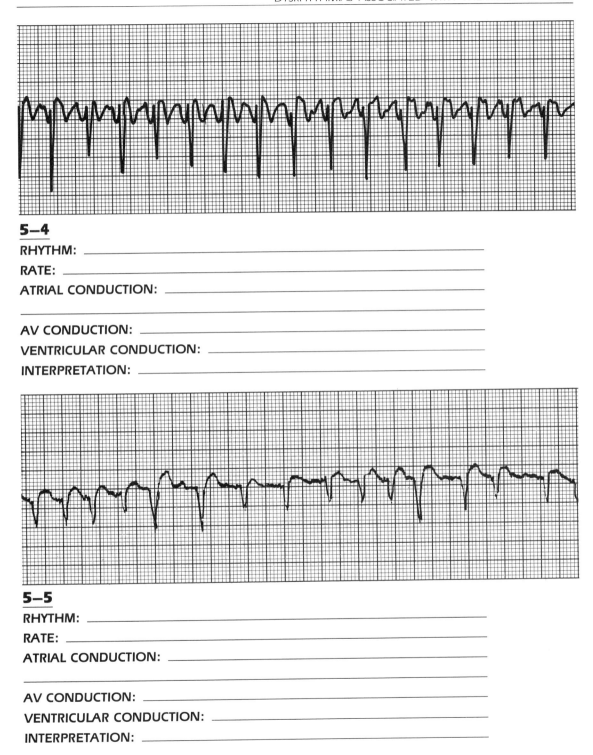

5–4

RHYTHM: _____

RATE: _____

ATRIAL CONDUCTION: _____

_____

AV CONDUCTION: _____

VENTRICULAR CONDUCTION: _____

INTERPRETATION: _____

5–5

RHYTHM: _____

RATE: _____

ATRIAL CONDUCTION: _____

_____

AV CONDUCTION: _____

VENTRICULAR CONDUCTION: _____

INTERPRETATION: _____

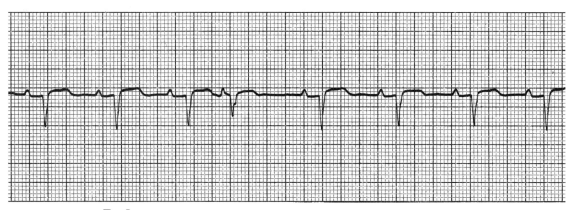

5–6

RHYTHM: _____

RATE: _____

ATRIAL CONDUCTION: _____

_____

AV CONDUCTION: _____

VENTRICULAR CONDUCTION: _____

INTERPRETATION: _____

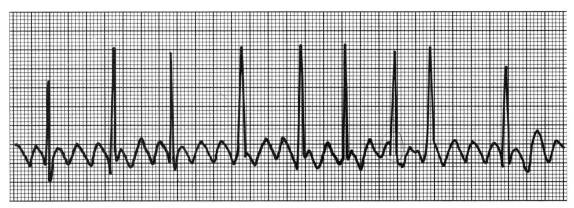

5–7

RHYTHM: _____

RATE: _____

ATRIAL CONDUCTION: _____

_____

AV CONDUCTION: _____

VENTRICULAR CONDUCTION: _____

INTERPRETATION: _____

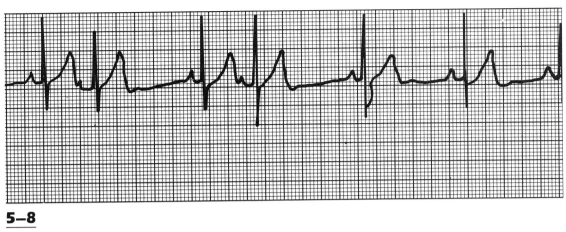

5—8

RHYTHM: _____

RATE: _____

ATRIAL CONDUCTION: _____

_____

AV CONDUCTION: _____

VENTRICULAR CONDUCTION: _____

INTERPRETATION: _____

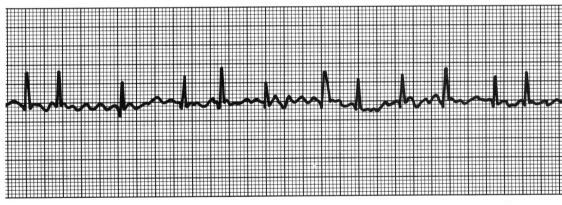

5—9

RHYTHM: _____

RATE: _____

ATRIAL CONDUCTION: _____

_____

AV CONDUCTION: _____

VENTRICULAR CONDUCTION: _____

INTERPRETATION: _____

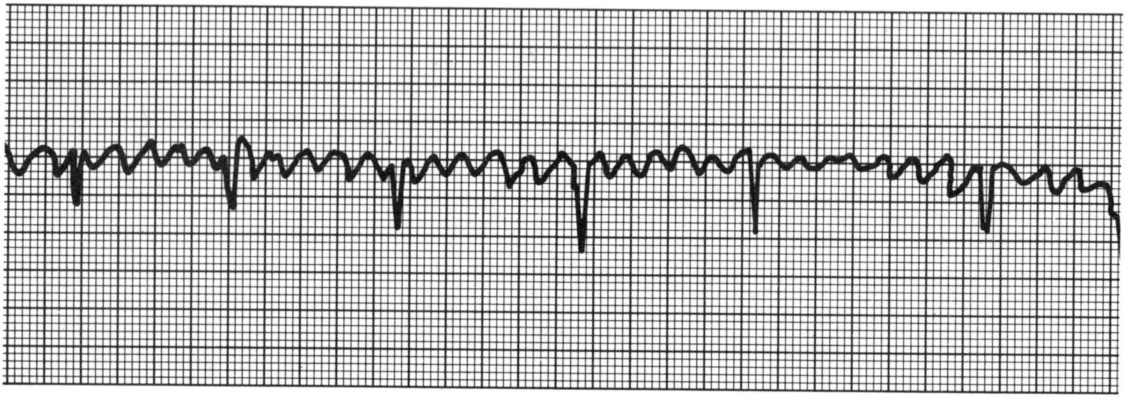

5–10

RHYTHM: _____

RATE: _____

ATRIAL CONDUCTION: _____

_____

AV CONDUCTION: _____

VENTRICULAR CONDUCTION: _____

INTERPRETATION: _____

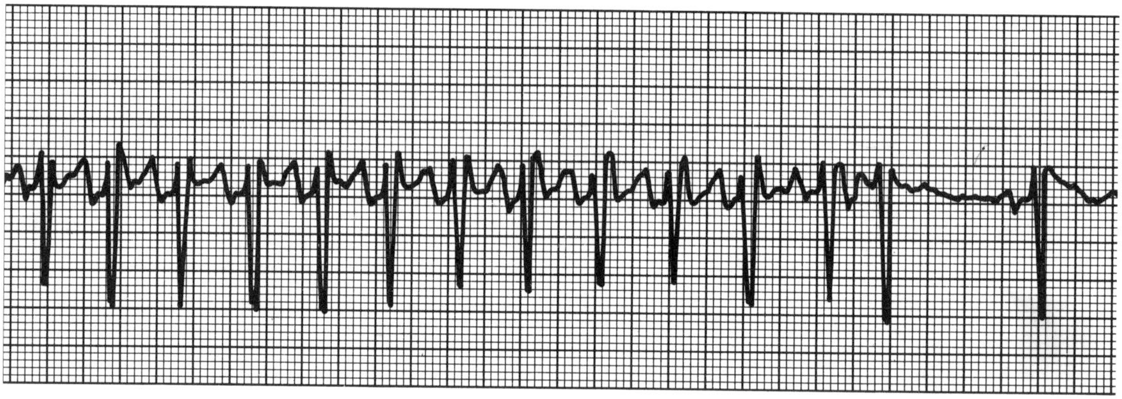

5–11

RHYTHM: _____

RATE: _____

ATRIAL CONDUCTION: _____

_____

AV CONDUCTION: _____

VENTRICULAR CONDUCTION: _____

INTERPRETATION: _____

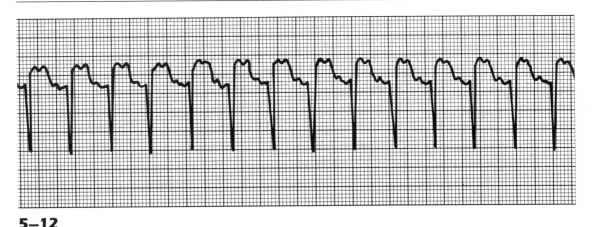

5–12

RHYTHM: _____

RATE: _____

ATRIAL CONDUCTION: _____
_____

AV CONDUCTION: _____

VENTRICULAR CONDUCTION: _____

INTERPRETATION: _____

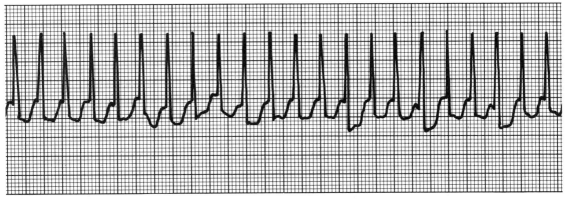

5–13

RHYTHM: _____

RATE: _____

ATRIAL CONDUCTION: _____
_____

AV CONDUCTION: _____

VENTRICULAR CONDUCTION: _____

INTERPRETATION: _____

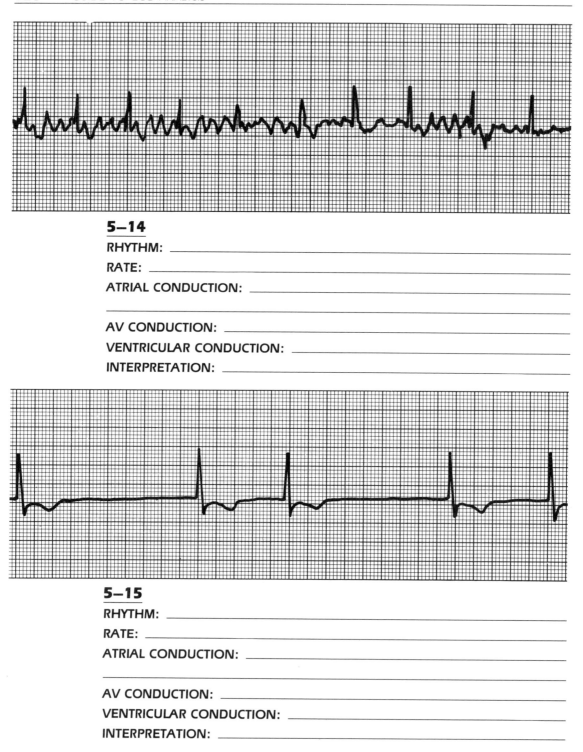

5-14

RHYTHM: _____

RATE: _____

ATRIAL CONDUCTION: _____

_____

AV CONDUCTION: _____

VENTRICULAR CONDUCTION: _____

INTERPRETATION: _____

5-15

RHYTHM: _____

RATE: _____

ATRIAL CONDUCTION: _____

_____

AV CONDUCTION: _____

VENTRICULAR CONDUCTION: _____

INTERPRETATION: _____

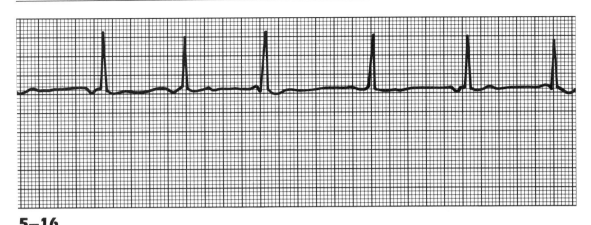

5—16

RHYTHM: _____

RATE: _____

ATRIAL CONDUCTION: _____

_____

AV CONDUCTION: _____

VENTRICULAR CONDUCTION: _____

INTERPRETATION: _____

CHAPTER

6

DYSRHYTHMIAS ASSOCIATED WITH THE AV JUNCTION

LEARNING OBJECTIVES

After studying this section, the learner will be able to:

1. Discuss the unique features of dysrhythmias that originate in the AV junction.
2. List the major causes for the junctional dysrhythmias.
3. Describe the physiologic mechanisms that produce the characteristic P waves associated with junctional dysrhythmias.
4. Name the key criteria for junctional dysrhythmias.
5. List the most common symptoms caused by junctional dysrhythmias.
6. Name the treatment and care methods for each of the junctional dysrhythmias.

The normal depolarization sequence for the heart begins in the sinoatrial (SA) node, travels through the atria, down through the atrioventricular (AV) node, and finally through the ventricular conduction system. This normal electrical activity in the heart produces the normal P-QRS-T sequence seen on the electrocardiogram (ECG) tracing. The normal sequence of cardiac electrical activity is disrupted when the depolarizing currents begin in the AV junction that is located in the center of the heart. The ventricles continue to be depolarized in the normal manner, but the atria are depolarized from a focus below their normal conduction system. The impulses from the AV junction must travel "backward" through the atria to cause their depolarization (Fig. 6-1). This backward depolarization is called *retrograde conduction*.

The most immediate effect of retrograde atrial conduction on the ECG tracing is that the P waves are produced backward or upside-down from the way they normally are produced. This retrograde conduction results in inverted P waves in a lead II, and sometimes in an MCL_1, although in an MCL_1, inverted P waves

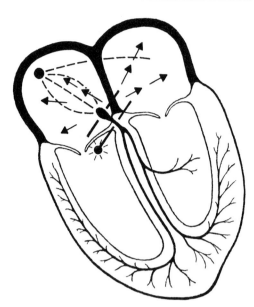

FIG. 6–1. RETROGRADE CONDUCTION OF THE ATRIA OCCURS WHEN THE DEPOLARIZING IMPULSE ORIGINATES BELOW THE ATRIA AND CAUSES THEM TO DEPOLARIZE FROM THE BOTTOM OF THE ATRIA TO THE TOP OF THEM. ATRIO-VENTRICULAR JUNCTION BECOMES IRRITABLE AND DISCHARGES EARLY IN THE CARDIAC CYCLE AT IRREGULAR INTERVALS. PREMATURE ECTOPIC BEATS ARE PRODUCED THAT HAVE INVERTED P WAVES BUT NORMAL QRS COMPLEXES, SINCE THE IMPULSES FOLLOW THE NORMAL PATHWAYS THROUGH THE VENTRICLES.

may be a normal variation. Inverted P waves are important indicators of AV junctional rhythms.

Another important effect of retrograde atrial conduction on the ECG tracing is that the normal sequence of wave forms is disrupted. With AV junctional rhythms, P waves can assume one of three locations in relationship to the QRS complex, depending on when the atria depolarize in relationship to the ventricles. If the atria and ventricles depolarize at the same time, the P wave is then hidden in the QRS complex. This relationship is probably the most common one. If the atria depolarize after the ventricles, the inverted P wave is seen after the QRS complex, often buried in the T wave. If the atria depolarize before the ventricles, the inverted P wave is seen before the QRS complex, but the PR interval is 0.11 second or less (Fig. 6-2).

The AV junction can become irritable and produce premature contractions, as do other areas in the heart that have the potential to produce depolarizing impulses. It is also one of the primary backup pacemaker sites for the heart that can assume pacemaker function if the SA node should fail to discharge impulses. As a backup pacemaker, the AV junction is slower than the sinus node (has an inherent rate of 40–60 beats/min) and is very regular but less reliable than the SA node.

Atrioventricular junctional rhythms are often misnamed AV nodal rhythms, or nodal rhythms. Through the process of myocardial electrophysiology studies where tiny wires are placed in or near a structure of the heart to measure the electrical activity of that structure, it has been discovered that the AV node does not have the ability to initiate cardiac impulses. The impulses that originate in the atria merely pass through the AV node to the ventricles. Some authors believe that the AV junctional tissues include the three parts of the AV node and the

FIG. 6–2. VARIOUS LOCATIONS FOR INVERTED P WAVES IN JUNCTIONAL DYSRHYTHMIAS.

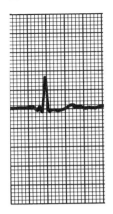

A P wave before the QRS complex (PRI < 0.11 second).

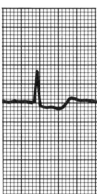

B P wave hidden in the QRS complex (PRI not measured).

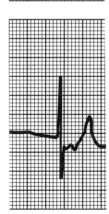

C P wave after the QRS complex (PRI not measured).

fibers of the bundle of His down to the bundle branch bifurcations. The potential pacemaker fibers of this structure are contained in the bottom section of the AV node and the upper fibers of the bundle of His. This area of tissue or fibers located at the point where the atria join with the ventricles is the AV junctional pacemaker site (Fig. 6-3).

FIG. 6–3. ATRIOVENTRICULAR JUNCTION AS PACEMAKER SITE.

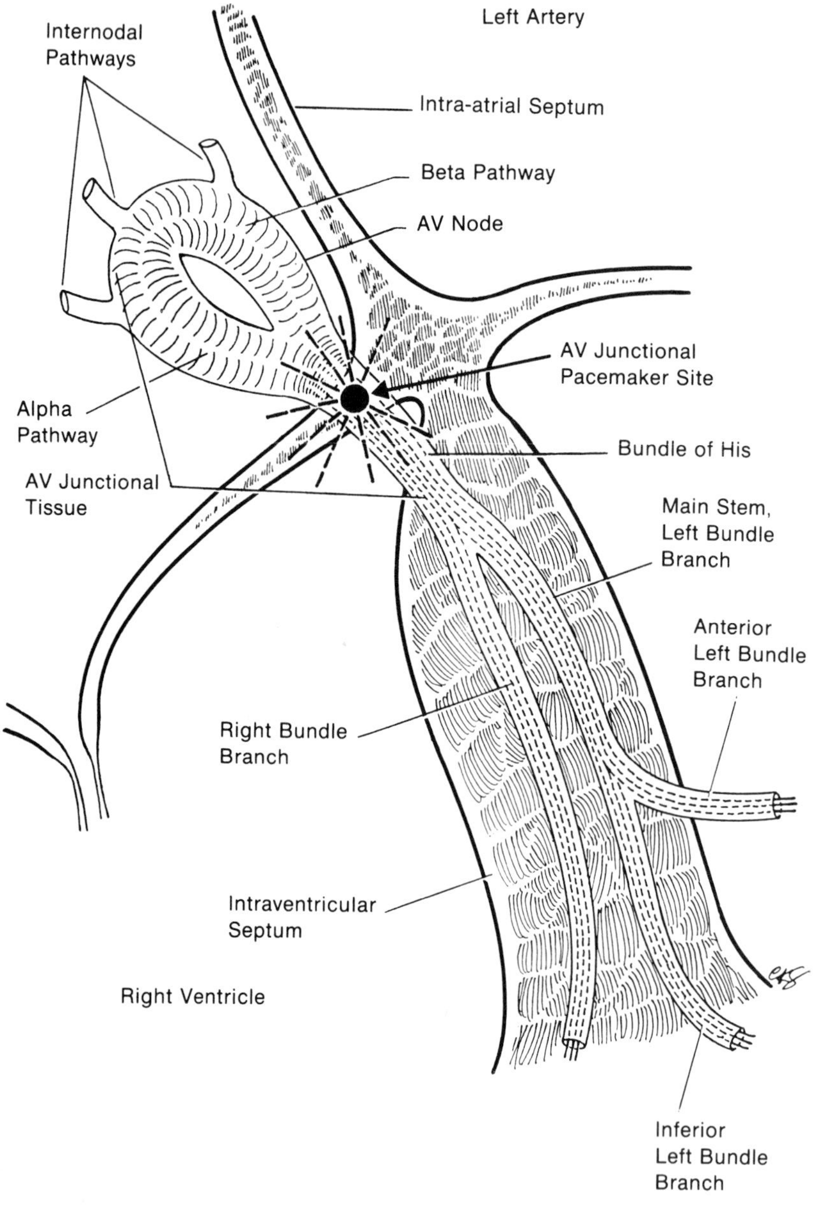

Internodal Pathways

Left Artery

Intra-atrial Septum

Beta Pathway

AV Node

AV Junctional Pacemaker Site

Alpha Pathway

AV Junctional Tissue

Bundle of His

Main Stem, Left Bundle Branch

Anterior Left Bundle Branch

Right Bundle Branch

Intraventricular Septum

Right Ventricle

Inferior Left Bundle Branch

PREMATURE JUNCTIONAL CONTRACTIONS

Premature junctional contractions (also called PJCs, premature nodal contractions, PNCs) (Fig. 6-1) occur when a single irritable area in the AV junction discharges an impulse before the next regular SA node impulse is due to be delivered. As with other types of premature beats, this early discharge interrupts the regularity of the underlying rhythm most of the time. Because the impulses are coming from an area other than the SA node, the P waves are abnormal. Since the area of impulse origination is in the center of the heart, the normal P-QRS-T sequence is disrupted. The P wave has the potential of coming after the QRS, of being hidden in the QRS, or coming before the QRS. The P wave is inverted in leads in which it is normally upright because of the retrograde conduction through the atria. In all junctional dysrhythmias, the QRS complex usually remains normal because the impulses follow the normal conduction pathways through the ventricles.

Premature junctional contractions are not very common. The AV junction is an area of the heart that does not becomes irritable easily. It is important to remember that these are just single beats that interrupt the regularity of the underlying rhythm. Interpretation of the PJC must include an analysis and interpretation of the underlying rhythm.

Premature junctional contractions have many characteristics in common with premature atrial contractions. An incomplete compensatory pause often follows premature junctional beats, although complete compensatory pauses are sometimes observed. It is possible to have *interpolated PJCs,* which fall between two normal beats without disrupting the underlying rhythm.

CAUSES

Although they are relatively rare when compared with other types of dysrhythmias, PJCs can occur from time to time in healthy individuals who have no history of heart disease. The factors that can cause PACs also have the potential to produce PJCs. Some of the more common causes are anxiety or fear, vigorous exercise, consumption of large amounts of caffeine, alcohol, tobacco, or use of central nervous system stimulant medications.

Cardiac diseases such as myocardial infarction (MI), congestive heart failure, rheumatic heart disease, congenital abnormalities, and generalized coronary heart disease are also responsible for the production of PJCs. Individuals who are having frequent PJCs and who have a history of heart disease require close monitoring because these ectopics may be a harbinger of significant changes in the person's cardiac status.

SYMPTOMS

Because PJCs cause only a minor, if any, decrease in total cardiac output, most patients who have them experience no symptoms. A small group of patients may complain of palpitations or feeling skipped beats in the chest, especially when the PJCs are frequent. Premature junctional contractions perfuse if they are late enough in the cycle to allow for ventricular filling.

TREATMENT

The goal of treatment for PJCs is usually aimed at eliminating the underlying cause. Reducing caffeine and tobacco intake, as well as reducing the stress and anxiety in the patient often eliminates the PJCs. In patients with pathologic heart disease that is responsible for the PJCs, cardiac medications, particularly quinidine sulfate, can be used to suppress their production (Fig. 6-4).

FIG. 6–4. EXAMPLE OF PREMATURE JUNCTIONAL CONTRACTION.

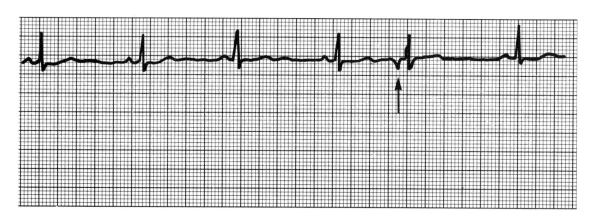

CRITERIA FOR PREMATURE JUNCTIONAL CONTRACTIONS

Rhythm: Basically regular rhythm that is interrupted by single premature ectopic beats. If the underlying rhythm is irregular, then the interpretation must be based on the abnormal P waves of the ectopic. The premature ectopic beat is most frequently followed by an incomplete compensatory pause.

Rate: The rate of the basic or underlying rhythm determines the overall rate of the pattern. Premature junctional contractions are counted in the total rate for the strip.

Atrial Conduction: The P wave of the premature beat is different from the P waves of the basic rhythm. Junctional P waves are characteristically inverted in lead II and are located after the QRS complex, hidden in the QRS complex, or before the QRS complex. There is one P wave for each QRS complex (unless it is hidden in the ectopic QRS). The P waves for the basic rhythm should be consistent.

AV Conduction: PRI 0.12–0.20 second for the underlying rhythm and consistent. If the P wave for the PJC comes after the QRS or is hidden in the QRS, the PR interval is not measured. If the inverted P wave of the PJC falls before the QRS, the PR interval should be 0.11 second or less.

Ventricular Conduction: QRS 0.06–0.10 second; QRS for the PJC should be the same as the QRSs for the basic rhythm.

JUNCTIONAL TACHYCARDIA

Junctional tachycardia is also called JT, paroxysmal junctional tachycardia, PJT, nodal tachycardia, NT, paroxysmal nodal tachycardia, and PNT (Fig. 6-5) It is a rapid dysrhythmia that arises from a single irritable area in the AV junction that has taken over the pacemaker function of the heart. It can be thought of as whole series of PJCs that occur one after the other.

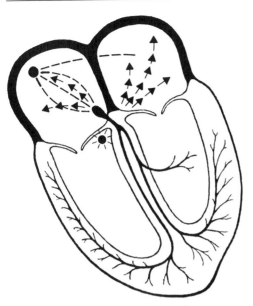

FIG. 6–5. THE AV JUNCTION BECOMES VERY IRRITABLE AND INITIATES IMPULSES RAPIDLY ONE AFTER ANOTHER, TAKING OVER THE PACEMAKER FUNCTION FROM THE SINOATRIAL NODE. ALL THE IMPULSES ARE CONDUCTED THROUGH THE NORMAL CONDUCTION PATHWAYS OF THE VENTRICLES.

Paroxysmal junctional tachycardia is a type of JT that begins suddenly and ends suddenly (paroxysmal = sudden onset). Paroxysmal junctional tachycardia has the potential to be faster than JT, with rates that sometimes reach the 180–250 beats/min range.

CAUSES

All the conditions and elements that produce PJCs are also capable of causing JT. The AV junction is not a structure that becomes irritable easily, and it is unlikely to produce a tachycardia unless there are significant causes. The majority of episodes of JT are associated with acute cardiac disease, especially MI or digoxin toxicity.

SYMPTOMS

In many individuals, particularly at rates below 150 beats/min, JT will produce no symptoms at all. At higher rates, there is the probability that some of the low cardiac output signs and symptoms will develop, including dizziness, weakness, syncope, chest pain or pressure, shortness of breath, or cardiac palpitations.

TREATMENT

Although there is no unique and specific treatment for JT, many of the medications used to treat atrial tachycardia help. The medications that are most successful are the calcium channel blockers, particularly diltiazem (Cardizem) and verapamil hydrochloride (Calan, Isoptin), digoxin (Lanoxin), and some of the central nervous system depressants. The dosages must be adjusted based on the severity of the signs and symptoms presented by the patient as well as his or her height and weight.

The other methods of treatment for atrial tachycardia are not often effective in the termination of JT. Because they are not harmful in themselves, vagal stimulation measures such as Valsalva's maneuver or coughing can be attempted while awaiting more definitive medical treatment. Patients who have frequent and long runs of JT, especially in the presence of an acute MI, need to be monitored closely, since the JT may indicate a generalized cardiac irritability. Tachy-ventricular dysrhythmias may develop secondary to the JT, particularly when digoxin toxicity is involved (Fig. 6-6).

FIG. 6–6. EXAMPLE OF JUNCTIONAL TACHYCARDIA.

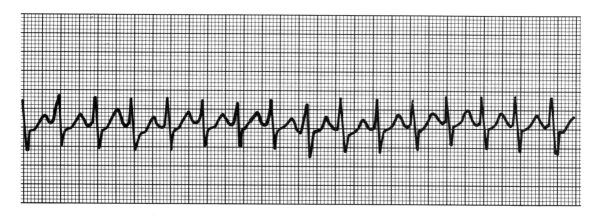

CRITERIA FOR JUNCTIONAL TACHYCARDIA

Rhythm: Regular—paroxysmal junctional tachycardia shows a sudden onset from the basic rhythm.

Rate: Usual rate is 100–180 beats/min. Paroxysmal junctional tachycardia may occur at rates of 180–250 beats/min.

Atrial Conduction: P waves are inverted in lead II either before the QRS, hidden in the QRS, or after the QRS. When the rate is above 150 beats/min, the P waves become very difficult to see.

AV Conduction: PR interval will be 0.11 second or less if the inverted P waves are before the QRS. The PR interval is not measured if the P waves come after the QRS or are hidden in the QRS.

Ventricular Conduction: QRS complexes should be normal for the entire rhythm; 0.06–0.10 second in duration and consistent.

JUNCTIONAL ESCAPE BEATS

Junctional escape beats (also called nodal escape beats) (Fig. 6-7) are produced when the normal pattern of atrial depolarization does not occur. Failure of the SA node to initiate an impulse or blockage of the SA nodal impulse high in the

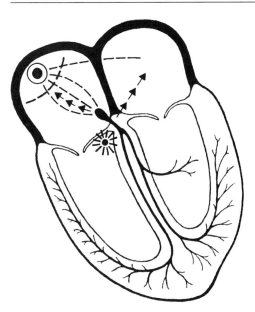

FIG. 6–7. THE SINOATRIAL NODE FAILS TO FIRE OR THE IMPULSE IS BLOCKED IN THE ATRIAL CONDUCTION SYSTEM FOR A SINGLE BEAT. THE ATRIOVENTRICULAR JUNCTION TAKES OVER THE PACEMAKER FUNCTION FOR THE ABSENT SINUS BEAT. THE IMPULSES FOLLOW THE NORMAL PATHWAYS THROUGH THE VENTRICLES SO THAT ALL THE QRS COMPLEXES ARE THE SAME.

atrial conduction system produces a pause in the cardiac cycle. The first backup pacemaker in the cardiac conduction system is the AV junction. It initiates a depolarizing current if the interval between the last sinus beat exceeds the inherent interval of the AV junction itself.

All escape beats come late in the cardiac cycle (see Chapter 3, Fig. 3-4). When the normal pacemaker of the heart does not produce an impulse, the escape or backup pacemakers protect the heart from stopping completely. Escape beats most commonly occur after normal beats that just stop, but they can also occur after premature beats that have long pauses after them or during episodes when the cardiac tissues are severely depressed by medications or disease. Escape beats may occur as isolated, individual beats that interrupt the underlying rhythm or in groups of beats.

As a backup pacemaker, the AV junction tends to produce regular beats but at a slower rate. The internal rate for the AV junction is 40–60 beats/min. The AV junction is less reliable than the SA node as a pacemaker site. This lack of reliability means that the AV junction has a higher probability of failure as a pacemaker, particularly when it has to function as the primary pacemaker over a long period of time. Also, the AV junction, at times, may fail to initiate an escape impulse, even after a long interval of no cardiac activity.

Junctional escape beats are recognizable by the location and shape of the P waves. As with the other junctional dysrhythmias discussed above, the P waves will be inverted in a lead II due to the retrograde conduction through the atria. They may fall in one of three locations in relationship to the QRS complex: hidden in the QRS, after the QRS, or before the QRS with a PR interval of 0.11 second or less. The QRS complexes should be normal in shape and duration and should be the same as the QRS complexes for the basic rhythm. As with other dysrhythmias that occur as single beats, both the basic rhythm and the ectopic beat must be analyzed and interpreted separately.

CAUSES

The most common factor that will produce junctional escape beats is suppression of the SA node or blockage of the impulses produced by the SA node either high in the atria or at the AV node. Those conditions that will produce sinus bradycardia, sinus block, or sinus arrest are responsible for the production of junctional escape beats. Primary conditions include vagal stimulation (vomiting, bronchial suctioning, and Valsalva's maneuver), inferior MIs, rheumatic heart disease, and atrial-septal defects.

Many of the cardiac depressant medications can also produce enough slowing or blockage of the SA node, resulting in junctional escape beats. Primary offenders in this group of medications include calcium channel blockers (particularly diltiazem), digoxin, and some of the beta blockers (propranolol and metoprolol). Large doses of central nervous system depressants, such as narcotic medications, sedatives, and sleeping aids, may slow the sinus rate enough to allow for junctional escape beats.

SYMPTOMS

The escape beats themselves produce few symptoms. Patients occasionally complain of feeling skipped beats because of the extra ventricular filling that takes place during the long pause preceding the junctional escape beat. More symptoms may be associated with the slow rhythm that precipitated the escape beats.

TREATMENT

There is no specific treatment for these beats. The goal of any treatment related to the elimination of escape beats would be to increase the inherent rate of the SA node to a point where the escape beats would not occur. Many of the treatments for sinus bradycardia would be effective in this situation (Fig. 6-8).

FIG. 6–8. EXAMPLE OF JUNCTIONAL ESCAPE BEAT.

Lead II

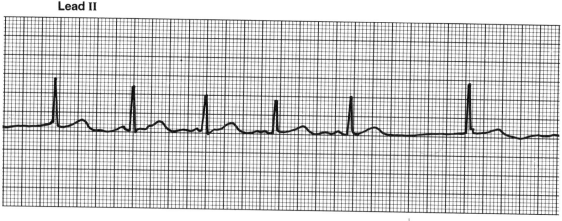

CRITERIA FOR JUNCTIONAL ESCAPE BEATS

Rhythm: The basic rhythm is usually regular to slightly irregular. It is interrupted by single late ectopic beats that follow a pause longer than the normal R to R interval.

Rate: The basic rhythm may be normal (60–100), faster than normal, or, more likely, slower than normal. The overall rate when the pause that is included is usually much slower than normal. Junctional escape beats are counted in the overall rate.

Atrial Conduction: P waves for the basic rhythm are in whatever form they are for that rhythm. The P waves from the ectopic are inverted in a lead II, and either before, hidden in, or after the QRS complex.

AV Conduction: PR interval for the basic rhythm is appropriate for that rhythm. PR interval for the ectopic is not measured if the P wave comes after the QRS or is hidden in the QRS. If the inverted P wave is before the QRS, then the PR interval will be 0.11 second or less.

Ventricular Conduction: QRS complexes for the basic rhythm and the ectopic is normal (0.06–0.10 second) and the same shape.

JUNCTIONAL ESCAPE RHYTHM

Junctional escape rhythm is also called junctional rhythm, passive junctional rhythm, idiojunctional rhythm, nodal escape rhythm, and nodal rhythm (Fig. 6-9). Probably the best way to understand a junctional escape rhythm is to picture it as a series of junctional escape beats that follow one after another. Most authors agree that when there are four or more escape beats in a row that the pattern can be called an escape rhythm. As discussed above, a junctional escape beat occurs when there is a temporary failure of the higher pacemaker to produce an

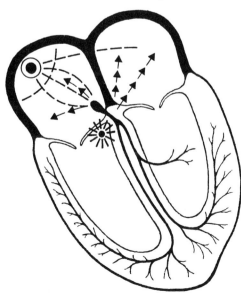

FIG. 6–9. WHEN THE SINOATRIAL NODE FAILS COMPLETELY OR ALL OF THE IMPULSES ARE BLOCKED FROM THE SINOATRIAL NODE, THE ATRIOVENTRICULAR JUNCTION BECOMES THE PRIMARY PACEMAKER. THE RATE IS SLOWER (40–60 BPM) BUT THE QRS COMPLEXES REMAIN NORMAL.

impulse. When that failure becomes more or less permanent, then a junctional escape rhythm may develop to keep the heart functioning even if it is at a somewhat reduced efficiency level.

The term *idiojunctional* is sometimes used in referring to this dysrhythmia. The prefix "idio" indicates the rhythm is self-initiating and self-contained. (The term *idio* is also used with slow dysrhythmias that are ventricular in origin.)

Because the AV junction has an inherent rate between 40 and 60 beats/min, the rate of junctional rhythms is slower than those of sinus rhythms. Also, junctional escape rhythms have the inverted P waves associated with other types of junctional dysrhythmias but maintain normal QRS complexes for the whole rhythm. The major decrease in cardiac output from a junctional escape rhythm is due to the slower rate, rather than from the junctional origin of the beats themselves. The ventricles usually contract normally in junctional rhythms. These beats should be palpable in the peripheral pulses.

CAUSES

As with the junctional escape beats, a junctional escape rhythm occurs when the higher pacemakers fail to discharge impulses. Suppression of the SA node due to vagal stimulation, cardiac medications, or heart disease is the most common cause of pacemaker failure. Blockage in the atrial conduction system or AV node also causes pauses long enough to trigger junctional escape rhythms.

SYMPTOMS

Many patients may experience no symptoms at all if the rate stays at 50 beats/min or above. Below this rate, the cerebral and cardiac perfusion decrease enough so that the patient begins to experience some signs and symptoms; activity intolerance, weakness, and syncope are commonly associated with slow heart rates, as are chest pain and pressure, shortness of breath, low blood pressure, and cool, moist skin. If the rate is extremely slow, unconsciousness may develop.

TREATMENT

There is no specific treatment for junctional escape rhythm. The main goal of treatment is to re-establish normal sinus node activity at a rate fast enough to prevent the escape rhythm. As with all of the dysrhythmia treatments, it is necessary to consider the clinical condition of the patient. In many cases where the patient is tolerating the junctional rhythm, a "wait and watch" approach may be appropriate. Close monitoring of patients who have experienced a recent MI and have developed a junctional rhythm secondary to the MI is important. Removal of the cause of the SA nodal suppression may be adequate to re-establish a normal sinus rhythm, particularly if it is due to medication toxicity or vagal stimulation.

More aggressive treatment of patients who are symptomatic with a junctional escape rhythm usually involves the use of atropine sulfate IV push for short-term emergency treatment. Atropine sulfate may cause one of two things to happen. It may cause stimulation of the SA node and a conversion to sinus rhythm, or it may cause an increase in the rate of the junctional rhythm to a point where the patient is no longer symptomatic. Use of sympathetic stimulating medications to increase the rate is also possible. Medications such as epinephrine, isoproterenol, or dopamine may accomplish this goal. These medications will increase the junctional rate even if there is no SA node activity.

If the patient does not respond to the medication treatments or if the junctional rhythm remains slow, an artificial pacemaker may be required. A temporary pacemaker may be used for short-term pacing in patients who recover normal sinus node activity in the near future. A permanent pacemaker may be required if the patient has little or no chance of regaining a normal rhythm at a normal rate (Fig. 6-10).

FIG. 6–10. EXAMPLE OF JUNCTIONAL ESCAPE RHYTHM.

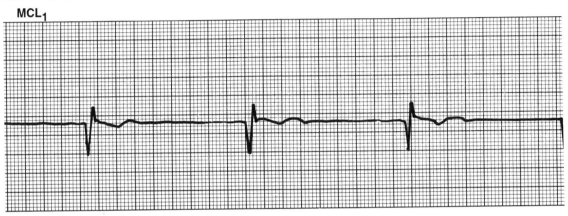

MCL₁

CRITERIA FOR JUNCTIONAL ESCAPE RHYTHM

Rhythm: Regular to slightly irregular.

Rate: Between 40 and 60 beats/min. Accelerated junctional rhythm takes place when the rate is between 60 and 100 beats/min. (Over 100 beats/min is tachycardia.)

Atrial Conduction: One P wave for each QRS complex. P waves will be inverted in a lead II and may come before the QRS, hidden in the QRS, or after the QRS complex.

AV Conduction: PR interval is not measured if the P wave comes after the QRS complex or is hidden in the QRS complex. If the inverted P wave is before the QRS complex, the PR interval should be 0.11 second or less.

Ventricular Conduction: QRS 0.06–0.10 second; uniform in shape.

PRACTICE ECG STRIPS FOR CHAPTER 6

Directions. On the following practice ECG strips, analyze each strip according to its rhythm, rate, atrial conduction, AV conduction, and ventricular conduction. Arrive at an interpretation of the strip based on the analysis and criteria for the dysrhythmias originating in the atria as learned in this chapter. (See Appendix II for interpretations.)

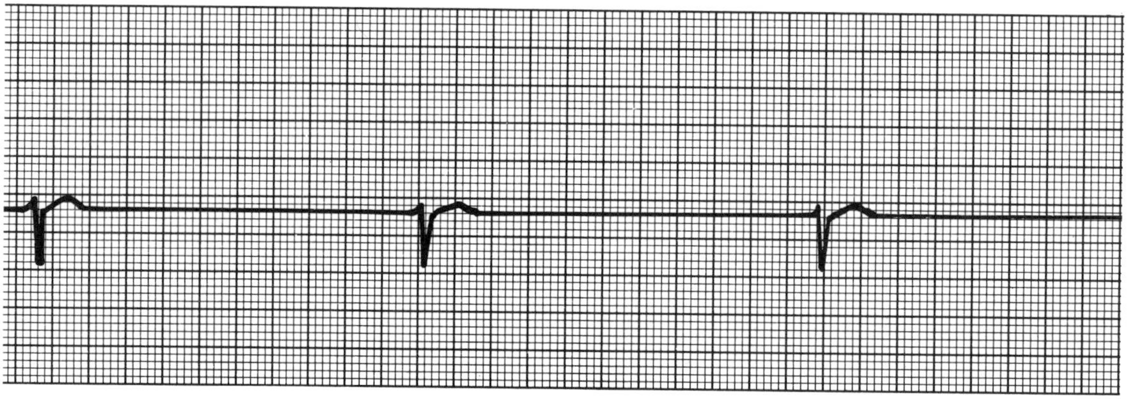

6–1

RHYTHM: _____

RATE: _____

ATRIAL CONDUCTION: _____

_____

AV CONDUCTION: _____

VENTRICULAR CONDUCTION: _____

INTERPRETATION: _____

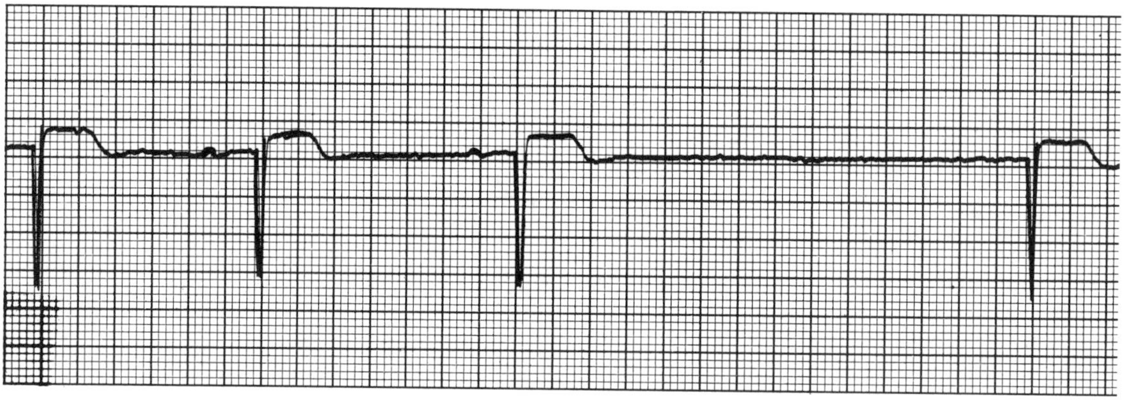

6–2

RHYTHM: _____

RATE: _____

ATRIAL CONDUCTION: _____

_____

AV CONDUCTION: _____

VENTRICULAR CONDUCTION: _____

INTERPRETATION: _____

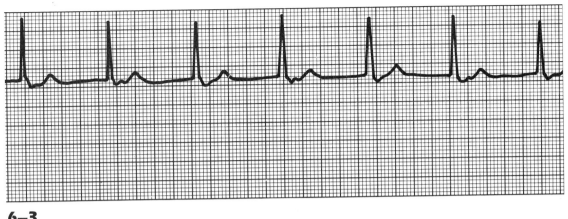

6–3

RHYTHM: _____

RATE: _____

ATRIAL CONDUCTION: _____

_____

AV CONDUCTION: _____

VENTRICULAR CONDUCTION: _____

INTERPRETATION: _____

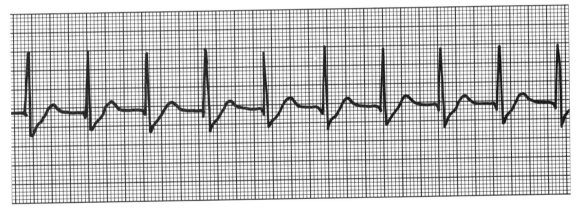

6–4

RHYTHM: _____

RATE: _____

ATRIAL CONDUCTION: _____

_____

AV CONDUCTION: _____

VENTRICULAR CONDUCTION: _____

INTERPRETATION: _____

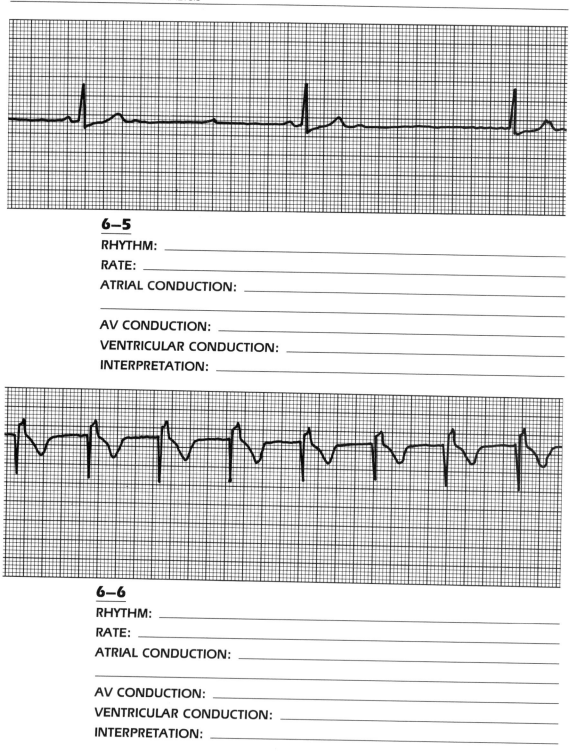

6—5

RHYTHM: _____

RATE: _____

ATRIAL CONDUCTION: _____

_____

AV CONDUCTION: _____

VENTRICULAR CONDUCTION: _____

INTERPRETATION: _____

6—6

RHYTHM: _____

RATE: _____

ATRIAL CONDUCTION: _____

_____

AV CONDUCTION: _____

VENTRICULAR CONDUCTION: _____

INTERPRETATION: _____

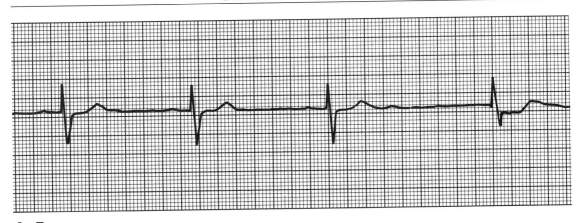

6–7

RHYTHM: _____

RATE: _____

ATRIAL CONDUCTION: _____

_____

AV CONDUCTION: _____

VENTRICULAR CONDUCTION: _____

INTERPRETATION: _____

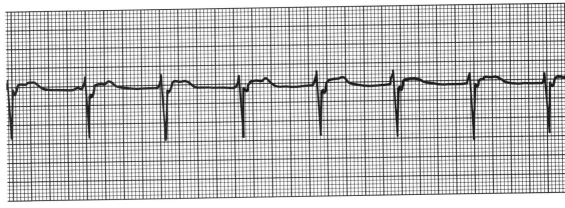

6–8

RHYTHM: _____

RATE: _____

ATRIAL CONDUCTION: _____

_____

AV CONDUCTION: _____

VENTRICULAR CONDUCTION: _____

INTERPRETATION: _____

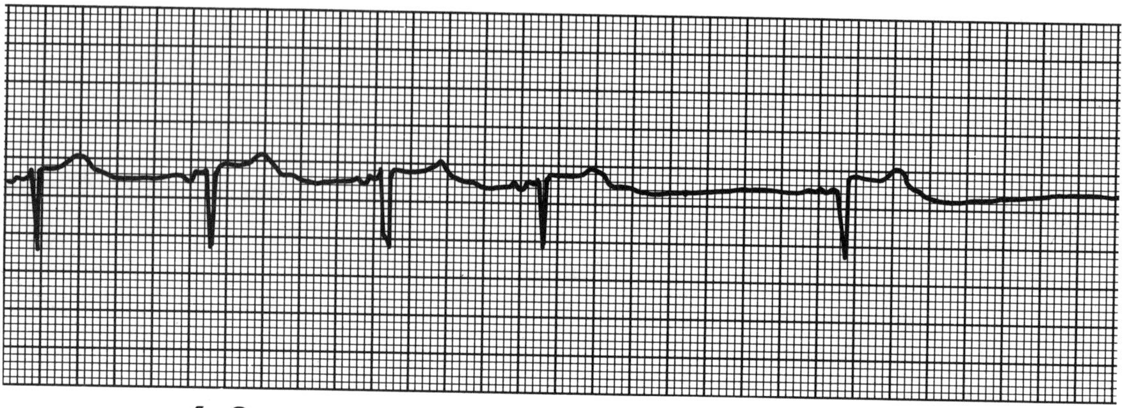

6—9

RHYTHM: _____

RATE: _____

ATRIAL CONDUCTION: _____

_____

AV CONDUCTION: _____

VENTRICULAR CONDUCTION: _____

INTERPRETATION: _____

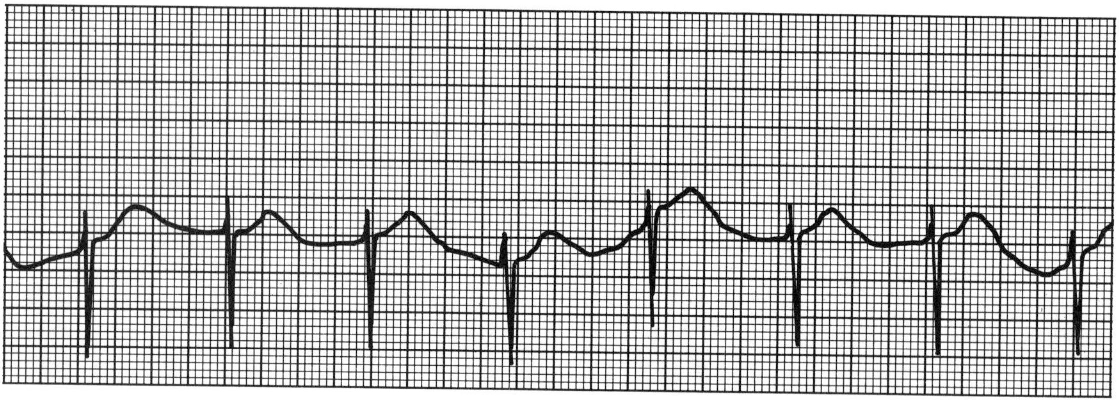

6—10

RHYTHM: _____

RATE: _____

ATRIAL CONDUCTION: _____

_____

AV CONDUCTION: _____

VENTRICULAR CONDUCTION: _____

INTERPRETATION: _____

7

DYSRHYTHMIAS ASSOCIATED WITH THE VENTRICLES

LEARNING OBJECTIVES

After studying this section, the learner will be able to:

1. Describe the abnormal mechanisms of conduction that produce abnormal QRS complexes in ventricular dysrhythmias.
2. Identify the factors that produce ventricular escape beats and escape rhythms.
3. List the most frequent elements that produce premature ventricular beats.
4. Identify the lethal ventricular dysrhythmias.
5. Name the appropriate treatments for ventricular dysrhythmias.
6. Analyze and interpret ECG rhythm strips that contain ventricular dysrhythmias.

The majority of the dysrhythmias discussed so far have been supraventricular dysrhythmias. These dysrhythmias have their origins above the conduction system of the ventricles. As noted in previous chapters, the only way a QRS complex of 0.10 second or less can be produced is if the impulses from the sinus node, atria, or atrioventricular (AV) junction follow the normal conduction pathways through the ventricles. Conditions (such as Wolff-Parkinson-White [WPW] or bundle branch block) that alter or delay the impulse as it is conducted through the ventricles produce QRS complexes that are wider than 0.12 second, with a PR interval less than 0.12 second for WPW.

As with other ectopic locations for cardiac impulse formation, ventricular impulses may be caused by irritable areas in the ventricle that produce premature or fast rhythms or by failure of higher pacemakers that produce escape rhythms. When the originating point for a dysrhythmia is in the ventricles, the conduction through the ventricles is abnormal. Because of this abnormal ventricular conduction, the QRS complex of ventricular dysrhythmias is usually wider than 0.12 second.

The repolarization of the ventricles is also abnormal in dysrhythmias that have a ventricular origin, therefore, the T wave after the QRS complex is usually attached to, and in the opposite direction of, the QRS complex. The combination of the wide QRS complex and the opposite direction T wave produce the characteristic wave forms observed in ventricular dysrhythmias (Fig. 7-1). It is some-

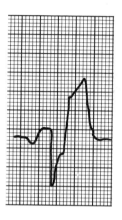

FIG. 7–1. COMMON CONFIGURATIONS OF QRS COMPLEXES IN VENTRICULAR DYSRHYTHMIAS.

A In ventricular complex A, the QRS complex (actually a QS or Q wave) is negative with the attached T wave, which is positive.

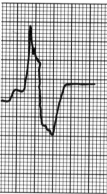

B In ventricular complex B, the QRS complex (R wave) is positively deflected with an attached, negatively deflected T wave.

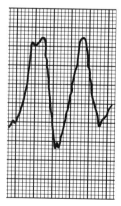

C In ventricular complex C, it is difficult to determine which is the QRS complex and which is the T wave. Identification is made primarily on the configuration and width of the QRS complex.

times difficult to identify the exact point at which the QRS complex ends and the T wave begins in ventricular dysrhythmias. This identification becomes even more difficult when analyzing ventricular dysrhythmias with rapid ventricular rates.

Because there is no conduction from the sinus node or atria producing ventricular beats, there are no conducted P waves before the ventricular ectopic beat (except for fusion beats). Incidental P waves may be seen before the ventricular ectopic but they are dissociated from it. Retrograde P waves may appear after the ventricular QRS complex if the impulse is conducted backward through the AV node to the atria.

Ventricular dysrhythmias are generally considered the most serious of all the dysrhythmias. When a depolarizing impulse starts in the ventricles, the normal depolarization and contraction pattern of the heart is completely changed. Normally, the atria contract before the ventricles, and the ventricles contract in a squeezing-type motion from the apex of the heart toward the base. This normal pattern of depolarization allows for the atria to empty into the ventricles and for the ventricles to contract in the most efficient pattern, producing blood flow to the pulmonary artery and the aorta. While other dysrhythmias alter this pattern, ventricular dysrhythmias usually produce little or no cardiac output, depending on the coupling interval length. Some ventricular beats do not perfuse if there is insufficient time to allow for ventricular filling and are sometimes not counted in the overall rate. In this book, all ventricular ectopics will be included in the rate analysis of the pattern.

Secondly, ventricular dysrhythmias are dangerous because, as a backup pacemaker site, the ventricles are slow and often do not produce depolarizations at a rate that is adequate to meet the metabolic and circulatory needs of the body. Ventricular pacemaker sites also tend to be less reliable than the higher pacemaker sites and may just stop initiating impulses at some point. If, for some reason, the ventricular pacemaker site should fail, there would be no other site left to take over.

Finally, ventricular dysrhythmias are dangerous because of their tendency to take over the pacemaker activity of the heart and become the established pattern. The probability of the ventricular pacemaker site taking over pacemaker function is much increased in rapid ventricular dysrhythmias. Although approximately 50% of these dysrhythmias stop spontaneously, the ones that do not stop produce low cardiac output symptoms and can lead to total circulatory failure, cardiac arrest, and death.

VENTRICULAR ESCAPE BEATS

Ventricular escape beats (VEBs) (Fig. 7-2) occur when the higher pacemaker sites fail to initiate impulses and normal atrial depolarization does not occur. Failure of the sinus node to initiate an impulse or a block of the sinoatrial (SA) nodal impulse high in the atrial conduction system produces a pause in the cardiac cycle. While the AV junction should be the first backup pacemaker site to take over the pacemaker function in case of SA node failure, it sometimes also fails to produce impulses. When the interval after the last sinus beat becomes longer than the inherent interval in the ventricular conduction system of the heart, the ventricles initiate an impulse. These impulses are generally from the Purkinje

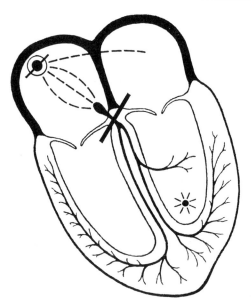

FIG. 7–2. VENTRICULAR ESCAPE BEATS OCCUR WHEN THERE IS FAILURE OF THE HIGHER PACEMAKER SITES TO INITIATE IMPULSES. AS A RESULT, SOME AREA IN THE VENTRICULAR CONDUCTION SYSTEM OR THE VENTRICULAR MYOCARDIUM BECOMES THE PACEMAKER SITE BY DEFAULT. COMPLETE AV BLOCKS AND SINOATRIAL NODE BLOCKS MAY ALSO CAUSE VENTRICULAR ESCAPE BEATS TO OCCUR. THE SAME CONDITIONS CAN ALSO PRODUCE A VENTRICULAR ESCAPE RHYTHM.

system of the ventricles but any area of the ventricular myocardium has the ability to initiate an impulse. These VEBs usually perfuse.

As noted above in the discussion of junctional escape beats, all escape beats come late in the cardiac cycle (see Chapter 3, Fig. 3-4). When the normal pacemaker of the heart does not produce an impulse, the escape or backup pacemakers protect the heart from asystole. Ventricular escape beats occur most commonly when normal beats just stop, but they can also occur after premature beats that have long pauses after them or during episodes when the cardiac tissues are severely suppressed by medication, hypoxia, or cardiac diseases. Ventricular escape beats can occur as isolated and separate beats that interrupt the regularity of the underlying rhythm or as groups of beats during intervals of atrial inactivity.

Ventricular escape beats are recognized by their location in the cardiac cycle and their QRS-T configuration. They are located late in the cardiac cycle, that is, they are preceded by a pause that is greater than the normal R to R interval of the basic pattern. Ventricular escape beats also have the characteristic wide QRS complex with the attached T wave, which deflects in the opposite direction of the QRS complex. As with the analysis of other single ectopic beats, both the underlying rhythm and the ectopic beat must be considered in the interpretation.

CAUSES

As in junctional escape beats, any condition that suppresses the sinus node or blocks the sinus impulses has the potential to produce VEBs. Factors that are responsible for slow sinus bradycardia, sinus block, or sinus arrest will produce R to R intervals long enough for VEBs to occur. As discussed above, conditions such as stimulation of the vagus nerve, myocardial infarction (MI), rheumatic heart disease, and atrial-septal defects are the primary producers of slow heart rates.

Cardiac depressant medications also have the potential to cause sufficient slowing of the heart rate for VEBs to occur. Included in this group are the usual medications such as digoxin, the beta blockers, and the calcium blockers. Suppression of the sinus node may also occur with large doses of central nervous system depressants, narcotic medications, sedatives, and sleeping aids, which results in the occurrence of VEBs.

SYMPTOMS

There are no specific symptoms from the escape beats themselves. Patients complain of feeling "skipped beats" during the long pause before the escape beat occurs. Although VEBs do produce some cardiac output, because of the slow rate, cardiac output is reduced from what would be produced by even a junctional escape beat. Patients with frequent VEBs may complain of the low cardiac output symptoms seen in slow dysrhythmias, although it is difficult to distinguish if the symptoms are caused by the escape beats or the slow underlying rhythm.

TREATMENT

There is no specific treatment for VEBs themselves. The goal of treatment is to increase the rate of the basic rhythm to a point that supports circulation and to have an R to R interval short enough for the VEBs not to occur. Many of the treatments for sinus bradycardia or AV block would be appropriate in this situation.

One caution when dealing with patients who are having VEBs or slow ventricular rhythms: *Never* administer intravenous (IV) lidocaine to a patient who is having VEBs. Because of the suppressing effect lidocaine has on ventricular ectopic sites, it effectively eliminates VEBs, leaving the patient with no functional backup pacemaker sites. Asystole and death are the remaining alternatives (Fig. 7-3).

FIG. 7–3. EXAMPLE OF A VENTRICULAR ESCAPE BEAT (IN A SECOND DEGREE AV BLOCK, TYPE I).

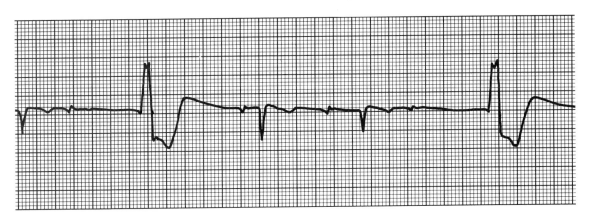

CRITERIA FOR VENTRICULAR ESCAPE BEATS

Rhythm: The rhythm may be regular or irregular depending on the underlying pattern. The pattern is interrupted by a single ectopic beat, which follows a pause that is longer than the normal R to R interval.

Rate: The basic rhythm may be normal but is frequently slower than normal. The overall rate when the pause is included is usually much slower than normal. Ventricular escape beats should be counted in the overall rate.

Atrial Conduction: P waves are totally dependent on the basic rhythm. They may or may not be present. The VEB does not have a conducted P wave before it but may have a retrograde P wave after or a dissociated P wave before it.

AV Conduction: PR interval is totally dependent on the basic rhythm. The VEB may have an incidental PR interval if a P wave occurs near it, but it does not indicate AV conduction.

Ventricular Conduction: QRS complex of the basic rhythm may be normal or wider than normal in the presence of bundle branch block. The QRS complex for the ectopic has a different shape than the rest of the rhythm and is wide (greater than 0.12 second). It has an attached T wave, which deflects in the opposite direction from the QRS.

VENTRICULAR ESCAPE RHYTHM

Ventricular escape rhythm is also called passive ventricular rhythm, idioventricular rhythm, and ventricular rhythm (Fig. 7-4).

A ventricular escape rhythm is a series of VEBs (usually four or more) together in a row. A ventricular escape *beat* occurs when there is a temporary failure of a higher pacemaker site. A ventricular escape *rhythm* occurs when the higher pacemaker failure becomes more or less permanent in duration. A ventricular escape rhythm can occur as an intermittent run of ventricular beats that is combined with longer runs of normal rhythms or as the sustained, predominant pattern of cardiac activity. The ventricular escape pattern keeps the heart functioning even if it is at a much less efficient level than it would normally function.

Because the inherent rate of impulse formation of the ventricular conduction and muscle tissue is 20–40 beats/min, ventricular escape rhythms are much slower than the normal cardiac rate. This much slower rate, combined with the abnormal depolarization that occurs in beats that originate in the ventricles, causes a significant decrease in cardiac output. In reality, the slower rate actually helps to increase the cardiac output because it allows for greater passive filling of the ventricles before they contract abnormally with the next ventricular beat. These beats should be palpable but may be much weaker than normal beats. Some patients tolerate ventricular escape rhythms for long periods of time if they remain at rest.

As a backup pacemaker site, the ventricles tend to produce regular to slightly irregular impulses. The ventricles are the least reliable of all the pacemaker sites. Although an alternate site in the ventricles may assume pacemaker function if a previous ventricular pacemaker site should stop, there is a high probability for total cardiac shutdown when a ventricular site is functioning as the primary or only pacemaker for the heart.

The characteristic ventricular QRS complex discussed above for escape beats is present in ventricular escape rhythms. Retrograde P waves may or may not be present, depending on the degree of conduction through the AV node causing an AV dissociation.

CAUSES

The same factors that produced VEBs have the potential to cause a ventricular escape rhythm. Any failure of the higher pacemakers caused by factors such as vagal stimulation, cardiac medication, or heart disease may produce conditions favorable for the production of a ventricular escape rhythm. A block in the atrial conduction system, sinus node, or AV node may produce an R to R interval long enough to have a ventricular escape rhythm occur. There must also be a failure of the AV junction to assume the pacemaker role in order to have a ventricular escape rhythm.

SIGNS AND SYMPTOMS

Sign and symptom production is very dependent on the basic rate of the ventricular escape rhythm. Rates that remain in the 35–40 beats/min range often support enough cardiac output to maintain cerebral perfusion while the patient is at rest. Increased activity is not tolerated even at these rates. Almost all patients are symptomatic at rates below 35 beats/min and require immediate intervention. Weakness, disorientation, syncope, and slow and weak regular pulses with a low blood pressure are commonly seen. Complaints of chest pressure or pain, and shortness of breath are also common with slow ventricular escape rhythms.

TREATMENT

The main goal of treatment is to maintain a ventricular rate sufficient to produce adequate cardiac output. If the patient has short, intermittent runs of ventricular escape rhythm without any symptoms, then he or she may not need treatment. If the basic slow rate is due to cardiac medications, then they must be reduced or eliminated. If the ventricular escape rhythm follows a recent MI, then the patient requires close monitoring and perhaps the insertion of an external temporary pacemaker. In instances where the patient is symptomatic and cannot wait for pacemaker insertion, atropine sulfate or a cardiac stimulant medication may be required.

Again, *never* administer IV lidocaine to a patient in a ventricular escape rhythm.

CRITERIA FOR VENTRICULAR ESCAPE RHYTHM

Rhythm: Regular to slightly irregular. The slower the rate, the less regular the rhythm tends to be.

FIG. 7–4. EXAMPLE OF VENTRICULAR ESCAPE RHYTHM.

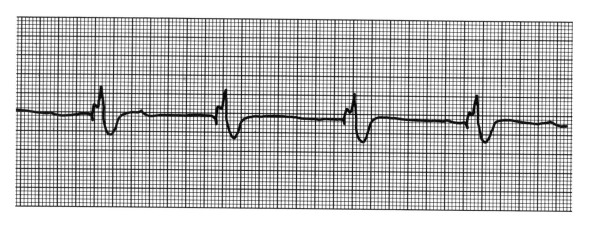

Rate: Between 20 and 40 beats/min. The name *accelerated ventricular escape rhythm* can be used if the rate is between 40 and 100 beats/min.

Atrial Conduction: P waves: if P waves are present before the QRS complexes, they are not associated with the complex (AV dissociation). Retrograde P waves may be present after the QRS complexes.

AV Conduction: PR interval if present, is incidental. Not measured.

Ventricular Conduction: QRS greater than 0.10 second: T wave is attached and in opposite direction from the QRS complex.

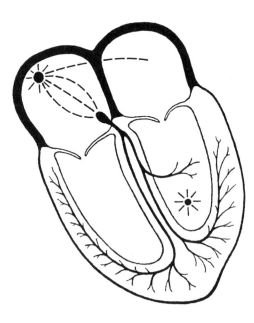

FIG. 7–5. PREMATURE VENTRICULAR CONTRACTIONS ARE PRODUCED WHEN AN AREA IN THE VENTRICLES BECOMES IRRITABLE AND BEGINS INITIATING IMPULSES EARLY IN THE CARDIAC CYCLE. THE SINOATRIAL NODE IS STILL FIRING AND P WAVES ARE PRESENT.

PREMATURE VENTRICULAR CONTRACTION

Premature ventricular contractions are also called PVCs, ventricular premature contractions, VPCs, premature ventricular beats, PVBs, ventricular premature beat, VPBs, and ventricular extrasystoles (Fig. 7-5).

Premature ventricular contractions occur when a single irritable area in one of the ventricles discharges an impulse before the next regular impulse is delivered from the sinus node. This early discharge interrupts the regularity of the underlying rhythm. It is possible to determine which ventricle is producing the PVC by the direction of the QRS complex of the PVC. The current flow in the ventricles when a PVC occurs is similar to the current flow in the ventricles when there is a bundle branch block. In the MCL_1 lead, the current from an irritable area in the right ventricle flows away from the positive electrode, producing a wave form that is primarily negative (Fig. 7-6). If the irritable area is in the left ventricle, the depolarizing current flow is toward the positive electrode, producing a wave form that is primarily positive (Fig. 7-7).

FIG. 7–6. CURRENT FLOW AND WAVE FORM FROM A RIGHT VENTRICULAR PVC.

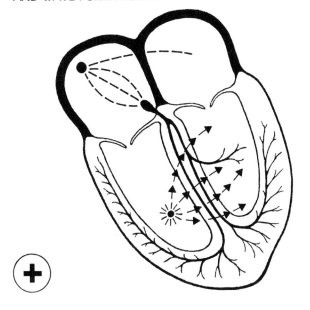

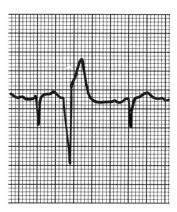

The current flow is away from the positive electrode in the MCL_1 lead, therefore, the wave form is in a negative in deflection.

As with other ventricular dysrhythmias, the ventricles are depolarized from an impulse arising in the ventricles in an abnormal manner, producing QRS complexes that are wide and have the characteristic ventricular shape. There may or may not be P waves before the PVC. If P waves are identified before the PVC, they are not associated with the abnormal QRS complex and most likely have originated from the sinus node. A way to discern if the P waves are from the sinus node is to analyze the P to P intervals. If all the P to P intervals are equal, including the one before the PVC, then that P wave is from the sinus

FIG. 7–7. CURRENT FLOW AND WAVE FORM FROM A LEFT
VENTRICULAR PVC.

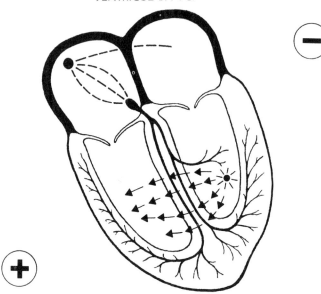

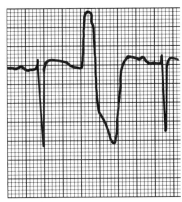

The current flow is toward
the positive electrode in the
MCL$_1$ lead, therefore, the
wave form is in a positive direction.

node. Retrograde P waves can occur after the PVC if the ventricular impulse has
been conducted backward through the AV node to the atria. In either case, the
PR interval does not indicate AV node activity and is not measured. It is an
incidental (accidental) PR interval.

Premature ventricular contractions are one of the most common of all the
dysrhythmias and *the* most common of all the ventricular dysrhythmias. Approximately 80% of all patients who have suffered an MI will have PVCs, making this
the most common dysrhythmia post MI. Like other premature beats, it is not a
rhythm in itself but an abnormal condition that occurs to another rhythm. Premature ventricular contractions may occur with any or all of the rhythms and
dysrhythmias discussed so far. In addition, PVCs may occur in a variety of
patterns and combinations. Remember to analyze and interpret the basic rhythm,
as well as the PVC and its pattern.

A complete compensatory pause follows a PVC most of the time, although
there are exceptions to this rule. Premature ventricular contractions may also be
followed by incomplete compensatory pauses or no pause at all in the case of
interpolated PVCs. As a rule of thumb, if a wide premature beat occurs that has
the characteristic ventricular shape and is followed by a complete compensatory
pause, the interpretation strongly favors a PVC.

The reason most PVCs have complete compensatory pauses after them is
because the depolarization of the ventricles from a ventricular focus is usually
isolated from the sinus node, that is, these ventricular impulses do not disrupt
the internal regular rhythm of the sinus node. The sinus beats after the PVC fall
back in cycle with the sinus beats preceding the PVC. This failure to disrupt the
internal regular rhythm of the sinus node is also the reason why sinus P waves

may appear near the PVC but are not associated with it. The exception to this rule occurs when there is retrograde conduction from the ventricles through the AV node to the atria that then disrupts the inherent regularity of the sinus node, much the same way it is disrupted by PACs or some PJCs.

Premature ventricular contractions, when they occur, produce little or no cardiac output. This lack of cardiac output from PVCs is due to the abnormal contraction pattern of the ventricles, as well as the lack of adequate filling of the ventricles due to the prematurity of the beat. Premature ventricular contractions may not perfuse (*i.e.*, are not palpable in peripheral pulses). Patients often complain of feeling "skipped beats" in their chests when they have PVCs. In reality, these patients are not feeling the PVC itself but the sinus beat that follows the PVC. During the long compensatory pause that follows the PVC, the ventricles actually overfill a little, increasing the cardiac output of the next sinus beat, and making it stronger. This increased output of the beat following a PVC may also be palpated in the peripheral pulse or even auscultated with a stethoscope over the left anterior chest.

CAUSES

Healthy individuals who have no history of heart disease may, from time to time, have PVCs. In general, any substance or condition that increases the irritability of the ventricles can cause PVCs. These causes include some common factors found in many individuals' lives, such as fear and anxiety, exercise, ingestion of beverages containing caffeine or alcohol, and use of tobacco. Use of a wide variety of nervous system stimulant medications ranging from therapeutic medications (such as aminophylline, epinephrine, and thyroid supplements) to street drugs (such as amphetamines and cocaine) may also produce PVCs. Cardiac medications, particularly digoxin and quinidine, may also produce PVCs if their levels become toxic.

Cardiac diseases, such as MI, congestive heart failure, and coronary heart disease, can produce PVCs. Because of the damage to the ventricular myocardial cells surrounding an infarcted area in patients who have had a myocardial infarction, post MI patients are particularly susceptible to PVCs and other types of ventricular dysrhythmias. These damaged cardiac cells tend to "leak" sodium and potassium through their damaged membranes, causing premature impulse formation.

Patients who have electrolyte imbalances, especially potassium, or hypoxia, frequently have PVCs. Many patients with chronic obstructive lung disease will have frequent and multiple PVCs due to the chronically low PO_2 levels they maintain.

SIGNS AND SYMPTOMS

Many individuals have no signs or symptoms at all when they are experiencing PVCs. The most common complaint is feeling "skipped beats" in the chest. If the PVCs are frequent, patients may complain of palpitations or "fluttering" in the chest.

TREATMENT

While the basic treatment for PVCs has not changed much over the years, the philosophy behind which PVCs get treatment has gone through major changes. Early in the evolution of coronary care, the philosophy of treatment was that all PVCs were to be considered dangerous and were treated aggressively in the attempt to eliminate them completely. As cardiology has evolved, the thinking has changed to consideration of the patient, the patient's clinical condition, and the underlying disease processes at work producing the PVCs. In patients who have long-term, irreversible disease processes such as chronic obstructive pulmonary disease and who are having many PVCs, it may be possible to eliminate the PVCs for the short run by aggressive IV medication therapy. But the underlying cause of the PVCs, lack of oxygen, does not change; therefore, the PVCs return when the medication is stopped. If these patients are not symptomatic from the PVCs and the PVCs are not what are considered dangerous, then benign neglect of the PVCs may be the most appropriate treatment, unless they also have myocardial ischemia.

Of course, if the cause of the PVCs can be traced to a specific medication or condition, then that medication must be eliminated or reduced. The combining of factors also increases the probability of PVCs occurring. A post MI patient who has a low potassium from diuretic therapy, is also on digoxin, and is extremely anxious about his or her condition is at very high risk for the occurrence of PVCs. Premature ventricular contractions are generally treated more aggressively when they occur following an acute MI, although even in this situation, the clinical condition of the patient must be taken into consideration.

The number of medications used to treat PVCs has increased dramatically in recent years. The following list of medications to treat PVCs is purposely brief but includes the most common medications used. These medications work to eliminate PVCs by altering the cell membranes of the myocardium and interfering with the autonomic control of the pacemaker cells. Basically, these medications disrupt the normal sodium/potassium ion exchange that takes place in all ventricular myocardial cells but especially in the damaged cardiac cells surrounding an infarcted area of the myocardium. This interruption effectively suppresses the ability of the ventricular myocardium to initiate impulses. In the classification system of antidysrhythmic medications, the majority of the medications used to treat PVCs fall into the class 1A, class 1B, class 1C, and class III medications. Class II medications can sometimes be used but are more appropriate for atrial dysrhythmias.

The first-line treatment of PVCs still relies upon the use of lidocaine hydrochloride (class 1B). This medication can only be given IV, but it works rapidly and is highly effective in the elimination of PVCs in most individuals. It has a low incidence of side effects, is compatible with many other medications, and does not decrease cardiac output. The initial dose after the IV has been started is a bolus of 50–100 mg, depending on the size and weight of the patient (mg/kg). A continuous IV infusion (drip) of the medication can then be initiated to run at 2–4 mg/min. Although some toleration to lidocaine may develop over time in some patients, long-term use has few serious consequences. In post MI patients, a lidocaine drip may be prophylactically administered for up to 72 hours, then tapered and discontinued.

The first-line backup antidysrhythmic medication that is used if lidocaine does not work or if the patient is becoming symptomatic with the lidocaine administration is procainamide hydrochloride (Procan, Pronestyl) (class 1A). Although this medication may be given orally, its IV administration is indicated when used as a backup medication for lidocaine. The initial IV bolus dose is somewhat higher than lidocaine and may range as high as 300–400 mg IV push (total bolus can be up to 1 g). The continuous infusion may have to run at 1–4 mg/min (or faster) to be effective. However, as with all drip medications, it is titrated to the clinical response desired, namely, elimination of the PVCs. Procainamide has a somewhat higher incidence of side effects than lidocaine because of its tendency to decrease the cardiac output. The blood pressure needs to be monitored closely during the initial infusion of procainamide because it has a tendency to drop drastically. This medication may also widen the QRS complexes of the normal beats.

A second backup medication to lidocaine that may be administered IV is bretylium tosylate (Bretylol) (class III). Although the popularity of bretylium's use has fluctuated dramatically in recent years, it is now in a cycle where its use is generally avoided unless all other medication treatments have failed. Its mechanism of action is somewhat different from the class 1 antidysrhythmic medications; it often increases the number of ventricular ectopic beats during the early stages of its administration. All the class III medications produce severe adverse reactions and are not among the first choice for antidysrhythmic therapy.

A third medication that may be used as a backup for IV lidocaine administration in the control of PVCs is phenytoin (Dilantin) (class 1B). While phenytoin is used primarily as an antiseizure medication and is most often administered orally, it can be given IV and is particularly effective for PVCs and other types of ventricular dysrhythmias caused by digoxin toxicity. The initial IV dose may be as high as 1000 mg administered IV push over an hour. Continuous IV administration of phenytoin is not recommended and seldom used but intermittent IV bolus administrations are possible for individuals who cannot take oral medications. Intravenous phenytoin is very alkaline, with a pH of approximately 11, and can only be administered with normal saline because dextrose and lactate solutions precipitate when exposed to it. Phenytoin is ideally administered through a central vein or large peripheral vein because of the irritating effect of the medication. Oral administration in dosages similar to what is used in seizure control is also effective in the control of PVCs.

Some of the common oral medications used to control PVCs that are taken long term outside of the hospital include the following: disopyramide phosphate (Norpace, Norpace CR—class 1A); procainamide hydrochloride (Procan, Procan SR—class 1A); tocainide hydrochloride (Tonocard—class 1B); mexiletine hydrochloride (Mexitil—class 1B); flecainide acetate (Tambocor—class 1C); encainide hydrochloride (Enkaid—class 1C); and amiodarone hydrochloride (Cordarone—class III). The dosages of these medications are individualized to the patient's needs. These medications have various side effects and the patient receiving them must be monitored for everything from urinary retention to bradycardia (Fig. 7-8).

CRITERIA FOR PREMATURE VENTRICULAR CONTRACTIONS

Rhythm: Basically regular rhythm is interrupted by a single premature ectopic beat. If the underlying rhythm is irregular, as in sinus dysrhythmia or atrial fibrillation, the pattern will be totally irregular, including the ectopic.

FIG. 7–8. EXAMPLE OF A PREMATURE VENTRICULAR CONTRACTION.

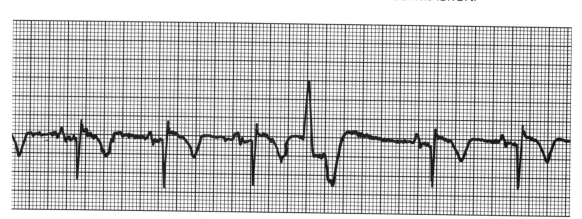

Rate: Determined by the rate of the basic rhythm. PVCs are counted into the overall rate.

Atrial Conduction: P waves are determined by the basic rhythm. The ectopic may have a P wave before it, but it is most likely a sinus P wave. Retrograde P waves may be present after the ectopic.

AV Conduction: PR interval is determined by the basic rhythm. Do not measure PR interval for the PVC.

Ventricular Conduction: QRS of the basic rhythm may be normal (0.06—0.10 second) or wider than normal if a bundle branch block is present. The ectopic is wider than 0.10 second and has the characteristic ventricular complex configuration. Premature ventricular contractions may appear in various shapes, patterns, and categories as demonstrated in Figures 7-9–7-22.

WHEN PVCs ARE DANGEROUS AND REQUIRE TREATMENT

Although the following list of types of PVCs are generally considered dangerous and require treatment, good clinical patient care practice demands that the patient's underlying disease processes as well as clinical condition be considered in the treatment of any dysrhythmia.
- Frequent PVCs
- Bigeminal pattern PVCs
- PVCs that are in the R on T pattern
- Multiformed PVCs
- PVCs that are in short runs or multiformed salvos

FIG. 7–9. CATEGORIES OF PVCs BY SHAPE: UNIFOCAL (UNIFORM) PVCs ORIGINATE FROM THE SAME SINGLE FOCUS IN THE VENTRICLES. THE ABNORMAL QRS COMPLEXES HAVE THE SAME SHAPE.

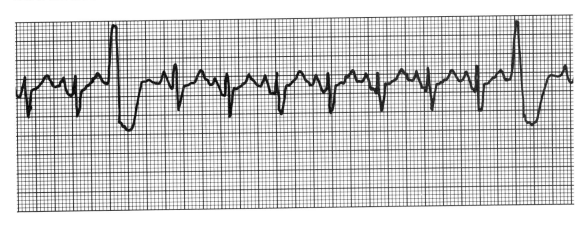

FIG. 7–10. CATEGORIES OF PVCs BY SHAPE: EXAMPLE OF MULTIFORMED PVCs.

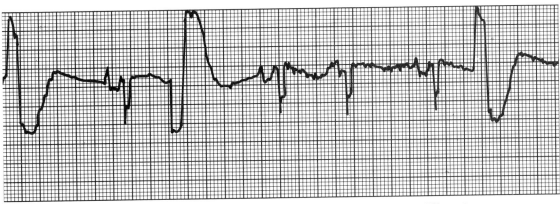

Multiform PVCs originate from different focal areas of one ventricle, from different ventricles, or from the same focal areas in the ventricle but are conducted differently. Because the current flow from the ectopic focus is different, the QRS complexes have different shapes.

FIG. 7–11. CATEGORIES OF PVCs BY PATTERN: EXAMPLE OF INTERPOLATED PVC.

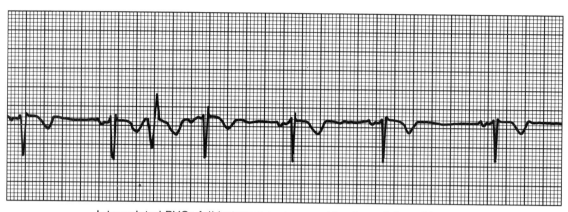

Interpolated PVCs fall between two normal beats and do not interrupt the underlying rhythm. They are not followed by any type of pause and are usually found in slower rates below 65 beats/min. In faster rates, there is not enough room to get the PVC between the two normal beats.

FIG. 7–12. CATEGORIES OF PVCs BY PATTERN: EXAMPLE OF BIGEMINAL PVCs.

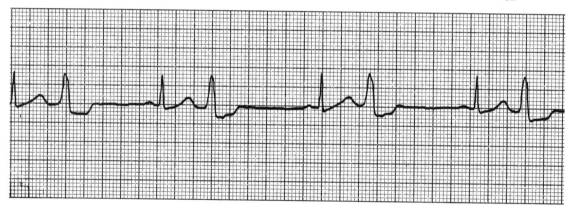

A bigeminal pattern (bigeminy) exists when one normal beat is followed by one ectopic beat in a repetitive pattern. Every other beat is an ectopic beat. Because every other beat is a PVC, the cardiac output may be cut in half during the time the patient is in a bigeminal PVC pattern, depending on the time of the coupling interval and if the ventricles have time to fill.

FIG. 7–13. CATEGORIES OF PVCs BY PATTERN: EXAMPLE OF TRIGEMINAL PVCs.

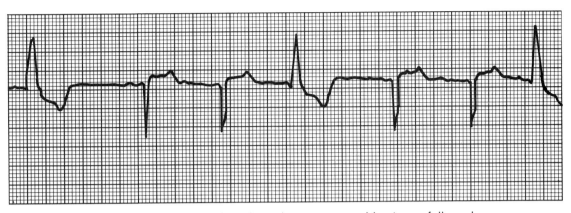

A trigeminal pattern (trigeminy) of PVCs exists when two normal beats are followed by an ectopic beat in a repetitive pattern. Every third beat is a PVC. The cardiac output decrease is much less in a trigeminal pattern than it would be in a bigeminal pattern and is often not treated. An alternate but rare pattern that may also be called trigeminal is a normal beat followed by two PVCs.

FIG. 7–14. CATEGORIES OF PVCs BY PATTERN: EXAMPLE OF QUADRIGEMINAL PVCs.

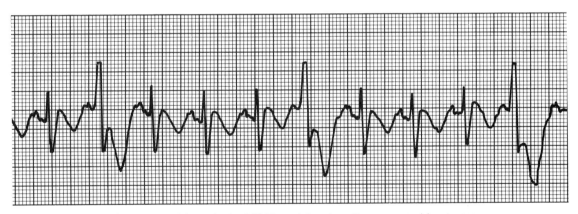

A quadrigeminal pattern (quadrigeminy) of PVCs exists when three normal beats are followed by an ectopic beat in a repetitive pattern. Every fourth beat is a PVC. This pattern produces only a minimal reduction in cardiac output. Also, because of the number of beats involved in the pattern, a 6-second strip may not be long enough to see the pattern clearly. An alternate but rare pattern that may also be called quadrigeminal is a normal beat folowed by three PVCs.

FIG. 7–15. CATEGORIES OF PVCs BY PATTERN: EXAMPLE OF PAIRS OF PVCs.

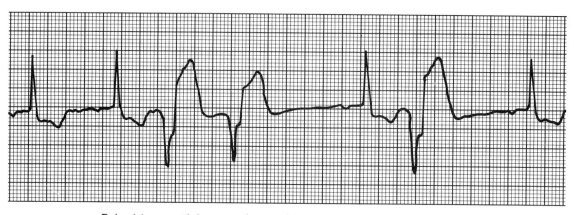

Paired (sequential—sometimes misnamed coupled) PVCs occur when there are two PVCs in a row. Occasionally, a PVC is followed by a long pause and then a ventricular escape beat. This pattern is different from bigeminal PVCs.

FIG. 7–16. CATEGORIES OF PVCs BY PATTERN: EXAMPLE OF PAIRED MULTIFORMED PVCs.

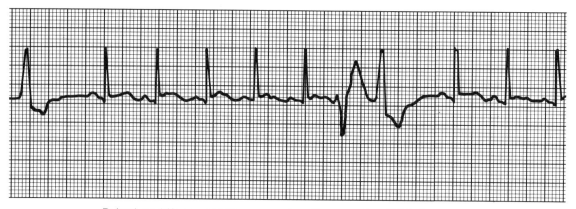

Paired, multiformed PVCs occur when there are two PVCs in a row that have different shapes or directions for their QRS complexes. This pattern is considered somewhat more serious than paired PVCs because it may indicate an increased irritability in several areas in the ventricles.

FIG. 7–17. CATEGORIES OF PVCs BY PATTERN: EXAMPLE OF A RUN OF PVCs.

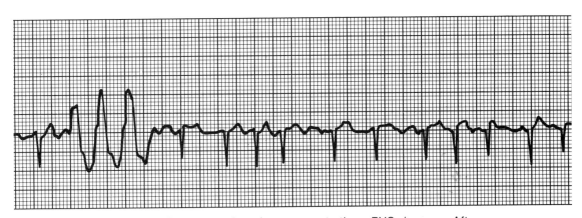

A run (salvo or volley) of PVCs occurs when there are up to three PVCs in a row. After three PVCs in a row, the pattern is usually called ventricular tachycardia. Because there is reduced cardiac output during the time that these runs are occurring, patients often become symptomatic and require treatment.

FIG. 7–18. CATEGORIES OF PVCs BY PATTERN: EXAMPLE OF MULTIFORMED RUN OF PVCs.

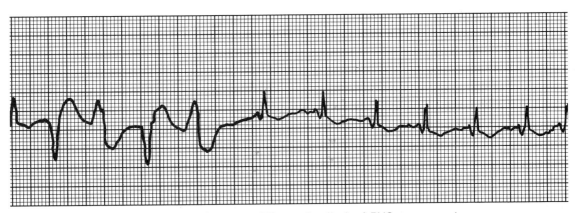

A multiformed run (multiformed salvo or multiformed volley) of PVCs occurs when there are up to three PVCs in a row that have different shapes or directions for their QRS complexes. All of the three beats do not have to be different from each other. If only one of the three beats is different, it is still a multiformed run of PVCs.

FIG. 7–19. CATEGORIES OF PVCs BY PATTERN: EXAMPLE OF AN R ON T PVC PATTERN.

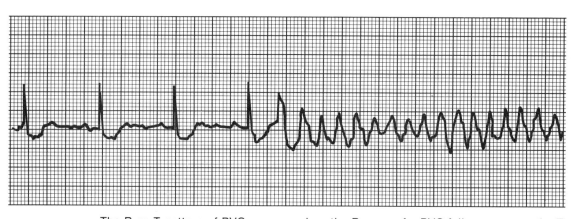

The R on T pattern of PVCs occurs when the R wave of a PVC falls near or on the T wave of the preceding normal beat. If this impulse should occur during the relative refractory period of the preceding beat, the patient may go into ventricular flutter (as shown above). This pattern is a particularly dangerous one and requires treatment.

FIG. 7–20. CATEGORIES OF PVCs BY PATTERN: VENTRICULAR FUSION BEATS.

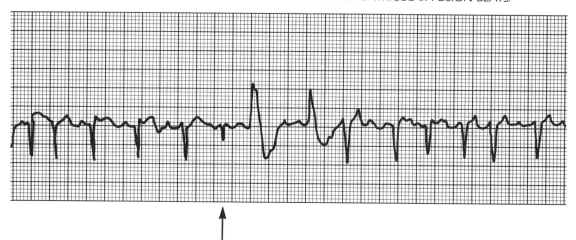

Ventricular fusion beats occur when a normal impulse from the sinus node has depolarized the atria and is beginning to depolarize the ventricles at the same time an irritable ventricular focus also initiates an impulse. The two impulses collide in their travels to depolarize the ventricles. The result is a beat that usually has a sinus P wave in front of it but looks neither like the normal beat nor the PVC. They are often much smaller in amplitude and are sometimes referred to as funny little beats (FLBs). They are not dangerous in themselves.

FIG. 7–21. CATEGORIES OF PVCs BY FREQUENCY: EXAMPLE OF RARE PVCs.

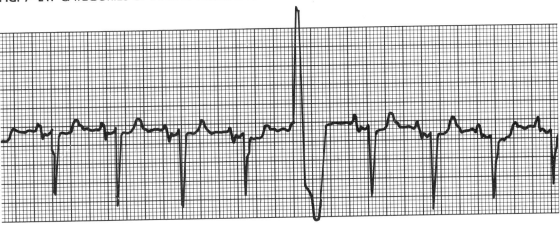

PVCs are called rare (isolated or occasional) when there are fewer than 6 per minute. Some authors believe that fewer than 10 PVCs per minute constitutes the category of rare. While the terms "rare" and "occasional" are synonomous, the term "isolated" has a different meaning. If a patient has one PVC all day, then it is isolated.

FIG. 7–22. CATEGORIES OF PVCs BY FREQUENCY: EXAMPLE OF FREQUENT PVCs.

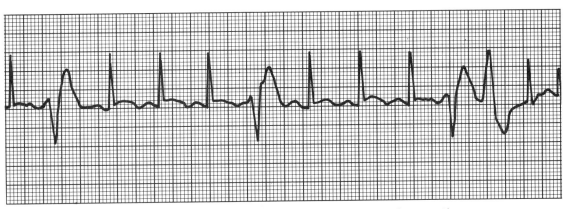

PVCs are frequent when they occur at a rate of more than 6 per minute. Some authors believe that there needs to be more than 10 per minute for PVCs to be frequent. Past automatic treatment of frequent PVCs has given way to a more conservative approach, which considers the patient's general status, as well as his or her clinical condition. A post myocardial infarction patient who has just begun having frequent PVCs and who is symptomatic from them will be treated much more aggressively than a long-term COPD patient who has chronic frequent PVCs and no symptoms.

VENTRICULAR TACHYCARDIA

Ventricular tachycardia (VT) (Fig. 7-23) is a rapid dysrhythmia that originates from a single, extremely irritable area in the ventricles. It can be thought of as a whole series of PVCs that occur one after the other. The cardiac output in VT is greatly decreased because of the rapid rate that limits the ventricular filling time and the abnormal depolarization of the ventricles found in all ventricular beats. Because the cardiac output produced by VT is often not adequate to maintain consciousness or even life, it is considered one of a group of dysrhythmias called *lethal dysrhythmias*. It quickly becomes the established rhythm and takes over the pacemaker functions of the heart.

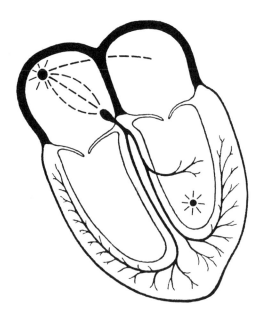

FIG. 7–23. VENTRICULAR TACHYCARDIA OCCURS WHEN ONE AREA OF THE VENTRICLES BECOMES SO IRRITABLE THAT IT TAKES OVER ALL THE PACEMAKER FUNCTIONS OF THE HEART. THE SINOATRIAL NODE MAY CONTINUE TO PRODUCE IMPULSES SO THAT P WAVES MAY BE MIXED IN WITH THE WIDE VENTRICULAR COMPLEXES BUT NOT BE ASSOCIATED WITH THEM.

The typical ventricular-shaped QRS complex, which is wider than normal and whose T wave goes in the opposite direction from the QRS, is present in VT. Because the QRS complexes in VT are produced rapidly one after the other, at times, the QRS complex and the T wave fuse together into one wave form. Nevertheless, the VT pattern is fairly easy to recognize even though exact measurement of the width of the QRS complexes may not be possible.

Because the activity of the sinus node may or may not be affected by impulses that arise in the ventricles, P waves may or may not be present on the electrocardiogram (ECG) strip that shows VT. If P waves are present during an episode of VT, they are not associated with the QRS complexes since they are not conducted to the ventricles. Ventricular tachycardia falls into the general category of AV dissociation as discussed above. For the same reason, PR intervals that may occur in VT are considered incidental and not measured.

CAUSES

In general, the factors that can cause cardiac irritability and PVCs may also cause VT. The causes of VT are sometimes subdivided into the following two general categories: intrinsic and extrinsic.

Intrinsic or internal causes. This category includes causes that arise from inside the body or heart itself, such as cardiac diseases (ischemia, MI, coronary heart disease, and congenital defects), ventricular aneurysms, R on T pattern PVCs, potassium imbalances, acidosis, and hypoxia.

Extrinsic or external causes. This category includes causes that are due to factors from outside the body. They include a large group of medications that may increase the irritability of the ventricles, such as epinephrine, thyroid medications, theophylline drugs; central nervous system stimulants such as amphetamines and cocaine; and cardiac medications such as digoxin and quinidine. Any type of invasive procedure that causes irritability to the heart may also cause VT. Common procedures that fit this category include pacemaker insertion; hemodynamic monitoring catheters such as central venous pressure lines and pulmonary artery catheters; left-sided cardiac catheterization procedures; and coronary angioplasty. Other external factors that may cause VT are electrical shock and sharp blows to the chest, such as precordial thump, that fall during the relative refractory period of the cardiac cycle.

These factors stimulate the heart to contract before it is completely ready, much as the R on T pattern does, and often produce VT.

SIGNS AND SYMPTOMS

Short runs of VT may be asymptomatic, although most patients experience some symptoms. To some degree, the production of symptoms in VT is rate-related. It is not uncommon for patients who have VT with a rate of 100–125 beats/min to be able to tolerate the dysrhythmia for a long time. Generally, these patients complain of "feeling funny," and experience a fluttering in the chest, some shortness of breath, and activity intolerance. Their blood pressure is low, with a rapid and weak pulse.

Ventricular tachycardia at rapid rates is seldom tolerated and produces the severe symptoms seen with major decreases in cardiac output. These symptoms include shortness of breath, diaphoresis, chest pressure and pain, changes in level of consciousness, unconsciousness, hypoxic type seizures, dilation of the pupils, no blood pressure, and no pulse. Patients with these symptoms require immediate treatment to terminate the VT.

TREATMENT

The treatment regimen is different, to some degree, depending on whether or not the patient is tolerating the dysrhythmia. If the patient is tolerating the VT, then the first-line IV medications used to treat PVCs may be administered IV push to terminate the dysrhythmia. As discussed above, these IV medications include lidocaine, procainamide, bretylium, and phenytoin. These medications are usually administered in an IV drip after the termination of the VT until the underlying cause is corrected or eliminated. The class 1A, 1B, 1C, and III oral antidysrhythmics may be used to prevent future episodes of VT but do not work rapidly enough to terminate current episodes of the dysrhythmia.

If the VT is not being tolerated and the patient is losing consciousness, then more aggressive treatment is indicated. While precordial thump may be used successfully if administered very early in the episode, electrical cardioversion is the treatment of choice for rapid termination of VT. If the VT lasts for longer than 4 or 5 minutes and the patient becomes acidotic, the VT may not convert to sinus rhythm unless the acidosis is corrected with sodium bicarbonate or hyperventilation. After termination of the VT and stabilization of the patient is achieved, the IV antidysrhythmic medications, particularly lidocaine, are administered in an IV drip.

Cardiopulmonary resuscitation (CPR) and cardioversion produce unique patterns on the ECG strip. Cardiopulmonary resuscitation, if it is being administered correctly, produces a wide, rounded-looking QRS complex in regular intervals on the ECG strip since the muscle tissue of the myocardium is being activated by external compressions (Fig. 7-24). This CPR pattern is similar to a pattern called

FIG. 7–24. EXAMPLE OF QRS COMPLEXES PRODUCED BY EFFECTIVE CARDIOPULMONARY RESUSCITATION.

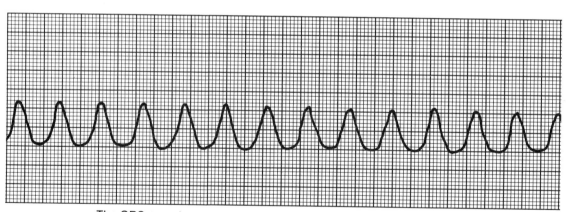

The QRS complexes produced by CPR are rounded, may be larger or smaller in size, and are regular if the chest compressions are being administered regularly. The best cardiac output from CPR is approximately 30% of normal.

agonal rhythm, which will be discussed later. Electrical cardioversion equipment produces relatively high electrical energy levels, which are much higher than the very small myocardial currents most ECG monitoring equipment is designed to detect. To prevent damage to the ECG monitoring equipment during cardioversion, there are built-in current suppressors in the monitor that prevent the high

FIG. 7–25. EXAMPLE OF ECG PATTERN PRODUCED BY ELECTRIC CARDIOVERSION.

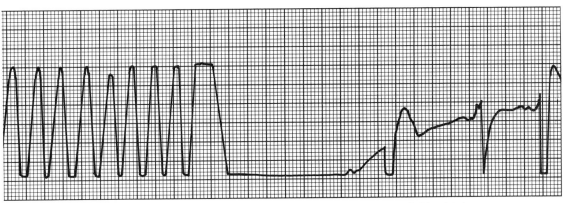

The electrical shock stops all cardiac activity for approximately 1 second. The high energy shock produced by the cardioverter appears as a flat line, which is off the paper at the top or bottom.

output energy from damaging it. Cardioversion on the ECG strip appears as a flat line that is either at the top or bottom of the strip for approximately 1–2 seconds (Fig. 7-25).

Other last-resort methods used to terminate VT when the usual methods have failed include the use of magnesium sulfate IV and the insertion of a temporary pacemaker to override the VT. Implantable defibrillators that detect VT or ventricular fibrillation and administer a strong impulse to terminate them can be used in the long-term prevention of VT in individuals who are particularly prone to this dysrhythmia (Fig. 7-26).

FIG. 7–26. EXAMPLE OF VENTRICULAR TACHYCARDIA.

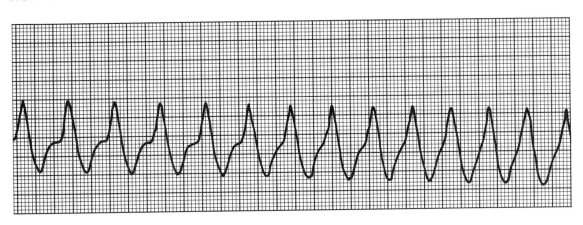

CRITERIA FOR VENTRICULAR TACHYCARDIA

Rhythm: Regular to slightly irregular.

Rate: Over 100 beats/min. Ventricular tachycardia may be in the 100–125 range, but the most common rate for VT is 130–170 beats/min.

Atrial Conduction: P waves usually not present. If P waves are seen, they may be sinus P waves that are dissociated from the VT or may be retrograde P waves.

AV Conduction: PR interval is not measured.

Ventricular Conduction: QRS complex is wide and in the typical ventricular beat configuration. May be difficult to identify the exact point at which the T wave begins.

VENTRICULAR FLUTTER

The same mechanisms that produce VT also produce ventricular flutter. This fact has led some experts in the field to believe that ventricular flutter is not really a separate dysrhythmia but a form of VT.

Ventricular flutter occurs when a single area in the ventricles becomes extremely irritable and takes over all the pacemaker functions of the heart. Ventricular flutter can be viewed as an intermediate stage between VT and ventricular fibrillation. It indicates more ventricular irritability than is found in VT and a decrease in cardiac functioning. One difficulty in discussing ventricular flutter is that there are two distinct ways of defining or identifying it.

The most common characteristic used to identify ventricular flutter is the shape of the QRS complexes. Rather than having the sharp pointed angular configuration that is usually found in VT, the QRS complexes in ventricular flutter begin to become rounded on both the top and bottom. This shape is sometimes referred to as a *sine wave* (pronounced "sign") shape. These QRS complexes are somewhat wider than those of VT and have the appearance of a spring, if looked at from the side, that has been stretched out. This rounding of the QRS complexes is probably caused by the decrease in ventricular contractility brought on by decreased perfusion and oxygenation of the myocardium. Ventricular flutter is also considered one of the lethal dysrhythmias.

The other characteristic used to identify ventricular flutter is the rate. Generally, if the rate is faster than 250 beats/min, the dysrhythmia is called ventricular flutter.

CAUSES

The causes are the same as the causes for VT.

SIGNS AND SYMPTOMS

This dysrhythmia is never tolerated, therefore, the signs and symptoms observed would be the same as those symptoms seen with nontolerated VT.

TREATMENT

The treatment is generally the same as for VT, except that it is started with electrical cardioversion. If not treated quickly, ventricular flutter rapidly degenerates into ventricular fibrillation (Fig. 7-27).

FIG. 7–27. EXAMPLE OF VENTRICULAR FLUTTER.

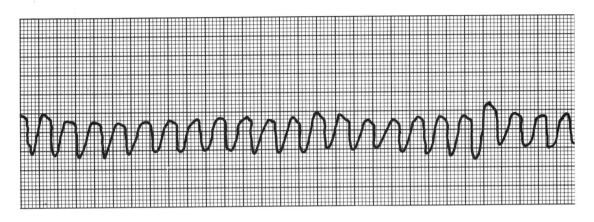

CRITERIA FOR VENTRICULAR FLUTTER

Rhythm: Regular to slightly irregular.

Rate: Faster than 250 beats/min.

Atrial Conduction: P waves usually not present. If P waves are seen, they may be sinus P waves that are dissociated from the dysrhythmia or may be retrograde P waves.

AV Conduction: PR interval is not measured.

Ventricular Conduction: QRS complexes are wide in the typical ventricular beat configuration. They have a rounded appearance in a sine wave shape. It is almost impossible to distinguish the T waves from the QRS complexes.

VENTRICULAR FIBRILLATION

Ventricular fibrillation (also called VF, V fib) (Fig. 7-28) occurs when there is uncoordinated, quivering activity of the ventricles, representing many ventricular areas contracting at the same time without any unified, effective contraction. This dysrhythmia indicates extreme irritability of the ventricular myocardium and is often considered one form of cardiac arrest because all circulation stops. It is also classified as one of the lethal dysrhythmias.

The QRS complexes produced by VF become disorganized and chaotic in

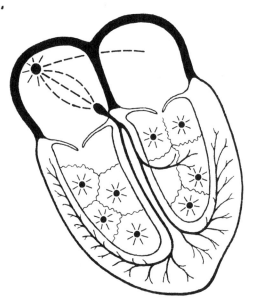

FIG. 7–28. VENTRICULAR FIBRILLATION OCCURS WHEN THE VENTRICLES OF THE HEART NO LONGER CONTRACT AS A UNIT. THERE ARE MULTIPLE AREAS OF THE VENTRICLES THAT ARE ALL CONTRACTING AT THE SAME TIME SO THAT THE MYOCARDIUM IS QUIVERING. THERE IS NO CIRCULATION WITH THIS DYSRHYTHMIA. THE SINOATRIAL NODE MAY CONTINUE TO PRODUCE IMPULSES FOR A SHORT TIME. P WAVES MAY BE PRESENT BUT ARE NOT ASSOCIATED WITH THE IRREGULAR, CHAOTIC QRS COMPLEXES.

configuration because there are no unified ventricular contractions taking place. These QRS complexes of VF may range in size from being rather larger and nearly the same size as the QRS complexes found in VT called *coarse VF* to very small, irregular undulations of the baseline called *fine VF*. The atria may continue to depolarize normally for a short time after the VF begins so that P waves may be present on the strip.

CAUSES

Most of the factors that produce VT also have the potential to produce ventricular fibrillation. It is often caused by activity that occurs during the relative refractory period of the cardiac cycle, such as R on T PVCs, precordial thump, or electrical shock; and by the use of invasive technology in the heart. Ventricular fibrillation is one of the worst complications of severe cardiac disease, especially MI. Ventricular fibrillation is often the terminal event in a variety of diseases.

SIGNS AND SYMPTOMS

When a patient goes into ventricular fibrillation, all circulation stops. There is no pulse, no blood pressure, and no respiration. The skin becomes cyanotic, cold and clammy; the pupils are fixed and dilated; and the patient becomes totally unresponsive in a short time. The picture is one of death.

TREATMENT

It is important to recognize this dysrhythmia immediately and begin CPR as soon as possible.

The precordial thump may be used if the patient is being monitored and the VF is witnessed. If the VF has been the dominant rhythm for more than 45 seconds, precordial thump probably is not effective. After this time frame, intubation and reversal of the acidotic state produced in cardiac arrest is required for successful conversion of the dysrhythmia. Use of electrical defibrillation in the unsynchronized mode is necessary. In general, fine VF will not convert even with electrical defibrillation. It must be changed to coarse VF by the use of IV epinephrine before defibrillation will be successful. After the ventricular fibrillation has been difibrillated, a lidocaine drip is started to prevent its recurrence. Patients who have had one episode of VF are highly susceptible to repeated episodes and must be monitored closely. Often these patients are placed on life support until their condition stabilizes (Figs. 7-29 and 7-30).

FIG. 7–29. EXAMPLE OF FINE VENTRICULAR FIBRILLATION.

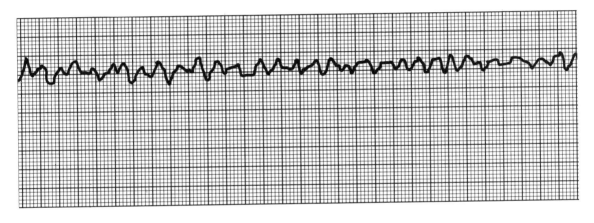

FIG. 7–30. EXAMPLE OF COARSE VENTRICULAR FIBRILLATION.

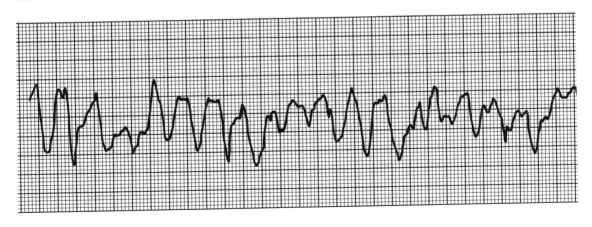

CRITERIA FOR VENTRICULAR FIBRILLATION

Rhythm: Totally irregular or chaotic. No recognizable QRS complexes.

Rate: Undetermined. The irregular complexes may be counted, but it has no significance since there is no cardiac output.

Atrial Conduction: P waves may be present but are not conducted.

AV Conduction: PR interval is not measured.

Ventricular Conduction: QRS complexes are indistinct, chaotic undulations of the baseline. Small undulations are called fine VF (see Fig. 7-29); large undulations are called coarse VF (see Fig. 7-30).

AGONAL RHYTHM

Agonal rhythm (also called dying heart pattern) is the name given to an ECG pattern that indicates progressive death of the ventricular myocardium. It is an intermediate stage between ventricular fibrillation or a slow idioventricular rhythm and asystole. As the ventricular myocardium becomes weaker from the progressive lack of oxygen, the QRS complexes produced become progressively wider while the amplitude decreases. The ventricular focus producing the rhythm also becomes slower and more irregular as the rhythm progresses. Left untreated, it always terminates in asystole. The atria are usually inactive during an agonal rhythm so that the appearance of P waves is extremely rare.

CAUSES

Agonal rhythm is a terminal event in the dying process that shows the death of the myocardium. It results from the degeneration of a ventricular dysrhythmia that has not been treated. It is rare that a patient proceeds from a sinus rhythm to an agonal rhythm. The causes include severe cardiac disease, such as massive MI, large pulmonary emboli that totally block circulation, and cardiogenic shock. Severe trauma to the heart from penetrating injuries, such as gun shot wounds and stabbing, also may produce an agonal rhythm.

SIGNS AND SYMPTOMS

There is no cardiac output with an agonal pattern. The depolarizations of the ventricles, although they do produce QRS complexes, do not produce any circulation. The patient has no pulse, no blood pressure, and no respirations. The pupils quickly become fixed and dilated, and the skin, cyanotic. The patient is totally unresponsive.

TREATMENT

An agonal rhythm does not respond to treatment. Advanced life support procedures with intubation and CPR may temporarily maintain circulation but do not convert the rhythm. Electric defibrillation of an agonal rhythm often results in asystole. One approach that is successful in a very small number of cases is to attempt to convert the agonal rhythm to ventricular fibrillation with CPR and IV epinephrine. Ventricular fibrillation does respond to electrical defibrillation. A temporary pacemaker may be inserted in an attempt to maintain a more effective ventricular pattern at a higher rate but may not be effective due to the underlying dying process of the heart that has already begun (Fig. 7-31).

FIG. 7–31. EXAMPLE OF AN AGONAL RHYTHM.

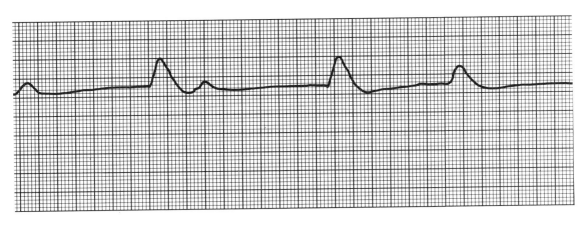

CRITERIA FOR AN AGONAL RHYTHM

Rhythm: Slightly irregular to totally irregular.

Rate: 20–40 beats/min, although it may be slightly faster. Pattern tends to slow as the myocardium progressively dies.

Atrial Conduction: P waves are usually not present.

AV Conduction: PR interval is not present and not measured.

Ventricular Conduction: QRS complexes are extremely wide and may exceed 0.60 second. They may be either positively or negatively deflected. Sometimes two distinct complexes representing the ventricles contracting separately may be present. The amplitude of the QRS complexes decreases as the myocardium continues to die.

ASYSTOLE

Asystole is also called cardiac arrest, cardiac standstill, ventricular standstill, straight line, and flat line (Fig. 7-32). Asystole is a type of ventricular dysrhythmia that exists when there is no electrical activity in the ventricular myocardium. It is the only true arrhythmia (without rhythm).

The pattern produced on the ECG strip will be an isoelectric line without any complexes, although it may not be absolutely straight. It is possible for atrial activity to continue for a short time after the ventricles stop, therefore, the strip may contain P waves without any QRS complexes. This pattern with the P waves is more appropriately named *ventricular standstill*.

In either case, there is no cardiac output and no circulation. The backup pacemakers fail to take over the pacemaker responsibility. Asystole is a lethal dysrhythmia that responds poorly to resuscitation efforts.

FIG. 7–32. EXAMPLE OF ASYSTOLE.

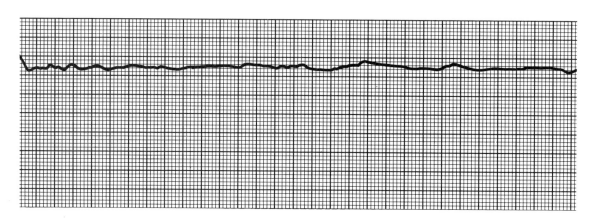

CAUSES

Occasionally a result of a complete heart block or a trifascicular block without a backup pacemaker site, asystole is more often the terminal event in the dying process. It is often used as one of the criteria for a determination of death. It may result from other ventricular dysrhythmias that are left untreated, particularly ventricular fibrillation and agonal rhythm. Asystole is usually preceded by other ventricular dysrhythmias, although some patients may have transient episodes of asystole during an otherwise normal sinus rhythm. There is often some history of heart disease underlying poor profusion of the myocardium.

SIGNS AND SYMPTOMS

The signs for death are observed in patients who go into asystole. No pulse, no blood pressure, no respiration, pupils fixed and dilated, cyanosis of the skin, and total unresponsiveness are all present in asystole. Transient episodes of asystole may produce Stokes-Adams Attack symptoms with transient syncope.

TREATMENT

It is important to verify asystole in at least two leads before initiating treatment. With some types of monitoring equipment, a disconnected lead may produce a *flat line.* Also, certain types of ventricular fibrillation may produce an asystole type pattern in one particular lead.

If the episode is witnessed on a monitored patient, a precordial thump delivered within 45 seconds of the onset sometimes brings about conversion to a more effective rhythm. If the asystole has continued for longer than approximately 1 minute or has not been witnessed, then the full Code Blue procedure with advanced life support measures, intubation, and chest compressions must be started. The treatment is similar to that used in fine ventricular fibrillation, including the use of epinephrine and defibrillation. If the asystole is a terminal event, the likelihood of it responding to treatment is poor. A temporary pacemaker may be inserted in the effort to initiate some ventricular activity.

CRITERIA FOR ASYSTOLE

Rhythm: If an atrial rhythm is present, it may be regular or irregular. The ventricles have an isoelectric line indicating electrical activity.

Rate: Atrial rate, if present, may be slow or fast. Ventricular rate is zero—no electrical activity.

Atrial Conduction: P waves may be present.

AV Conduction: PR interval not measured.

Ventricular Conduction: QRS not present. (Be sure to verify this absence of a QRS in a second lead and by assessing the absent pulse.) There is an isoelectric line indicating no electrical activity in the ventricles.

PRACTICE ECG STRIPS FOR CHAPTER 7

Directions. On the following practice ECG strips, analyze each strip according to its rhythm, rate, atrial conduction, AV conduction, and ventricular conduction. Arrive at an interpretation of the strip based upon the analysis and criteria for the dysrhythmias originating in the atria as learned in this chapter. (See Appendix II for interpretations.)

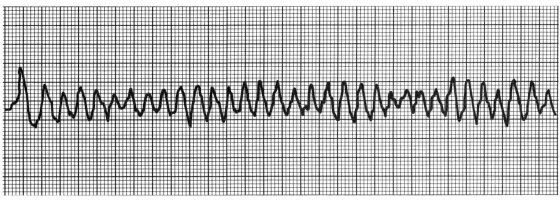

7–1

RHYTHM: _____

RATE: _____

ATRIAL CONDUCTION: _____

_____

AV CONDUCTION: _____

VENTRICULAR CONDUCTION: _____

INTERPRETATION: _____

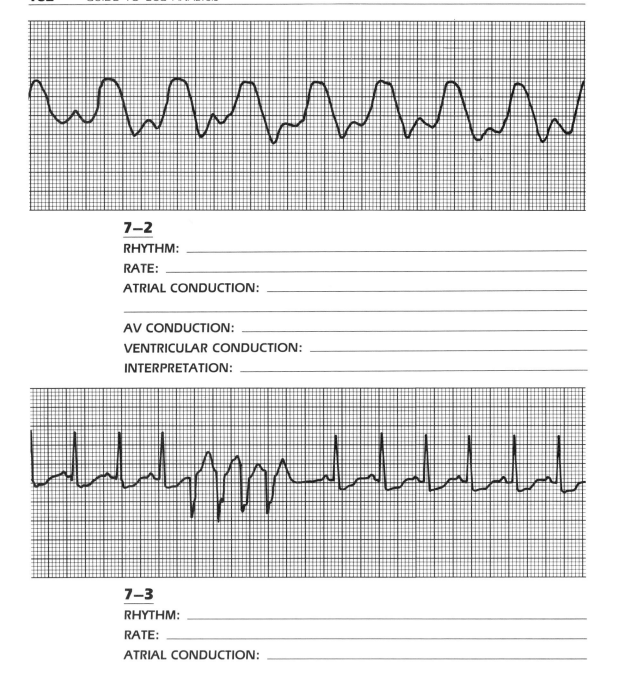

7–2
RHYTHM: _____

RATE: _____

ATRIAL CONDUCTION: _____

_____

AV CONDUCTION: _____

VENTRICULAR CONDUCTION: _____

INTERPRETATION: _____

7–3
RHYTHM: _____

RATE: _____

ATRIAL CONDUCTION: _____

_____

AV CONDUCTION: _____

VENTRICULAR CONDUCTION: _____

INTERPRETATION: _____

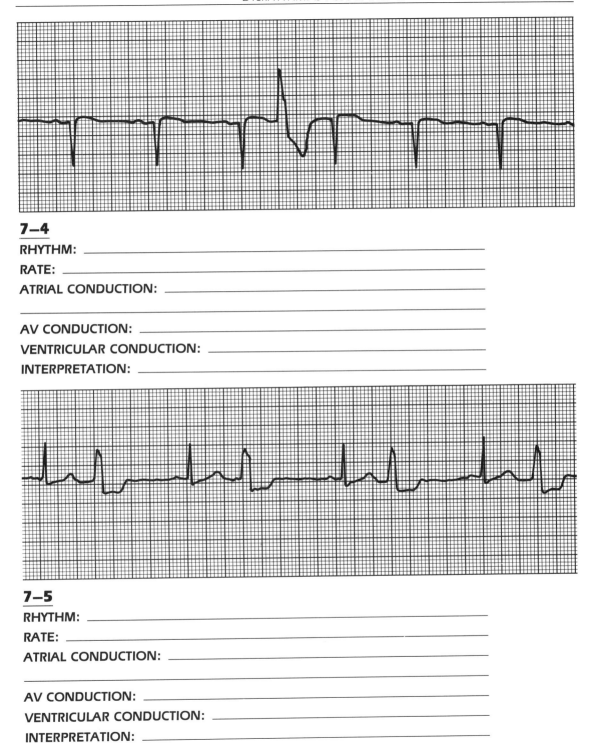

7–4

RHYTHM: _____

RATE: _____

ATRIAL CONDUCTION: _____

_____

AV CONDUCTION: _____

VENTRICULAR CONDUCTION: _____

INTERPRETATION: _____

7–5

RHYTHM: _____

RATE: _____

ATRIAL CONDUCTION: _____

_____

AV CONDUCTION: _____

VENTRICULAR CONDUCTION: _____

INTERPRETATION: _____

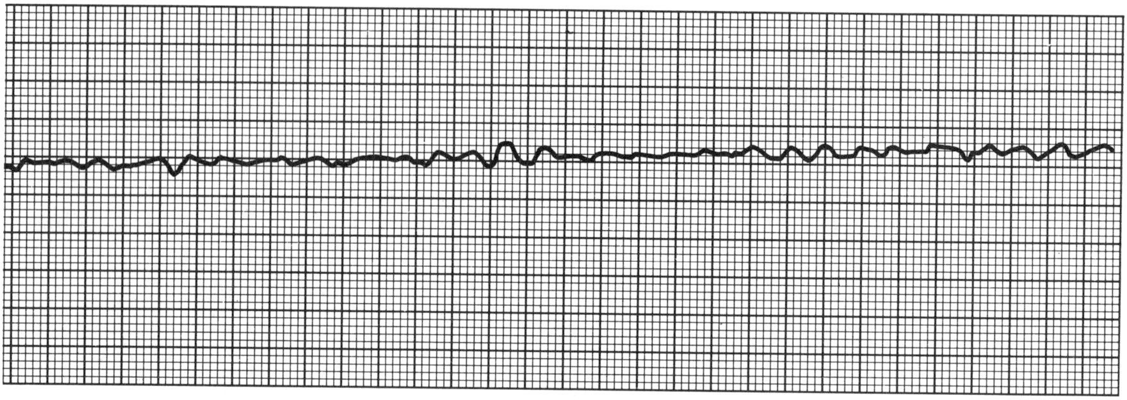

7–6

RHYTHM: _____

RATE: _____

ATRIAL CONDUCTION: _____

_____

AV CONDUCTION: _____

VENTRICULAR CONDUCTION: _____

INTERPRETATION: _____

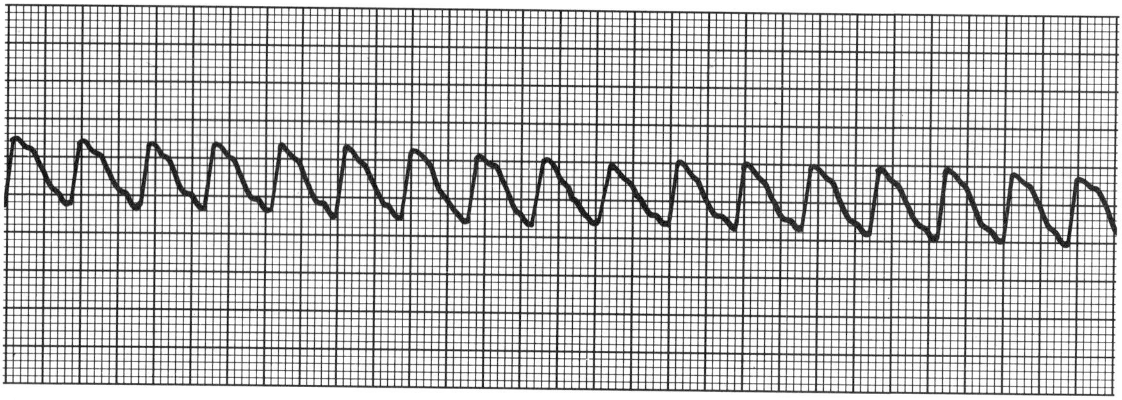

7–7

RHYTHM: _____

RATE: _____

ATRIAL CONDUCTION: _____

_____

AV CONDUCTION: _____

VENTRICULAR CONDUCTION: _____

INTERPRETATION: _____

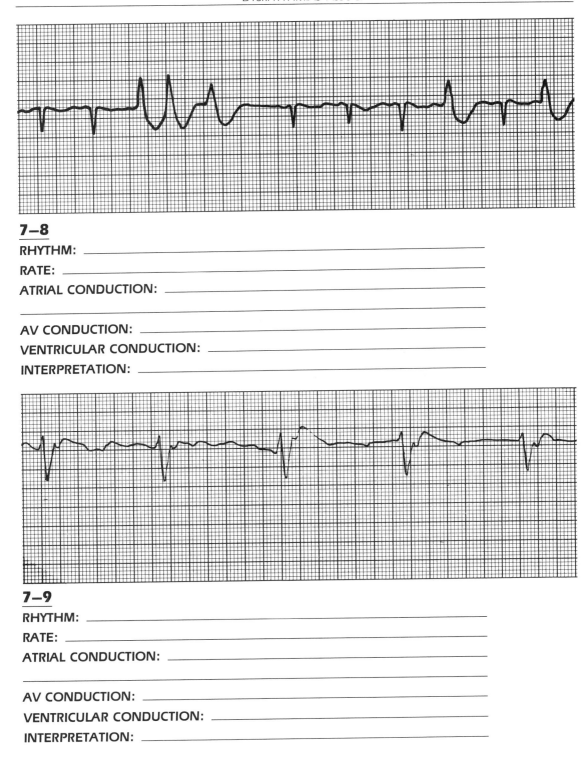

7–8

RHYTHM: _____

RATE: _____

ATRIAL CONDUCTION: _____

_____

AV CONDUCTION: _____

VENTRICULAR CONDUCTION: _____

INTERPRETATION: _____

7–9

RHYTHM: _____

RATE: _____

ATRIAL CONDUCTION: _____

_____

AV CONDUCTION: _____

VENTRICULAR CONDUCTION: _____

INTERPRETATION: _____

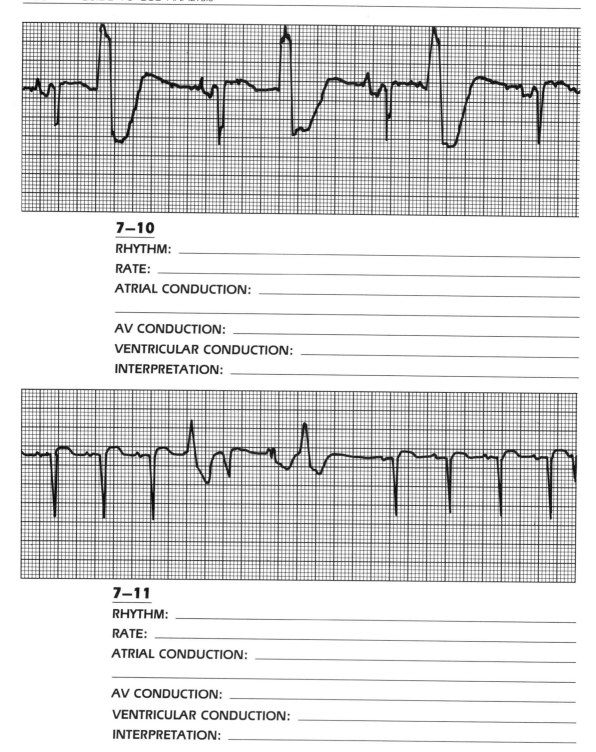

7-10

RHYTHM: _____

RATE: _____

ATRIAL CONDUCTION: _____

_____

AV CONDUCTION: _____

VENTRICULAR CONDUCTION: _____

INTERPRETATION: _____

7-11

RHYTHM: _____

RATE: _____

ATRIAL CONDUCTION: _____

_____

AV CONDUCTION: _____

VENTRICULAR CONDUCTION: _____

INTERPRETATION: _____

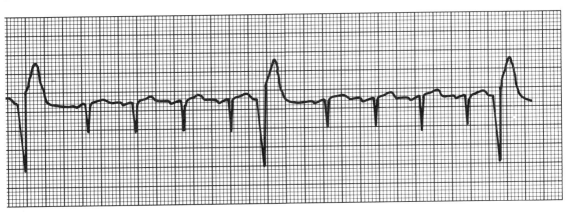

7–12

RHYTHM: _____

RATE: _____

ATRIAL CONDUCTION: _____

_____

AV CONDUCTION: _____

VENTRICULAR CONDUCTION: _____

INTERPRETATION: _____

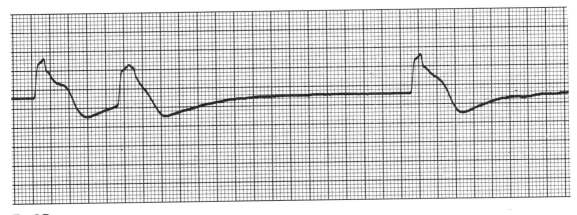

7–13

RHYTHM: _____

RATE: _____

ATRIAL CONDUCTION: _____

_____

AV CONDUCTION: _____

VENTRICULAR CONDUCTION: _____

INTERPRETATION: _____

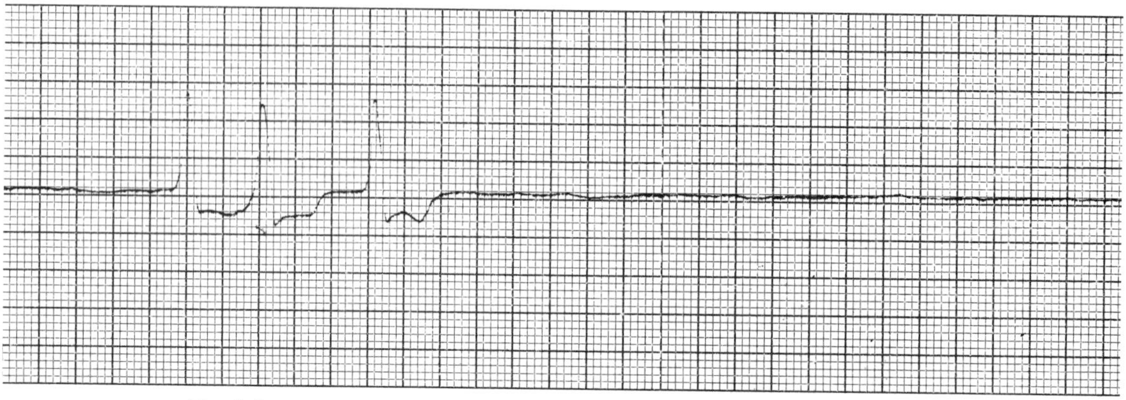

7–14

RHYTHM: _____

RATE: _____

ATRIAL CONDUCTION: _____

_____

AV CONDUCTION: _____

VENTRICULAR CONDUCTION: _____

INTERPRETATION: _____

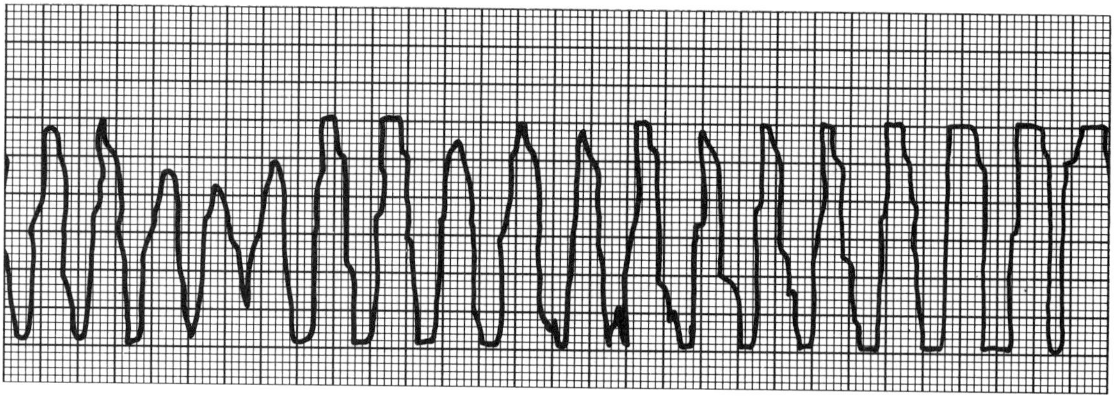

7–15

RHYTHM: _____

RATE: _____

ATRIAL CONDUCTION: _____

_____

AV CONDUCTION: _____

VENTRICULAR CONDUCTION: _____

INTERPRETATION: _____

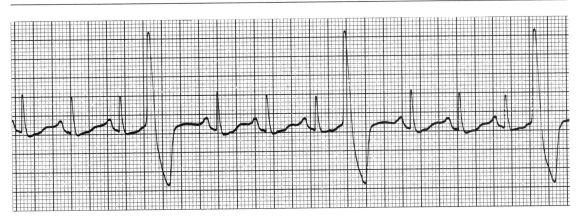

7–16

RHYTHM: _____

RATE: _____

ATRIAL CONDUCTION: _____

_____

AV CONDUCTION: _____

VENTRICULAR CONDUCTION: _____

INTERPRETATION: _____

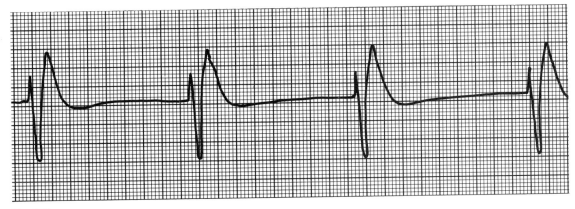

7–17

RHYTHM: _____

RATE: _____

ATRIAL CONDUCTION: _____

_____

AV CONDUCTION: _____

VENTRICULAR CONDUCTION: _____

INTERPRETATION: _____

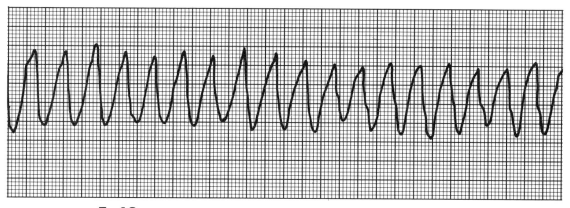

7–18
RHYTHM: _____

RATE: _____

ATRIAL CONDUCTION: _____

_____

AV CONDUCTION: _____

VENTRICULAR CONDUCTION: _____

INTERPRETATION: _____

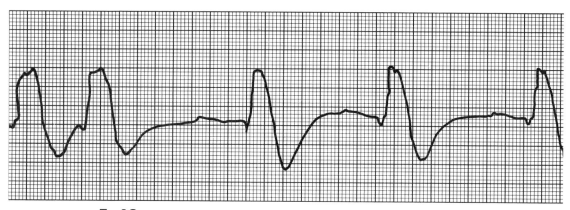

7–19
RHYTHM: _____

RATE: _____

ATRIAL CONDUCTION: _____

_____

AV CONDUCTION: _____

VENTRICULAR CONDUCTION: _____

INTERPRETATION: _____

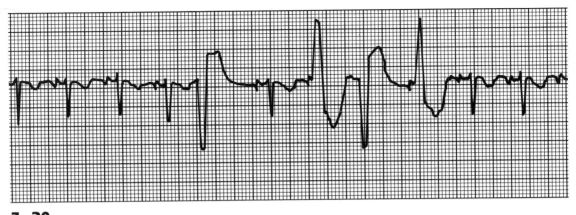

7–20

RHYTHM: _____

RATE: _____

ATRIAL CONDUCTION: _____

_____

AV CONDUCTION: _____

VENTRICULAR CONDUCTION: _____

INTERPRETATION: _____

DYSRHYTHMIAS ASSOCIATED WITH BLOCKS IN THE AV NODE

LEARNING OBJECTIVES

After studying this section, the learner will be able to:

1. Describe the underlying pathology in AV blocks.
2. List the AV blocks according to the categories and describe the identifying features of each category.
3. Discuss the common causes for AV blocks.
4. List the most serious symptoms associated with AV blocks.
5. Name the common treatments for AV blocks.
6. Identify AV blocks on ECG strips based on the criteria learned in the chapter.

Whenever a depolarizing impulse is obstructed somewhere in the conduction system of the heart, a conduction block exists. Atrioventricular (AV) blocks are the most common of all conduction abnormalities in the heart. Atrioventricular blocks can occur anywhere between the sinoatrial (SA) node and the Purkinje fibers, although the most common site is the AV node itself.

Identifying AV blocks is somewhat easier than identifying some of the other dysrhythmias. The key factor in identifying AV blocks is the PR interval. Another important analysis factor is the presence of more P waves than QRS complexes in the higher degree blocks. Atrioventricular blocks have the potential to be very serious dysrhythmias, therefore, it is important to make accurate interpretations when they are present.

Traditionally, three different types of AV blocks have been classified: *first degree AV block, second degree AV block,* and *third degree AV block*. Second degree AV block is further subdivided into two categories based on the pattern of the block. Some authors disagree with this traditional classification and add a fourth degree (advanced block). The major area of conflict centers on the traditional classification system, which implies that higher degree blocks are more serious and dangerous than lower degree blocks. This belief is not always true. Some second degree AV blocks can be potentially more dangerous and decrease cardiac output more than some third degree AV blocks. Other systems of classification have been proposed based on the actual clinical potential of the block. These classes are referred to as *low grade blocks* and *high grade blocks*. However, they also include the traditional classification system. The learner must have a thorough understanding of the traditional classification system of AV blocks to understand the newer classification systems.

FIRST DEGREE AV BLOCK

First degree AV block, also called first degree block and prolonged PR interval (Fig. 8-1), is not a dysrhythmia in and of itself. It is not a true block. Rather, first degree AV block is a condition that is imposed on an electrocardiogram (ECG) pattern. This fact is important because the analysis involves identifying both the basic or underlying pattern and the AV block itself.

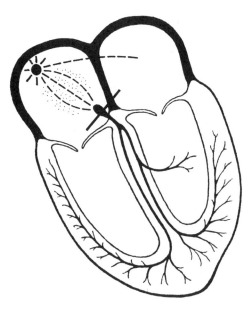

FIG. 8–1. IN FIRST DEGREE AV BLOCK, THE IMPULSES FROM THE SINUS NODE ARE DELAYED IN THEIR CONDUCTION THROUGH THE AV CONDUCTION SYSTEM AND AV NODE. EVENTUALLY, THE IMPULSES ARE CONDUCTED TO THE VENTRICLES SO THERE IS ONE P WAVE FOR EVERY QRS COMPLEX.

In first degree AV block, the depolarizing impulse is delayed somewhere between the atrial and the Purkinje fibers, but none of the impulses are really blocked. The impulses that originate in the SA node or atria depolarize the atria normally, producing normal P waves, but the impulse is delayed longer than the usual one tenth of a second. The result is that the PR interval is longer than normal. Even though it is delayed, all the impulses eventually pass through to the ventricles, so that every QRS complex has a P wave before it. Since the impulses are following the normal conduction pathways through the ventricles, the QRS complexes appear normal.

A question occasionally arises about how long an impulse can be delayed in the AV node and still be conducted to the ventricles. Rule-of-thumb and conventional thinking hold that a PR interval of more than 0.44 second indicates a nonconducted impulse. In practice, intervals of 0.44 second and longer have been observed to remain consistent with every P wave followed by a QRS complex; this would indicate that the impulses were indeed being conducted to the ventricles. The difficulty that arises when the PR interval exceeds 0.80 second is that the overall rate becomes so slow that the P waves either become hidden in the preceding T wave or junctional escape beats may start to appear. There is no good answer for this question of long PR intervals except to consider each pattern individually as well as the patient's clinical condition, and make a determination based upon both factors.

CAUSES

First degree AV block can occur in individuals who have no history of cardiac disease; it can be normal for young, healthy adults. First degree AV block is commonly seen in older individuals and may be part of the aging effect on the heart or an early sign of degenerative disease of the conduction system of the heart. Myocarditis, arteriosclerotic heart disease, and myocardial infarction (MI) are common causes of first degree AV block.

One of the most common causes is the effect of cardiac medications, particularly digoxin. Other medications that have the potential to produce first degree AV block include the calcium-channel blockers and the beta blockers. Rarely will quinidine sulfate be responsible for a first degree AV block.

SYMPTOMS

There are no symptoms caused by first degree AV block since it has little or no effect on the cardiac output by itself. If the block is imposed upon a dysrhythmia that is capable of producing symptoms, such as a very slow sinus bradycardia, the symptoms would be those seen with that particular dysrhythmia.

TREATMENT

If the first degree AV block has been caused by cardiac medication, reducing the dosage of those medications or eliminating them from the treatment regimen will return the PR interval to normal. There are no other specific treatments for first degree AV block.

A first degree AV block that develops after a patient has had an MI must be monitored closely because there is a tendency for the block to progress to a higher level, particularly within the first 72 hours post MI. First degree AV blocks not associated with MI tend not to progress to a higher degree block (Fig. 8-2).

FIG. 8–2. AN EXAMPLE OF SINUS RHYTHM WITH FIRST DEGREE AV BLOCK.

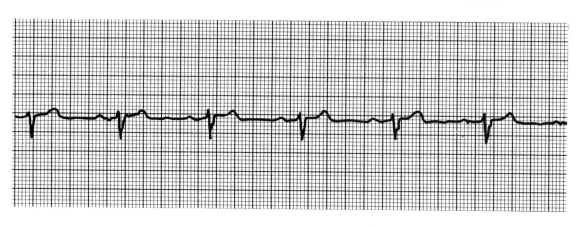

CRITERIA FOR FIRST DEGREE AV BLOCK

Rhythm: May be regular or irregular depending on what the pattern of the underlying rhythm is.

Rate: Depends on the underlying rhythm.

Atrial Conduction: P waves generally are normal, upright, and rounded—one P wave for each QRS complex.

AV Conduction: PR intervals are greater than 0.20 second; they are the same for all beats.

Ventricular Conduction: QRS complexes 0.06–0.10 second; same shape across the whole strip.

SECOND DEGREE AV BLOCK

Second degree AV block, also called second degree block, is a true block because impulses from the SA node or atrial sites are prevented from passing through the conduction system to the ventricles. The end result is that there are P waves (atrial depolarization) on the ECG strip that have no QRS complexes after them (no ventricular depolarization). Second degree heart block is usually divided into two types, depending on the pattern of P waves and QRS complexes produced on the ECG strip. One of the keys to distinguishing between these two types of second degree AV block is the analysis of the PR interval.

AV WENCKEBACH

AV Wenckebach is also called Mobitz type I, second degree AV block; Mobitz I, type I second degree AV block (Fig. 8-3). Although Wenckebach blocks may occur in the sinus nodes or the bundle branches, AV Wenckebach is the most

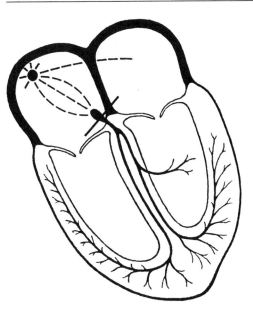

FIG. 8–3. IN AV WENCKEBACH, THE CONDUCTION DEFECT IS USUALLY IN THE AV NODE AND BEGINS TO BLOCK SOME OF THE IMPULSES FROM THE SINUS NODE. A PATTERN OF PROGRESSIVELY LONGER PR INTERVALS WITH DROPPED QRS COMPLEXES IS CHARACTERISTIC OF THIS TYPE OF BLOCK.

common form of this block. AV Wenckebach is the less serious of the two types of second degree AV block because it is usually transient and does not progress to a third degree AV block. The physiologic mechanism that produces the blocked beats is similar to the mechanism that produces a first degree AV block. The top portion of the AV node is the area that most commonly interferes with conduction of the impulses through to the ventricles. The speed at which the impulses are conducted through the AV node are gradually decreased so that the impulse takes longer and longer to get through. This progressive slowing of impulse conduction appears on the ECG as a PR interval that gets longer and longer. At some point in the series of increasingly slow impulses, one of the conduction impulses is completely blocked. That impulse appears on the ECG as a P wave without a QRS complex after it.

The blocked beat (or missed or dropped beat) most often occurs every fourth or fifth beat but can be as frequent as every second beat or as infrequent as every seventh or eighth beat. During the interval when the impulse is not conducted to the ventricles, the AV node recovers its conduction ability, and the PR interval of the first beat following the blocked impulse returns to normal. As the pattern repeats itself and impulses through the AV node gradually slow, a pattern of a progressively lengthening PR interval is reproduced again until another impulse is blocked. This pattern can be in a fixed ratio of, for example, five P waves to four QRS complexes (5:4) that occurs over and over again. The pattern can also occur as a variable ratio that changes periodically, for example, from a 5:4 ratio to a 4:3 ratio, then to a 6:5 ratio and then back to a 5:4 ratio again. With the higher ratio patterns, an ECG strip longer than 6 seconds may be required to visualize the blocked beat and the repetition of the pattern of progressively longer PR intervals.

It is important to remember that the SA node is a regular pacemaker and is not affected by blocks in the lower conduction system. The SA node continues to produce impulses at regular intervals no matter how that impulse is blocked later in its travels through the heart. This regular production of SA nodal impulses appears on the ECG as P waves with regular P to P intervals. Because the P to P intervals remain the same while the PR intervals are increasing in length, the QRS complexes tend to become further and further apart. The R to R interval in an AV Wenckebach pattern is irregular in a progressively shorter pattern before the pause. When a slow basic rhythm such as a sinus bradycardia is combined with AV Wenckebach, the pause produced by the blocked beat may become long enough to have a junctional escape beat occur. Even if there is a junctional escape beat as the terminating beat of the pause, the PR interval of the following beat is shorter than the PR interval of the conducted beat before the pause.

CAUSES

Any of the factors that can cause a first degree AV block also can cause an AV Wenckebach. AV Wenckebach does not occur in individuals who do not have some type of heart disease. It is commonly seen in post MI patients as a transitory conduction defect. Myocarditis and other types of inflammatory heart disease, as well as coronary heart disease and congenital conditions, can produce an AV Wenckebach.

Cardiac medications, especially digoxin, are fairly common causes of this type of block. Combination of beta blockers with calcium-channel blockers also have the potential to produce this type of block.

SIGNS AND SYMPTOMS

If the overall rate of the underlying rhythm and block remains near normal, as it does in the majority of cases, the patient is asymptomatic. If the rate of the underlying rhythm is slow to begin with and the block decreases it even lower, then low cardiac output symptoms may appear. These include complaints of dizziness and weakness, transient syncopal episodes, chest pressure or pain, slow irregular pulse, and a low blood pressure. Occasionally, a patient complains of being able to feel "skipped beats" when the blocked beat occurs.

TREATMENT

There is no specific treatment for this block since it tends to be asymptomatic, transient, and does not progress to a higher degree block. If the cause of the block has been traced to cardiac medications, these medications must be reduced or eliminated from the patient's treatment regimen. In the few cases where the rate is very slow and the patient is symptomatic, atropine sulfate, as a short-term treatment, can be given intravenously to increase the overall rate. Sympathetic stimulating medications, such as isoproterenol or dopamine, may be used to maintain an adequate rate until the rate returns to normal on its own. As a last and drastic measure, a permanent demand pacemaker may be inserted (Fig. 8-4).

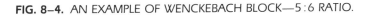

FIG. 8–4. AN EXAMPLE OF WENCKEBACH BLOCK—5 : 6 RATIO.

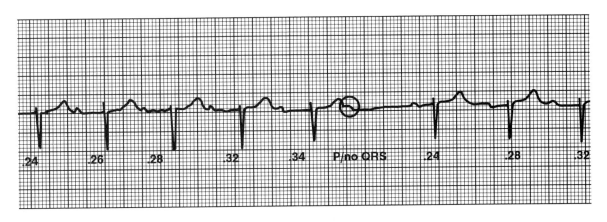

CRITERIA FOR AV WENCKEBACH

Rhythm: Regular—P to P intervals; irregular—R to R intervals that become shorter before the pause. Overall, the pattern appears irregular.

Rate: Atrial rate: 60–100 beats/min (may be faster or slower).
Ventricular Rate: Slower than the atrial rate. It will partially depend on the atrial rate and partially depend on the ratio of P waves to QRS complexes. (A 3 : 1 ratio will be slower than a 5 : 4 ratio, given the same atrial rates.)

Atrial Conduction: P waves should be normal, same shape with a regular P to P interval across the whole strip.

AV Conduction: PR interval becomes progressively longer until there is a P wave without a QRS complex after it. After the dropped beat, the gradually lengthening PR interval pattern repeats itself.

Ventricular Conduction: QRS complexes 0.06–0.10 second; same shape across the whole strip.

CLASSIC SECOND DEGREE AV BLOCK

Classic second degree AV block is also called Mobitz type II second degree AV block, second degree AV block Mobitz, Mobitz II, type II second degree AV block (Fig. 8-5).
   Although less common, classic second degree AV block tends to be a more serious type of block than AV Wenckebach because it progresses to a higher degree block more frequently. The bundle of His or the bundle branches are commonly affected and produce conduction abnormalities in the classic second degree AV block. The further down the conduction difficulty is in the conduction system, the more likely a prolonged QRS complex will develop.
   The pattern produced with this type of block is quite different from the pattern produced by AV Wenckebach. In classic second degree AV block, the AV node

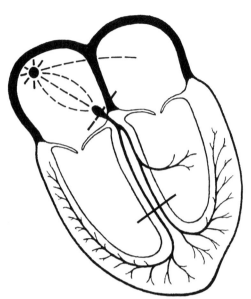

FIG. 8–5. CLASSIC SECOND DEGREE AV BLOCK IS RECOGNIZED BY THE PATTERN OF BLOCKED IMPULSES FROM THE SINUS NODE. WHEN IMPULSES ARE CONDUCTED, THE TIME IT TAKES THEM TO GET THROUGH THE BLOCKED AREA IN THE AV CONDUCTION SYSTEM IS THE SAME; THEREFORE, THE PR INTERVALS ARE THE SAME ON ALL CONDUCTED BEATS. IF THE BLOCK IS IN THE BUNDLE BRANCH REGION, THE QRS COMPLEXES ARE PROLONGED.

either blocks impulses or conducts impulses, but it does not slow them down. The impulses that are conducted are all conducted at the same velocity through the AV node so that the PR interval remains consistent in the conducted beats. First and second degree AV block can coexist in the same patient at the same time. In the classic second degree AV block, the PR interval may be normal (0.12–0.20 second) or it may be combined with a first degree AV block and be longer than normal. (Rather than naming this abnormality a second degree AV block with a first degree AV block, it is better to name it a second degree AV block with a long PR interval.) In either case, the PR interval will remain the same across the whole strip where P waves precede the QRS complexes.

Because some of the impulses from the SA node are not conducted to the ventricles after the atria are depolarized, the ECG strip shows a P wave without QRS complex after it. There will be two or more P waves for each QRS complex. As observed in Chapter 5, particularly with atrial flutter, when there are more P waves than QRS complexes, the rhythm and rate of the atria and the ventricles must be considered separately. Because the SA node is a very regular pacemaker, the P waves produced in a classic second degree AV block commonly have a regular P to P interval and often a normal rate (60–100 per minute). Sinus dysrhythmia can occur in this type of block, producing irregular P to P intervals and making the blocks identification more difficult. The depolarization of the ventricles is dependent upon the impulses passing through the AV node. In classic second degree AV block, some or many of the SA node impulses are blocked, with the result that the ventricular rate is slower than the atrial rate. The regularity of the ventricles depends upon the pattern of impulses that the AV node allows to be conducted through to the ventricles. If it is a fixed or unchanging pattern of conduction, for example, every other beat is allowed to pass through (2:1 ratio), then the ventricular rhythm will be regular. If the pattern of AV conduction is variable or changing, then the ventricular rhythm is irregular.

CAUSES

The same factors that cause first degree AV block or AV Wenckebach can also cause classic second degree AV block. It is more often associated with acute cardiac disease such as anterior MI or inflammatory heart disease but can also be produced by toxic blood levels of digoxin, diltiazem, or propranolol.

SYMPTOMS

Depending on the ventricular rate, the common low cardiac output symptoms may occur and range from the very mild, such as activity intolerance and lethargy, to the most severe, such as syncope and respiratory arrest. Although a small group of patients with this dysrhythmia remain asymptomatic, most will experience some level of discomfort.

TREATMENT

Classic second degree AV block is generally considered dangerous and is treated aggressively even in patients with few or no symptoms. If the cause is cardiac medications, then these must be stopped. The major danger with this dysrhythmia, particularly in patients who have suffered a recent MI, is that it often progresses to a third degree heart block. If nothing else, even asymptomatic patients demand close monitoring until the block has resolved itself or is treated with a pacemaker.

The usual methods to treat a slow heart rate can be used to treat patients with slow ventricular rates as a result of classic second degree AV block. Atropine sulfate IV will increase the rate of the SA node and indirectly increase the rate of the ventricles. For example, if Mr. X's atrial rate is 90 beats/min with a block ratio of 2:1, the ventricular rate will be 45 beats/min—hardly enough to maintain adequate tissue perfusion. Giving Mr. X atropine sulfate increases his atrial rate to 100 beats/min and will result in an increase of the ventricular rate to 50 beats/min with the same 2:1 ratio. Atropine sulfate also acts as a positive dromotropic medication and actually increases the speed at which impulses pass through the conduction system. This effect sometimes "opens up" the block in the AV node and allows more impulses to be conducted to the ventricles (i.e., it will reduce the conduction ratio). If the atropine does not help increase the ventricular rate, then medications that directly stimulate the ventricles can be used. These include the sympathetic stimulating medications listed above, as well as medications such as norepinephrine, epinephrine, and dobutamine.

A temporary pacemaker is indicated if the classic second degree AV block has developed post MI and is producing symptoms. If the block does not go away by itself in 72–96 hours after developing, then a permanent demand pacemaker can be implanted (Fig. 8-6).

FIG. 8–6. AN EXAMPLE OF CLASSIC SECOND DEGREE AV BLOCK—2:1 RATIO, LONG PRI.

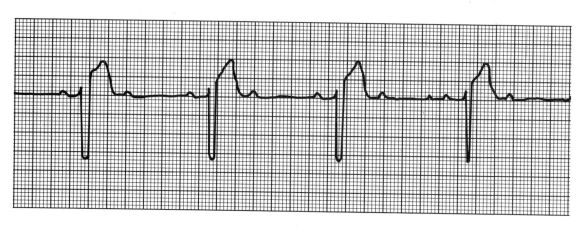

CRITERIA FOR CLASSIC SECOND DEGREE AV BLOCK

Rhythm: Regular P to P intervals. R to R intervals may be regular if the conduction ratio is fixed or irregular if the conduction ratio is variable.

Rate: Atrial rate usually normal 60–100 beats/min but may be faster or slower depending on the SA node. Ventricular rate will be slower than the atrial rate. Its exact rate depends on the conduction ratio of the AV node.

Atrial Conduction: P waves normal, more P waves than QRS complexes.

AV Conduction: PR interval where conducted can be normal (0.12–0.20 second) or may be longer than normal. In all conducted beats, the PR interval will be the *same*.

Ventricular Conduction: QRS 0.06–0.12 second if the block is higher in the AV conduction system. QRS complex may be greater than 0.12 second if the conduction defect is in the bundle branches; same shape where present.

THIRD DEGREE AV BLOCK

Third degree AV block is also called complete heart block, CHB, complete AV block, high degree AV block, high grade block, advanced block, type I & type II, AV dissociation, AVD (Fig. 8-7).

From the multiple names for this dysrhythmia, it is evident that there is disagreement by experts in cardiac dysrhythmias about what exactly comprises this dysrhythmia. While the different names are used to identify more or less the same dysrhythmia, they are not totally synonymous. Third degree AV block is the oldest name used for an abnormal condition that exists in the conduction system of the heart when no impulses from the SA node and atrial conduction system are conducted through the AV node to the ventricles. This name is also consistent with the other "degree" classifications of AV blocks. The AV node completely blocks all impulses from the SA node on their way to the ventricles. Complete heart block is a good description of this condition.

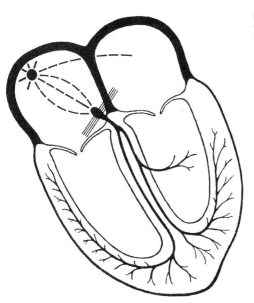

FIG. 8–7. IN THIRD DEGREE AV BLOCK, THE AV NODE BLOCKS *ALL* THE IMPULSES THAT COME FROM THE SA NODE. WITHOUT A BACKUP PACEMAKER SITE BELOW THE BLOCK, NO VENTRICULAR ACTIVITY WILL TAKE PLACE.

Atrioventricular dissociation is a general category into which third degree AV block falls. Atrioventricular dissociation exists when there are two pacemaker sites in the heart (one for the atria and one for the ventricles) that are discharging impulses at the same time independently of each other. The heart is functioning as two completely separate halves that have nothing to do with each other. Atrioventricular dissociation, as a general category, is not limited to third degree AV block. Other examples of AV dissociation include PVCs, ventricular tachycardia, atrial fibrillation with block, and certain types of junctional rhythms. To further complicate the issue, AV dissociation may be described as a temporary or transient condition. Third degree AV block may be transient and temporary or it may be a permanent conduction defect of the AV node. There is also a question about whether AV dissociation exists if the ventricular rate is the same or faster than the atrial rate. Given these various questions concerning the term or concept of AV dissociation, it would probably be best to avoid using it as a descriptor for the dysrhythmia called third degree AV block.

The terms *high degree AV block, high grade AV block,* or *advanced AV block* are used in the newer classification system of AV blocks. Some third degree blocks are included in these categories and others are not. The key element in determining a high grade AV block is the presence of multiple, nonconducted, consecutive P waves during which there is a long interval with no ventricular contractions. When a ventricular contraction does occur, it may be due to a conducted impulse from the SA node or from an escape beat. The main differentiating feature of high degree AV block from third degree AV block is that in high degree AV block some of the impulses from the AV node are conducted to the ventricles. While it is possible to have multiple, nonconducted, consecutive P waves with long pauses between ventricular complexes in third degree AV block, *none* of the atrial impulses are conducted through the AV node. To further complicate the usage of the term *high degree AV block,* dysrhythmias such as atrial flutter or atrial fibrillation with a very slow ventricular rate may also be considered a high degree AV block, even though the AV node is functioning as it should. In the newer system of classification, the atrial rate is critical in diagnosing advanced or high grade blocks.

In this text, the terms *third degree AV block* or *complete heart block* will be used exclusively when describing AV blocks in which no impulses from the SA node are conducted through the AV conduction system. If none of the impulses are being conducted through the AV node to the ventricles, then a backup pacemaker site is needed to produce ventricular contractions. The two most common sites for a backup pacemaker for the ventricles are the AV junction and the Purkinje system of the ventricles (often called a ventricular site).

There are two factors that help distinguish these backup pacemaker sites from each other. First, the duration of the QRS complex is the most accurate way to distinguish between a junctional site and a ventricular site. With a junctional pacemaker, the impulses follow the normal conduction system through the ventricles and the QRS will be a normal 0.06–0.11 second in duration (Fig. 8-8). When the backup pacemaker site is in the ventricles, the impulse which depolarizes the ventricles does not follow the normal conduction pathways so that the QRS complex produced is wider than 0.12 second (Fig. 8-9).

The second factor to consider in distinguishing between a junctional and a ventricular pacemaker site is the rate of the ventricular rhythm. The inherent rate of the AV junction is 40–60 beats/min. Ventricular pacemaker sites initiate impulses at the rate of 20–40 beats/min. This second method is less accurate in distinguishing the origin of the backup pacemaker because of the fact that there is the possibility for accelerated junctional or ventricular rhythms or even for the possibility of a junctional rhythm slowing below a rate of 40 beats/min. It is important to identify the backup pacemaker site (or escape rhythm) in a third

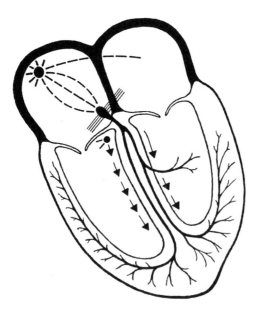

FIG. 8–8. A JUNCTIONAL BACKUP PACE-MAKER SITE IS THE MOST COMMON ONE. SINCE THE IMPULSES ARE FOLLOWING THE NORMAL CONDUCTION PATHWAYS THROUGH THE VENTRICLES, THE QRS COMPLEXES ARE NORMAL. INHERENT RATE OF THE AV JUNCTION IS 40–60 BEATS/MIN BUT THIS MAY VARY.

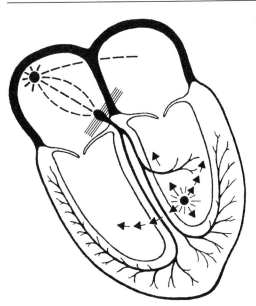

FIG. 8–9. A VENTRICULAR BACKUP PACE-MAKER SITE IN A THIRD DEGREE AV BLOCK PRODUCES QRS COMPLEXES THAT ARE WIDER THAN NORMAL. IMPULSES THAT ORIGINATE IN THE VENTRICLES DO NOT FOLLOW THE NORMAL PATHWAYS AND DEPOLARIZE THE VENTRICLES IN AN UNUSUAL MANNER. INHERENT RATE OF A VENTRICULAR PACEMAKER SITE IS 20–40 BEATS/MIN BUT MAY BE FASTER.

degree AV block because the urgency and type of treatment will vary somewhat. If the AV junction is the pacemaker site, the rate will usually be faster and if it should fail, the ventricles could take over pacemaker function. If the pacemaker site is the ventricles, the rate will most likely be slower and if it should fail, there are no backup pacemaker sites left.

Analysis of the PR interval in third degree AV block is important in distinguishing it from other degrees of AV blocks. The PR interval in third degree AV block will be variable *without* any repeating pattern (as seen in AV Wenckebach). Because the P waves are being produced randomly in relation to the QRS complexes, occasionally a PR interval appears to be "normal." This pattern is called an incidental or coincidental PR interval and does *not* indicate a conducted beat. Keep in mind that different degrees of AV block can occur in the same patient at the same time. A patient may have a transient third degree AV block that alternates with a second degree AV block.

Because the SA node is such a regular pacemaker, the P to P intervals are usually regular and at the normal SA node rate of 60–100 per minute. There are also more P waves than QRS complexes, although in certain patterns where the rate of the backup pacemaker is near to that of the SA node, there may be almost as many P waves as QRS complexes. The R to R intervals are also regular but may be slightly irregular due to the slower rate. The major reason why third degree AV block is considered to be a serious dysrhythmia is because the backup pacemaker sites of the AV junction and ventricles are unreliable in comparison to the SA node. Unreliable means that these backup pacemaker sites have a tendency to just stop all impulse production, leaving the patient in a state of ventricular asystole. When the ventricles do not contract, no circulation takes place and brain death will occur in 4–6 minutes unless cardiopulmonary resuscitation is started or the heart is made to function.

CAUSES

While all those factors that have the potential to produce first or second degree AV block can also produce third degree AV block, third degree AV block indicates a high degree of damage to the AV conduction system. This damage is usually caused by MI or long-term degenerative heart disease such as congestive heart failure or coronary heart disease. It can also develop as a result of extreme digoxin toxicity or toxic blood levels of the beta blockers or calcium-channel blockers. Certain types of cardiac surgical procedures, such as valve replacements, may also damage the AV node sufficiently to produce a third degree heart block.

SIGNS AND SYMPTOMS

Some patients who have third degree AV block with a ventricular rate high enough to produce adequate cardiac output may have no symptoms while at rest. They usually cannot tolerate any type of activity increase. Most patients will experience some degree of the decreased cardiac output symptoms, including weakness, dizziness, syncope, chest pressure or pain, and shortness of breath. The pulse will be slow and the blood pressure low.

A condition called Stokes-Adams syndrome or Stokes-Adams attacks can be caused by transient third degree AV blocks. The Stokes-Adams attacks consist of transient fainting spells that are marked by low blood pressure, slow regular pulses, and Cheyne-Stokes respirations. The difficulty in diagnosing these attacks lies in their transient nature. By the time the patient is brought to the hospital and placed on a cardiac monitor, he or she is no longer in the third degree AV block. Unless the block occurs during the course of the hospitalization, it will not be identified as the cause of the syncopal episode.

TREATMENT

In general, third degree AV block is considered a cardiac emergency and is treated aggressively. The exception to this treatment is if the patient is tolerating the dysrhythmia and if the escape pattern is junctional with an adequate rate and if it is transitory after an acute MI. In these cases, close monitoring with emergency medications close at hand may be sufficient.

The first-line treatment for slow rhythms of IV atropine sulfate is usually attempted in third degree heart block. It may or may not help because the primary effect atropine exerts is to increase the rate of the SA node. In a third degree AV block where none of the impulses are being conducted to the ventricles, increasing the atrial rate often only produces more P waves on the strip. Atropine sometimes increases the conduction through the AV node and helps eliminate the block or at least decrease its degree.

A temporary pacemaker may be inserted if the physician determines that the block is transient or temporary. Otherwise, a permanent pacemaker is inserted to maintain an adequate rate.

Isoproterenol administered in an IV drip is the third choice of treatment for patients with third degree AV blocks. If not actually administered, it is kept at the bedside ready to be started (on standby) should the rhythm become slower. Because of its suppressing effect on ventricular pacemaker sites, in all cases of third degree AV block, lidocaine should *never* be used (Figs. 8-10 and 8-11).

FIG. 8–10. AN EXAMPLE OF ST WITH THIRD DEGREE AV BLOCK WITH A JUNCTIONAL BACKUP PACEMAKER SITE.

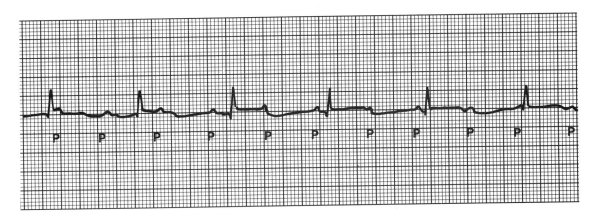

FIG. 8–11. AN EXAMPLE OF SB WITH THIRD DEGREE AV BLOCK WITH A VENTRICULAR BACKUP PACEMAKER SITE.

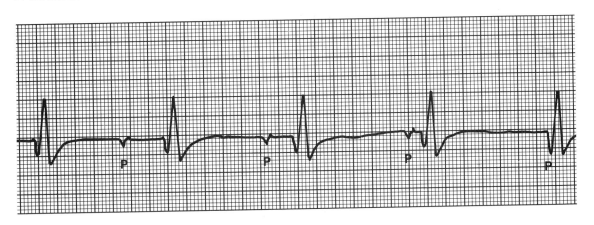

CRITERIA FOR THIRD DEGREE AV BLOCK

Rhythm: Regular P to P intervals; irregular R to R intervals.

Rate: Atrial 60–100 beats/min (may be faster or slower). Ventricular: Junctional site—40–60 beats/min (may be faster or slower). Ventricular site: 20–40 beats/min (may be faster).

Atrial Conduction: P waves normal, more P waves than QRS complexes.

AV Conduction: PR intervals vary, all different, no pattern. Incidental PR intervals may appear normal.

Ventricular Conduction: QRS complexes: Junctional site: 0.06–0.10 second. Ventricular site: greater than 0.12 second.

PRACTICE ECG STRIPS FOR CHAPTER 8

Directions. On the following practice ECG strips, analyze each strip according to its rhythm, rate, atrial conduction, AV conduction, and ventricular conduction. Arrive at an interpretation of the strip based upon the analysis and criteria for the dysrhythmias due to conduction abnormalities in the AV node as learned in this chapter. (See Appendix II for interpretations.)

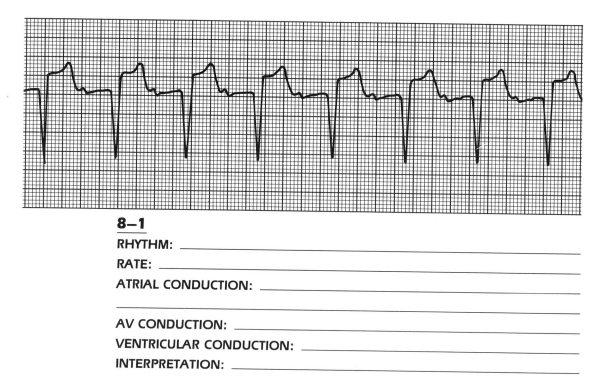

8–1

RHYTHM: _____

RATE: _____

ATRIAL CONDUCTION: _____
_____

AV CONDUCTION: _____

VENTRICULAR CONDUCTION: _____

INTERPRETATION: _____

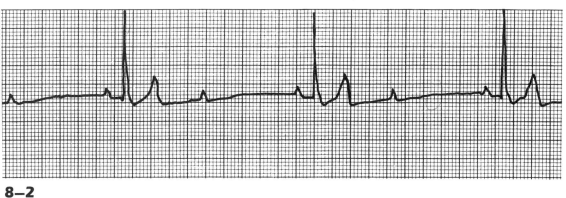

8–2

RHYTHM: _____

RATE: _____

ATRIAL CONDUCTION: _____

_____

AV CONDUCTION: _____

VENTRICULAR CONDUCTION: _____

INTERPRETATION: _____

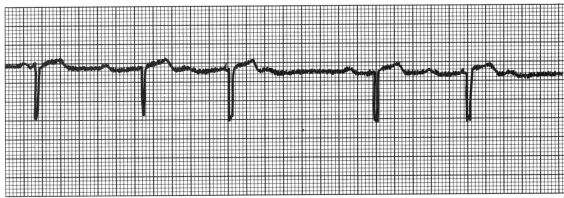

8–3

RHYTHM: _____

RATE: _____

ATRIAL CONDUCTION: _____

_____

AV CONDUCTION: _____

VENTRICULAR CONDUCTION: _____

INTERPRETATION: _____

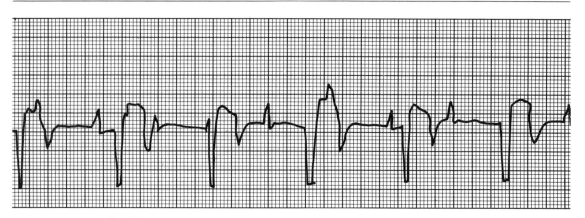

8–4

RHYTHM: _____

RATE: _____

ATRIAL CONDUCTION: _____

_____

AV CONDUCTION: _____

VENTRICULAR CONDUCTION: _____

INTERPRETATION: _____

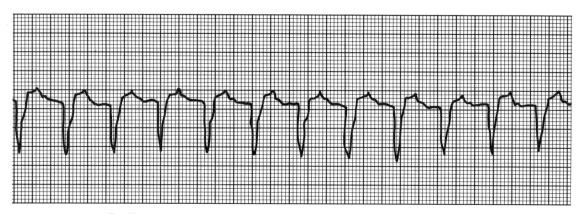

8–5

RHYTHM: _____

RATE: _____

ATRIAL CONDUCTION: _____

_____

AV CONDUCTION: _____

VENTRICULAR CONDUCTION: _____

INTERPRETATION: _____

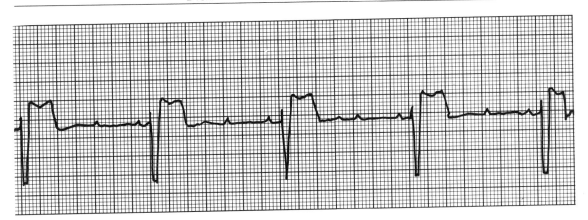

8–6

RHYTHM: _____

RATE: _____

ATRIAL CONDUCTION: _____

_____

AV CONDUCTION: _____

VENTRICULAR CONDUCTION: _____

INTERPRETATION: _____

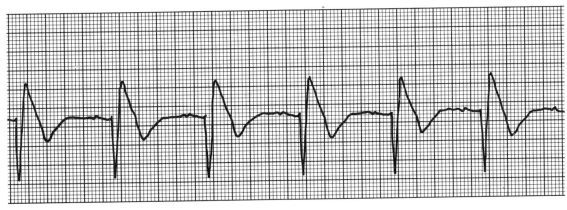

8–7

RHYTHM: _____

RATE: _____

ATRIAL CONDUCTION: _____

_____

AV CONDUCTION: _____

VENTRICULAR CONDUCTION: _____

INTERPRETATION: _____

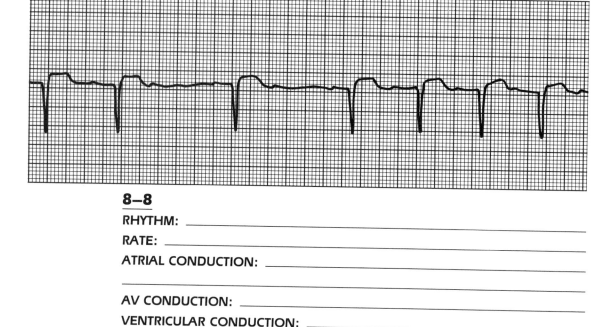

8–8

RHYTHM: _____

RATE: _____

ATRIAL CONDUCTION: _____

_____

AV CONDUCTION: _____

VENTRICULAR CONDUCTION: _____

INTERPRETATION: _____

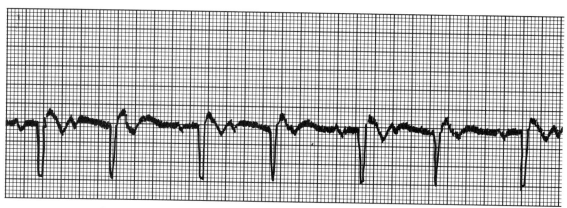

8–9

RHYTHM: _____

RATE: _____

ATRIAL CONDUCTION: _____

_____

AV CONDUCTION: _____

VENTRICULAR CONDUCTION: _____

INTERPRETATION: _____

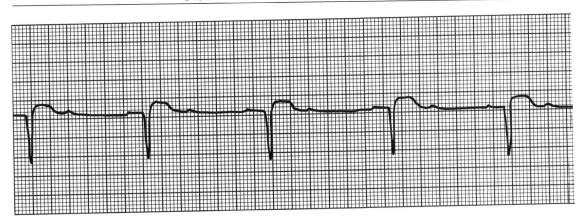

8–10

RHYTHM: _____

RATE: _____

ATRIAL CONDUCTION: _____

_____

AV CONDUCTION: _____

VENTRICULAR CONDUCTION: _____

INTERPRETATION: _____

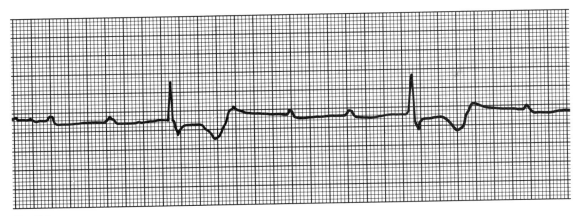

8–11

RHYTHM: _____

RATE: _____

ATRIAL CONDUCTION: _____

_____

AV CONDUCTION: _____

VENTRICULAR CONDUCTION: _____

INTERPRETATION: _____

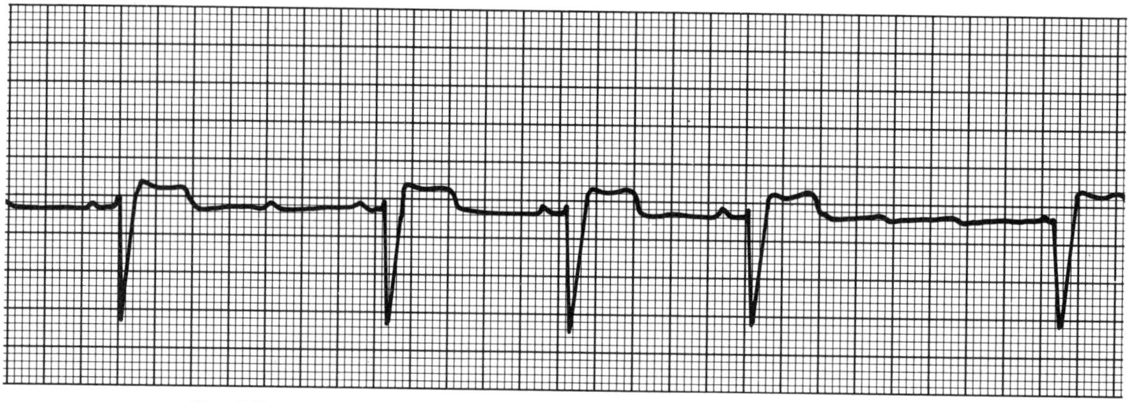

8–12

RHYTHM: _____

RATE: _____

ATRIAL CONDUCTION: _____

_____

AV CONDUCTION: _____

VENTRICULAR CONDUCTION: _____

INTERPRETATION: _____

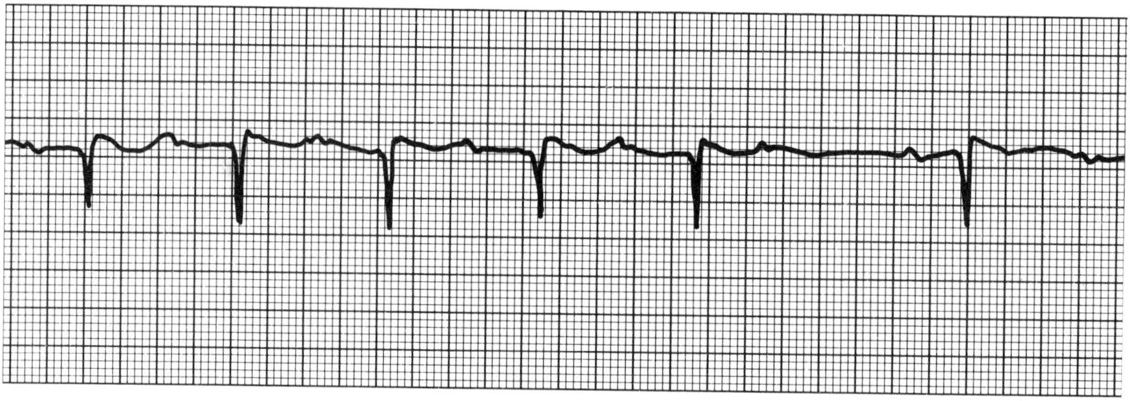

8–13

RHYTHM: _____

RATE: _____

ATRIAL CONDUCTION: _____

_____

AV CONDUCTION: _____

VENTRICULAR CONDUCTION: _____

INTERPRETATION: _____

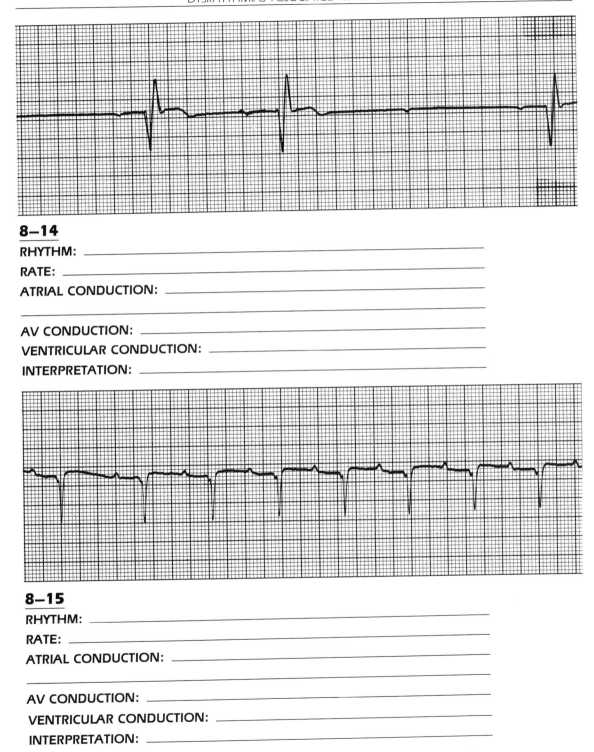

8–14

RHYTHM: _____

RATE: _____

ATRIAL CONDUCTION: _____

AV CONDUCTION: _____

VENTRICULAR CONDUCTION: _____

INTERPRETATION: _____

8–15

RHYTHM: _____

RATE: _____

ATRIAL CONDUCTION: _____

AV CONDUCTION: _____

VENTRICULAR CONDUCTION: _____

INTERPRETATION: _____

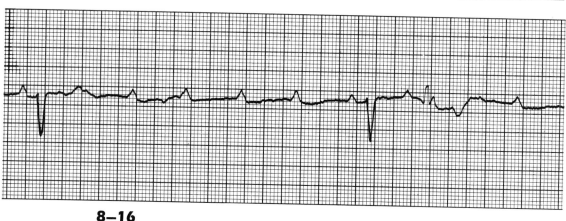

8–16

RHYTHM: _____

RATE: _____

ATRIAL CONDUCTION: _____

_____

AV CONDUCTION: _____

VENTRICULAR CONDUCTION: _____

INTERPRETATION: _____

9

SUPRAVENTRICULAR TACHYCARDIA DYSRHYTHMIAS

LEARNING OBJECTIVES

After studying this section, the learner will be able to:

1. Describe the mechanisms that produce supraventricular tachycardia.
2. List the various tachy dysrhythmias that can fall into the category of supraventricular tachycardia.
3. Identify the key features of supraventricular tachycardia.
4. Name the elements that comprise tachy-brady syndrome.
5. List appropriate interventions for supraventricular tachycardia and tachy-brady syndrome.
6. Analyze and correctly identify supraventricular tachycardia and tachy-brady syndrome from the criteria learned in this chapter.

SUPRAVENTRICULAR TACHYCARDIA

Supraventricular tachycardia is also called SVT, paroxysmal supraventricular tachycardia, and PSVT (Fig. 9-1).

Supraventricular tachycardia is not a specific dysrhythmia but a group of dysrhythmias that originate above the ventricles and are usually conducted normally through the conduction system of the ventricles. Supraventricular tachycardia is one of the ''catch-all'' categories that is used when the rhythm under analysis is not clearly identifiable based on the usual criteria for specific dysrhythmias. The main difficulty in analysis of these dysrhythmias is identification of the P waves. When rhythms that are sinus, atrial, or junctional in origin become very rapid (usually 150 beats/min or more), the P waves tend to become hidden in the T wave or even the QRS complex of the preceding beat. This loss

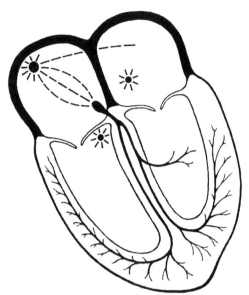

FIG. 9–1. MULTIPLE IRRITABLE SITES IN THE ATRIA, INCLUDING THE SA NODE AND THE AV JUNCTION, CAN PRODUCE THE RAPID TACHYCARDIA WITH UNIDENTIFIABLE P WAVE THAT MARK SUPRAVENTRICULAR TACHYCARDIA. THE IMPULSES FOLLOW THE NORMAL CONDUCTION PATHWAYS THROUGH THE VENTRICLES SO THE QRS COMPLEXES ARE NORMAL.

of the visible P waves makes determination of the origin of the dysrhythmia very difficult if not impossible.

Because the impulses usually follow the normal conduction pathways through the ventricles, the QRS complexes are normal in duration and shape. The PR interval is not always measurable because of the lack of distinct P waves.

Some of the tachycardias that can be included in the determination of SVT are the following:

1. Sinus tachycardia: usual ventricular rate 100–160 beats/min.
2. Atrial tachycardia: usual ventricular rate 150–250 beats/min.
3. Junctional tachycardia: usual ventricular rate 100–250 beats/min.
4. Uncontrolled atrial fibrillation: usual ventricular rate 150–200 beats/min.
5. Atrial flutter with a 2:1 conduction: usual ventricular rate 150 beats/min.

Supraventricular tachycardia may occur in relatively short episodes that begin and end suddenly, or it may be a sustained rhythm that lasts for several hours or even days. It may be possible to determine the origin of an SVT if the first beat of the run of rapid beats can be seen and identified. For example, if the first beat is a premature atrial contraction, then the rhythm that follows is most likely atrial tachycardia, even though the P waves cannot be identified.

Supraventricular tachycardia tends to be a very regular rhythm. These regular rhythms also include atrial fibrillation, which is usually identified by its irregularity. At very rapid rates, atrial fibrillation may be regular. The one element that may interrupt the regularity of SVT is the presence of other ectopic beats in the dysrhythmia. While it is not very common, it is possible to have premature atrial contraction (PAC) mixed in with a run of junctional tachycardia.

CAUSES

Since this category of dysrhythmia includes several rapid dysrhythmias, there is no single, unique cause for it. In general, any of those factors discussed above that cause sinus tachycardia, atrial tachycardia, atrial fibrillation, atrial flutter, or junctional tachycardia can produce SVT. The factors most frequently associated with SVT include fear and anxiety, intake of caffeine, tobacco and alcohol, use of central nervous system stimulants such as cocaine and amphetamines, medications such as theophylline or even thyroid preparations, or toxic levels of cardiac medications, particularly digoxin. Supraventricular tachycardia may be a complication of MI or other severe cardiac disease states.

SYMPTOMS

Most patients will experience some signs and symptoms with SVT because of the lowered cardiac output that the rapid rates produce. The signs and symptoms may range from mild, such as feeling palpitations or fluttering in the chest, to more severe, such as dizziness, weakness, shortness of breath, chest pain or pressure, and low blood pressure. At extremely fast rates, the patient may become unconscious, cyanotic, and diaphoretic. The main element to monitor these patients for is a change to ventricular tachycardia.

TREATMENT

Treatment of SVT is difficult because it may be one of several dysrhythmias that have different treatments. Unless the origin of the dysrhythmia has been identified (in which case it would no longer be called SVT), a generic treatment approach must be used. This approach includes the use of vagal stimulation techniques, cardiac suppressant medications (negative chronotropic), particularly IV digoxin and IV verapamil, central nervous system depressants, and sedation. If a specific cause for the rapid rhythm has been determined, then removal of that cause would be essential. As a last resort, electrical cardioversion can be used to stop the tachycardia and convert it to a sinus rhythm (Fig. 9-2).

FIG. 9–2. AN EXAMPLE OF SUPRAVENTRICULAR TACHYCARDIA.

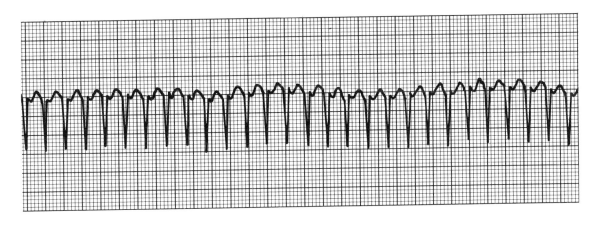

CRITERIA FOR SUPRAVENTRICULAR TACHYCARDIA

Rhythm: Regular to slightly irregular.

Rate: 150 beats/min or faster. (In rates under 150 beats/min, the P waves are usually identifiable.)

Atrial Conduction: P waves are not always visible and are most likely hidden in the T wave or QRS complex of the preceding beat.

AV Conduction: PR interval cannot always be measured.

Ventricular Conduction: QRS 0.06–0.10 second; uniform shape.

TACHY-BRADY SYNDROME

Tachy-brady syndrome is also called tachycardia-bradycardia syndrome, TBS, Brady-Tachy syndrome, BTS, sick sinus syndrome, SSS, sluggish sinus node syndrome, sinoatrial syncope (Fig. 9-3).

Tachy-brady syndrome is a dysrhythmia in which there are episodes of SVT that alternate with episodes of bradycardia, sinus arrest, or sinus block. The tachycardia can be from several supraventricular origins including sinus tachycardia, atrial tachycardia, atrial fibrillation or flutter, or even junctional tachycardia. When the tachycardia component of the dysrhythmia terminates, it is sometimes followed by a long (4 or more seconds) pause. The bradycardia component of this dysrhythmia may be a sinus bradycardia, a junctional escape rhythm, or some other supraventricular rhythm that is interspersed with short episodes of asystole (pauses) usually caused by sinus block or sinus arrest.

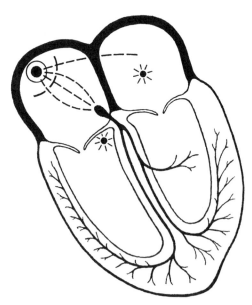

FIG. 9–3. TACHY-BRADY SYNDROME IS A COMBINATION OF DYSRHYTHMIAS THAT INVOLVE MULTIPLE AREAS OF THE HEART AND ITS CONDUCTION SYSTEM. TACHYCARDIA CAN ORIGINATE FROM ANY SUPRAVENTRICULAR AREA. BRADYCARDIA IS PRODUCED BY A DAMAGED SA NODE OR ATRIAL CONDUCTION SYSTEM. THE IMPULSES THAT ARE PRODUCED FOLLOW THE NORMAL CONDUCTION SYSTEM THROUGH THE VENTRICLES.

Sick sinus syndrome is a special type of tachy-brady syndrome that exists only when episodes of sinus tachycardia alternate with episodes of sinus bradycardia. The term *sick sinus syndrome* is often used inaccurately to name a variety of dysrhythmias that would be more accurately named *tachy-brady syndrome* because the tachycardia is often not identifiable as a sinus tachycardia. Sick sinus syndrome is also used in referring to dysrhythmias that would be more accurately described as irregular, slow wandering pacemakers, sinus bradycardia with episodes of sinus arrest, or sinus block because they do not have any component that can be called a tachycardia (rate above 100 beats/min).

In either case, this dysrhythmia indicates significant damage to the normal pacemaker system of the heart. The tendency of tachy-brady syndrome to eventually proceed to asystole or other serious dysrhythmias is well documented and individuals who have been identified with this dysrhythmia receive rather aggressive treatment.

CAUSES

Most commonly, this dysrhythmia is found in patients who have suffered a recent myocardial infarction (MI). As many as 5% of individuals who have inferior MIs develop tachy-brady syndrome. It can also be caused by rheumatic heart disease, severe, prolonged hypertension, and by congenital cardiac defects such as atrial septal defects that affect the SA node and atrial conduction system of the heart. Less commonly, tachy-brady syndrome can be caused by toxic levels of cardiac medications, especially digoxin.

SYMPTOMS

While the same symptoms may develop from either the tachycardia component or the bradycardia component of this dysrhythmia, it is usually the long pauses and slow rates that decrease the cardiac output most. Weakness, dizziness, and transient syncope are the most common symptoms of this dysrhythmia. Low blood pressure and slow, irregular pulses also mark the bradycardia component of this dysrhythmia.

TREATMENT

This dysrhythmia is difficult to treat because of the conflicting nature of the components. The usual treatments to slow a fast rate, such a digoxin, verapamil, or other cardiac depressants, tend to make the bradycardia even slower when it occurs. Medications commonly used to increase the rate in bradycardia make the tachycardia component even faster. A common and effective treatment for tachy-brady syndrome is to give the patient cardiac depressant medications to control the SVT and to implant a permanent artificial demand pacemaker to insure a minimum cardiac rate and adequate cardiac output (Fig. 9-4).

CRITERIA FOR TACHY-BRADY SYNDROME

Rhythm: Irregular overall, but while the rhythm is in a prolonged run of either tachycardia or bradycardia, it may appear regular.

FIG. 9–4. AN EXAMPLE OF TACHY-BRADY SYNDROME.

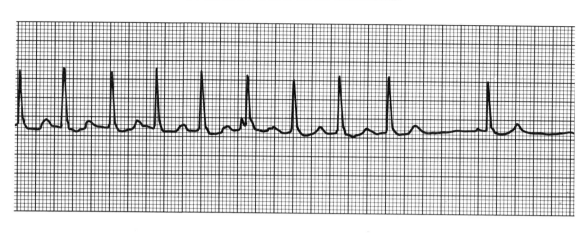

Rate: 20–59 beats/min in the bradycardia phase; 100–250 beats/min while in the tachycardia phase. (The designation sick sinus syndrome is sometimes used even if the rate of the faster rhythm never exceeds the 100 beats/min criteria for tachycardia) (Fig. 9-5).

Atrial Conduction: P waves are visible only in the bradycardia phase of the dysrhythmia. May be normal P waves if the rhythm is sinus bradycardia or the P waves may be abnormal if the slow rhythm is junctional in origin.

AV Conduction: PR interval is present only when the P waves are visible. PR interval may vary from normal to longer than normal.

Ventricular Conduction: QRS 0.06–0.10 second; same shape for both phases of the dysrhythmia.

FIG. 9–5. AN EXAMPLE OF WHAT IS SOMETIMES CALLED SICK SINUS SYNDROME.

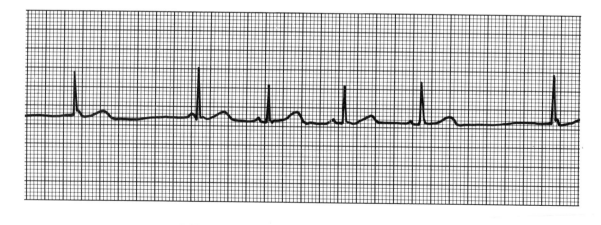

PRACTICE ECG STRIPS FOR CHAPTER 9

Directions. On the following practice ECG strips, analyze each strip according to its rhythm, rate, atrial conduction, AV conduction, and ventricular conduction. Arrive at an interpretation of the strip based upon the analysis and criteria for the dysrhythmia as learned in this chapter. (See Appendix II for interpretations.)

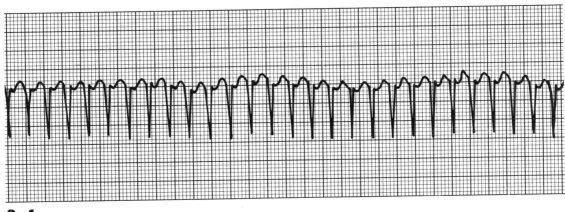

9–1

RHYTHM: _____

RATE: _____

ATRIAL CONDUCTION: _____

_____

AV CONDUCTION: _____

VENTRICULAR CONDUCTION: _____

INTERPRETATION: _____

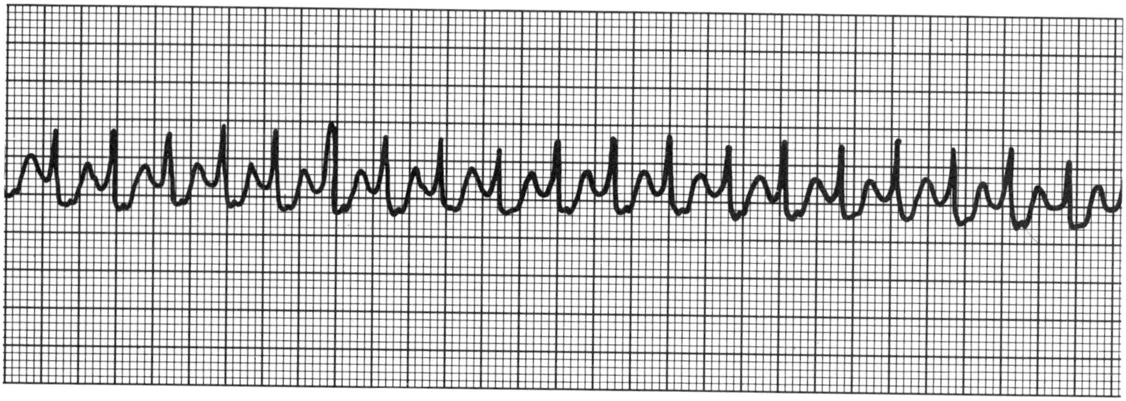

9–2

RHYTHM: _____

RATE: _____

ATRIAL CONDUCTION: _____

_____

AV CONDUCTION: _____

VENTRICULAR CONDUCTION: _____

INTERPRETATION: _____

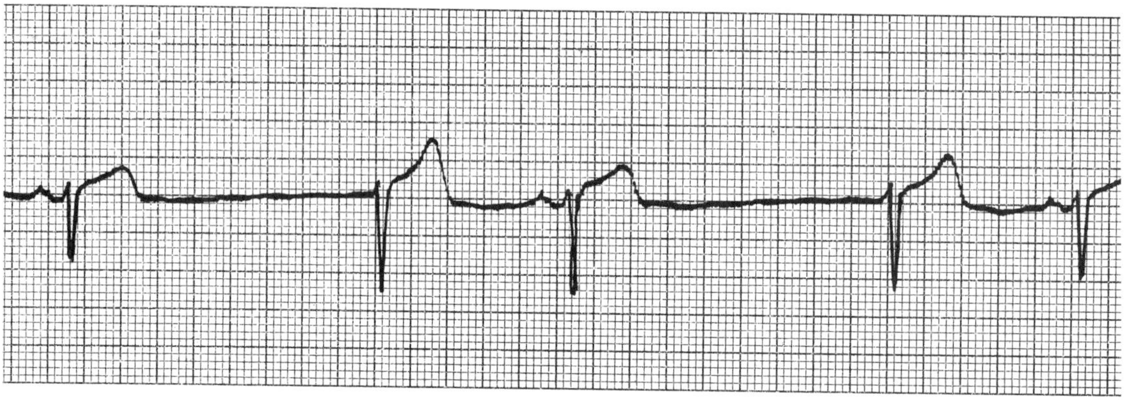

9–3

RHYTHM: _____

RATE: _____

ATRIAL CONDUCTION: _____

_____

AV CONDUCTION: _____

VENTRICULAR CONDUCTION: _____

INTERPRETATION: _____

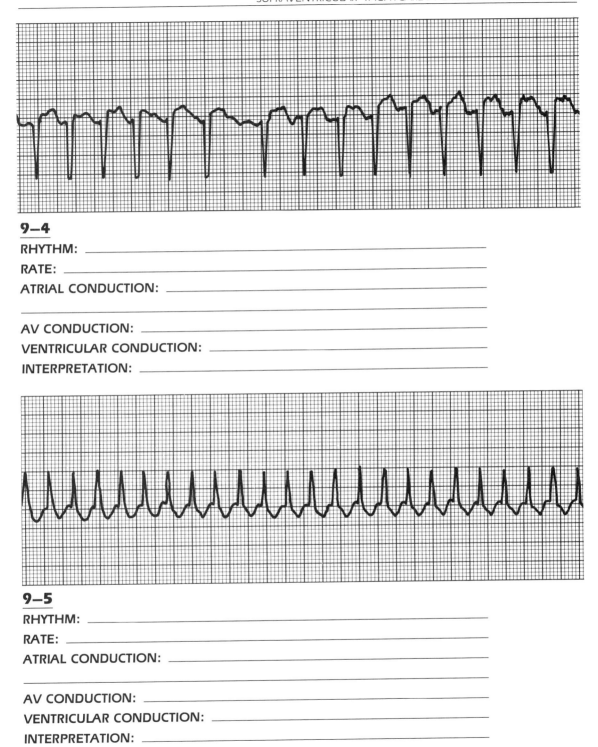

9—4

RHYTHM: _____

RATE: _____

ATRIAL CONDUCTION: _____

_____

AV CONDUCTION: _____

VENTRICULAR CONDUCTION: _____

INTERPRETATION: _____

9—5

RHYTHM: _____

RATE: _____

ATRIAL CONDUCTION: _____

_____

AV CONDUCTION: _____

VENTRICULAR CONDUCTION: _____

INTERPRETATION: _____

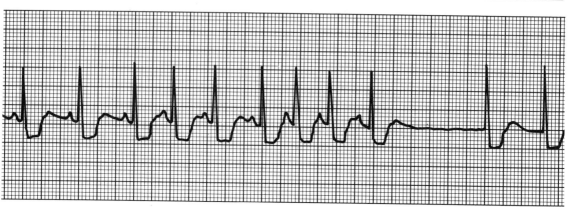

9–6

RHYTHM: _____

RATE: _____

ATRIAL CONDUCTION: _____
_____

AV CONDUCTION: _____

VENTRICULAR CONDUCTION: _____

INTERPRETATION: _____

10

CONDUCTION ABNORMALITIES IN THE BUNDLE BRANCHES

LEARNING OBJECTIVES

After studying this section, the learner will be able to:

1. Identify the mechanisms of conduction defects that produce bundle branch blocks.
2. Distinguish between a right bundle branch block and a left bundle branch block.
3. List the elements fundamental to hemiblocks.
4. Analyze and interpret ECG rhythm strips that contain bundle branch blocks.

Although most basic electrocardiogram (ECG) dysrhythmia interpretation books do not include a presentation of bundle branch blocks, these blocks are very common and frequently observed in the patient population of intensive care units. A bundle branch block is not a dysrhythmia; rather, it is a condition that is imposed on another rhythm. The interpretation must include identification of the underlying rhythms, such as "sinus rhythm with a right bundle branch block." The physiologic mechanisms that produce bundle branch block patterns are similar to the mechanisms that produce other types of conduction blocks, such as the atrioventricular (AV) blocks. The differentiating feature of bundle branch blocks is the potential multiple locations for the block.

A bundle branch block occurs when the conduction through one or more of the branches of the trifascicular conduction system of the ventricles becomes altered or completely blocked. The term *trifascicular* literally means "three parts." The three part bundle branch conduction system of the ventricles is composed of the right bundle branch (RBB), the main stem left bundle branch (LBB), and the two subdivisions of the LBB (posterior branch and anterior branch of the LBB).

In a normal heart beat, the impulse from the sinus node is conducted through the AV node and then down through both bundle branches at the same time so the right and left ventricles depolarize simultaneously. This simultaneous depolarization is also called *synchronized depolarization.*

When one of the bundle branches of the system becomes blocked, the impulse is conducted through the nonblocked branch first. After the ventricle on the nonblocked side depolarizes, the impulse must travel secondary pathways across the intraventricular septum so that the ventricle on the side with the blocked bundle branch can also depolarize. The result of this type of ventricular depolarization is two separate ventricular contractions at different times. This type of depolarization is called *sequential depolarization* or *dyssynchronous depolarization.*

Because the ECG monitoring equipment combines the two separate depolarizations of the right and left ventricles, sequential depolarization of the ventricles produces a QRS complex that is wider than the normal QRS complex (Fig. 10-1). In general, any time an impulse does not follow the normal conduction pathways through the ventricles, a wider than normal QRS complex is produced. The wide QRS complex is the distinguishing feature of the bundle branch block.

A conduction abnormality that produces a pattern similar to the bundle branch block is called aberrant ventricular conduction. Aberrant ventricular conduction occurs when the bundle branches do not repolarize at the same time. Because the RBB is longer and narrower, it normally has a slightly longer refractory period than the LBB; this period usually does not affect the conduction time or prevent the simultaneous depolarization of the ventricles in normal hearts.

In the presence of atrial premature beats, very rapid supraventricular rhythms, or Ashman type patterns, the RBB may not be completely repolarized before the

FIG. 10–1. SEQUENTIAL VENTRICULAR DEPOLARIZATION IN BUNDLE BRANCH BLOCK

Lead MCL₁

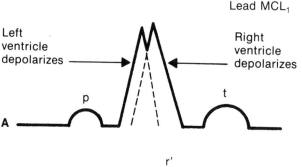

Left ventricle depolarizes ⟶   Right ventricle depolarizes ⟵

In a bundle branch block, the ventricles depolarize one after the other. The ECG monitoring equipment combines the two depolarizations into one QRS complex.

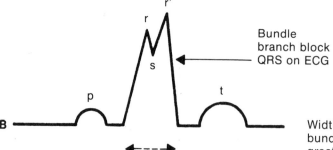

Bundle branch block QRS on ECG

Width of QRS complex in a bundle branch block is greater than 0.12 second.

next impulse arrives. Because the RBB is still in its refractory period when the impulse arrives, its depolarization is delayed, producing a type of sequential depolarization in which the left ventricle depolarizes first, followed by the right ventricle. The result is a wider than normal QRS complex. While involvement of the RBB is most common in aberrant ventricular conduction, longer than normal repolarization may involve the LBB, particularly in the presence of cardiac disease, myocardial infarction (MI), or toxic levels of negative-inotropic cardiac medications. Even though the patterns may appear identical, strictly speaking, this type of abnormal conduction should not be called a bundle branch block because, although late, every impulse is conducted through both bundle branches. Aberrant ventricular conduction with rapid rhythms is one of the most difficult rhythm interpretations nurses must make and is discussed in detail in advanced ECG dysrhythmia interpretation books.

Although both RBB and LBB blocks produce wider than normal QRS complexes in all monitoring leads, leads MCL_1 and MCL_6 are the most useful in distinguishing a RBB from a LBB block. Because of the location of the positive electrode in these two leads, the direction of the electrical currents producing ventricular depolarization is either toward the positive electrode or away from it when a bundle branch block is present (Figs. 10-2 and 10-3). For the purposes of this book, all ECG strips with a bundle branch block pattern will be MCL_1 unless indicated otherwise.

FIG. 10–2. ELECTRICAL PATTERN FLOW IN LBBB.

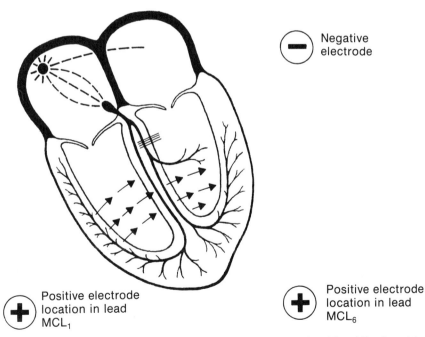

Negative electrode

Positive electrode location in lead MCL_1

Positive electrode location in lead MCL_6

The depolarizing currents in an LBBB flow from the right side of the heart to the left side. This flow will be toward the positive electrode in MCL_6 and away from the positive in MCl_1.

FIG. 10–3. ELECTRICAL PATTERN FLOW IN RBBB.

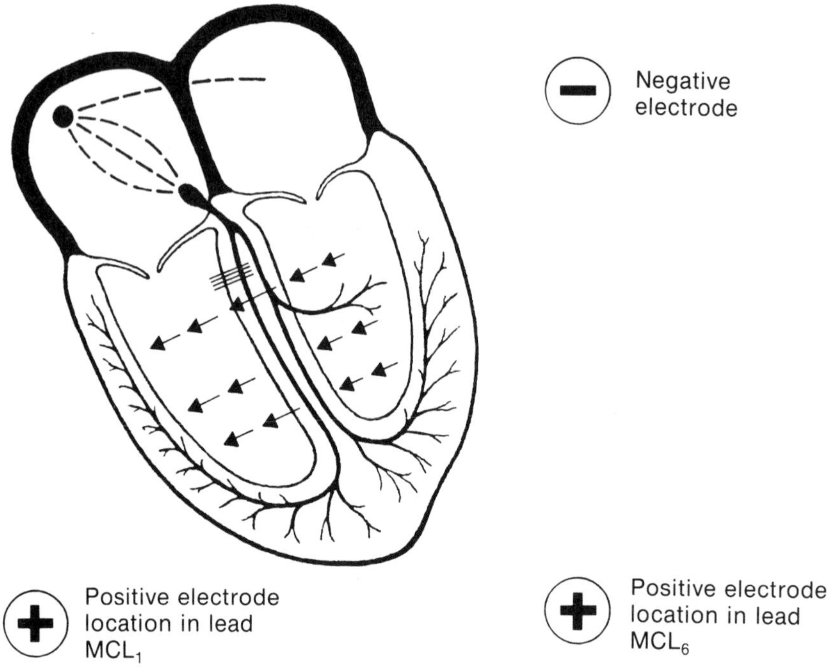

The depolarizing currents in a RBBB flow from the left side of the heart to the right side. This flow will be toward the positive electrode in MCL$_1$ and away from the positive electrode in MCL$_6$.

A bundle branch block may be a temporary or transient conduction abnormality in some individuals. There is a tendency to identify these intermittent abnormal patterns as ventricular extrasystoles. When the underlying rhythm is atrial fibrillation, its inherent irregularity negates some of the basic criteria for ventricular premature beats.

RIGHT BUNDLE BRANCH BLOCK

When the RBB becomes blocked, the depolarizing impulse travels down the LBB first, depolarizes the left ventricle and the intraventricular septum, then crosses over and depolarizes the right ventricle. The movement of the electrical activity that is depolarizing the ventricles in a right bundle branch block (RBBB) is toward the positive electrode in the MCL$_1$ lead and produces an upright or positive wave form (Fig. 10-4).

Because the bulk of the ventricular muscle tissue is located in the left ventricle, the QRS complexes produced in a RBBB often have three parts or are *triphasic*. These triphasic QRS complexes are designated by the direction and location of the wave form and its relative size. For example, the designation rsR' (read r, s, R prime) means that there is an initial small r wave, followed by a small s wave, followed by a larger R wave, all in the same QRS complex (Fig. 10-5). The rsr' and rsR' are the most common configurations observed in the MCL$_1$ lead with a

FIG. 10–4. RIGHT BUNDLE BRANCH BLOCK.

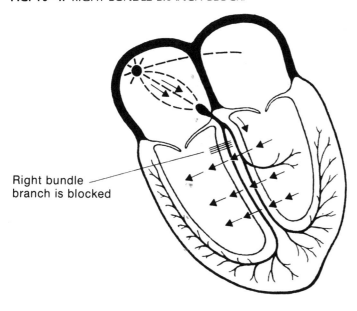

Right bundle branch is blocked

Impulses originating in the SA node or atria are conducted through the AV node to the ventricles. The impulse is unable to pass through the right bundle branch so it depolarizes the left ventricle first and then the right ventricle. This sequential depolarization produces a wider than normal QRS complex.

FIG. 10–5. POSSIBLE QRS COMPLEX PATTERNS WITH RBBB IN LEAD MCL

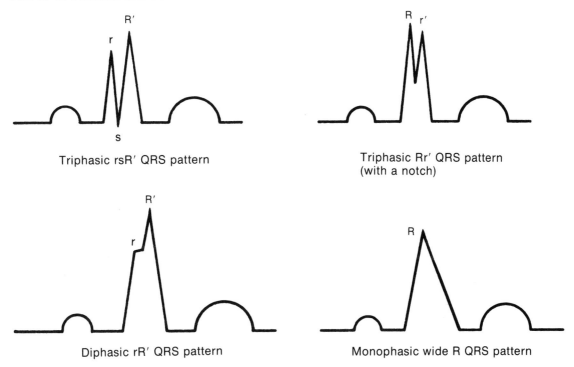

Triphasic rsR' QRS pattern

Triphasic Rr' QRS pattern (with a notch)

Diphasic rR' QRS pattern

Monophasic wide R QRS pattern

No matter what the configuration of the QRS complex, in a RBBB in lead MCL$_1$, the QRS will always be upright and wider than 0.12 second.

RBBB, although any type of wide upward or positive QRS complex in MCL$_1$ lead may be called a RBBB, even if it lacks the characteristic triphasic pattern. This pattern is sometimes simply referred to as "rabbit ears" with either a taller right rabbit ear or left rabbit ear with the rabbit looking away from the reader (Fig. 10-6).

FIG. 10–6. *RABBIT EAR PATTERN IN RBBB (LEAD MCL).*

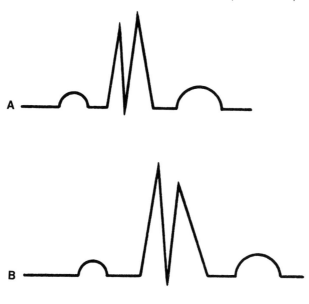

This rsR′ pattern of a RBBB is sometimes referred to as a rabbit ear pattern with a taller right rabbit ear.

This Rsr′ pattern of a RBBB is sometimes referred to as a rabbit ear pattern with a taller left rabbit ear.

CAUSES

Congenital heart diseases that affect the right side of the heart are the principle causes for RBBB in children and teenagers. Right ventricular hypertrophy produced by chronic obstructive pulmonary disease is the principle cause of RBBB in patients in the 20–40-year age range. Right bundle branch block in patients over 50 years of age is often caused by cardiac diseases, such as long-term coronary heart disease, hypertension, congestive failure, and right ventricular MI. Transient RBBB is rare but may develop after acute MI or secondary to cardiac medications such as digoxin, beta blockers or calcium blockers. Development of RBBB secondary to antidysrhythmic therapy with either lidocaine or procainamide IV may be an indication of medication sensitivity or the development of toxicity.

SIGNS AND SYMPTOMS

Although the mechanical results of RBB block are sequential or dyssynchronous ventricular contraction, the condition rarely has much clinical significance. Cardiac output is compromised minimally or not at all and cardiac function remains normal. There are no symptoms associated with RBBB by itself. Symptoms may develop secondary to dysrhythmias in which RBBB is occurring.

TREATMENT

If the cause of RBBB can be attributed to the use of cardiac medications, then elimination of those medications from the regimen eliminates the block. Right bundle branch block has a low potential to progress to a complete block, although, in the presence of an acute MI, this potential is increased. There is no specific treatment for RBBB (Fig. 10-7).

FIG. 10-7. AN EXAMPLE OF A RIGHT BUNDLE BRANCH BLOCK PATTERN.

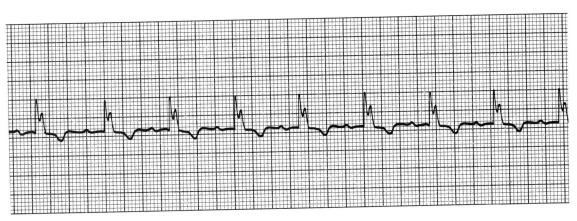

CRITERIA FOR RIGHT BUNDLE BRANCH BLOCK

Rhythm: Regular or irregular depending on the basic rhythm.

Rate: Dependent on the basic rhythm.

Atrial Conduction: P waves: may or may not be present depending on whether the basic rhythm has P waves.

AV Conduction: PR interval: may or may not be present depending on whether basic rhythm has any P waves. May be normal or longer than normal.

Ventricular Conduction: QRS complex: will be greater than 0.12 second; will be upright or positive in an MCL_1 lead; may be triphasic in configuration.

LEFT BUNDLE BRANCH BLOCK

Although the LBB has the potential to become blocked in one of three locations (main stem LBB, left anterior branch of the LBB, or left posterior branch of the LBB), blocks in the main stem LBB produce the characteristic QRS complex observed in left bundle branch block (LBBB) (Fig. 10-8). When the main stem

FIG. 10–8. LEFT BUNDLE BRANCH BLOCK.

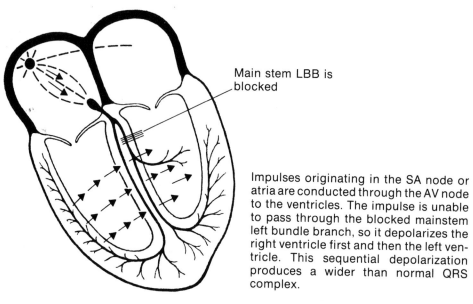

Main stem LBB is blocked

Impulses originating in the SA node or atria are conducted through the AV node to the ventricles. The impulse is unable to pass through the blocked mainstem left bundle branch, so it depolarizes the right ventricle first and then the left ventricle. This sequential depolarization produces a wider than normal QRS complex.

LBB becomes blocked, the depolarizing impulse from the atria travels down the RBB first, depolarizes the right ventricle and the intraventricular septum, then travels to the left ventricle to produce its depolarization. The movement of the electrical activity in the heart that produces depolarization in a LBBB is away from the positive electrode in an MCL$_1$ lead. The pattern produced in this lead is downward (inverted) or negative. In a LBBB, the complexes produced may be triphasic but are predominantly diphasic (two parts to the complex) or monophasic (only one part to the wave form) (Fig. 10-9).

CAUSES

Long-term cardiac disease in older adults is the most common cause of LBBB. Hypertension is a usual common denominator for LBBB, especially when associated with ischemic heart disease, congestive heart failure, mitral valve disease, acute left-sided MI, and general conduction system degeneration. The same medications that produce RBBB also cause LBBB.

SIGNS AND SYMPTOMS

Generally, there are no symptoms associated with the block itself.

TREATMENT

If caused by the use of cardiac medications, these should be eliminated from the medical regimen. A recently developed LBBB in association with acute MI has an increased incidence of progression to a type of complete block and a higher mortality rate. While there is no treatment for the LBBB itself, patients in this latter situation require close monitoring and perhaps the insertion of a temporary pacemaker (Fig. 10-10).

FIG. 10–9. POSSIBLE QRS COMPLEX PATTERNS WITH LBBB IN LEAD MCL$_1$.

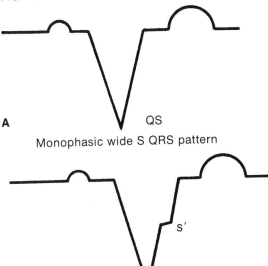

A   QS
Monophasic wide S QRS pattern

B   S'   S
Diphasic Ss' QRS pattern

No matter what the configuration of the QRS complex in a LBBB in lead MCL$_1$, the QRS will always be downward (negative) and wider than 0.12 second.

FIG. 10–10. AN EXAMPLE OF LEFT BUNDLE BRANCH BLOCK PATTERN.

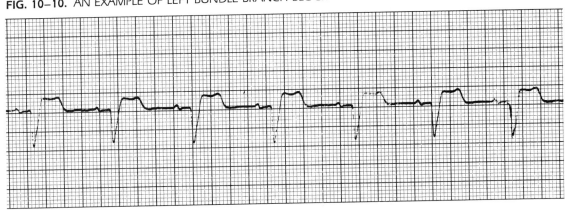

CRITERIA FOR LEFT BUNDLE BRANCH BLOCK

Rhythm: Regular or irregular depending on the basic rhythm.

Rate: Dependent on the basic rhythm.

Atrial Conduction: P waves: may or may not be present depending on whether the basic rhythm has P waves.

AV Conduction: PR interval: may or may not be present depending on whether the basic rhythm has P waves; may be normal or longer than normal.

Ventricular Conduction: QRS complex: greater than 0.12 second; downward or negative in an MCL$_1$ lead; usually will be monophasic.

HEMIBLOCKS AND MULTIFASCICULAR BLOCKS

Because there are three separate segments to the ventricular bundle branch conduction system, a possibility of some 11 types of blocks exist. The majority of these blocks are only marginally distinguishable on the 12 lead ECG and not at all on a single lead rhythm strip. Their study more appropriately belongs in a book explaining 12 lead ECG interpretation.

ALTERNATING AND INTERMITTENT BUNDLE BRANCH BLOCKS

An alternating bundle branch block exists when the block in the ventricular conduction system switches back and forth from one bundle branch to the other. The switching of blocks may occur in alternating beats but most commonly occurs in groups of beats. Depending on the lead, the ECG pattern produced has wide positive QRS complexes that alternate with wide negative QRS complexes. These alternating QRS complexes may be present in any type of underlying rhythm but seem to be more common in atrial fibrillation. It is relatively easy to confuse these alternating beats with ventricular extrasystoles.

An intermittent bundle branch block occurs when one or the other of the bundle branches becomes blocked temporarily for one or more beats. The ECG pattern shows wide QRS complexes that alternate with normal QRS complexes. Like the alternating bundle branch block, these wide beats are sometimes confused with ventricular extrasystoles. The main feature that distinguishes beats with a bundle branch block from ventricular beats is the otherwise normal parts of the ECG pattern in the bundle branch block beats. The beats that have a bundle branch block have the same P wave, PR interval, and T wave as the beats in the nonbundle branch block portion of the ECG strip. In addition, the wide bundle branch block beats will fall on time or in cycle with the rest of the ECG pattern. Ventricular beats generally do not have these characteristics.

CAUSES

The same factors which produced either a RBBB or LBBB also cause alternating or intermittent bundle branch blocks.

SYMPTOMS

No symptoms are produced by these blocks.

TREATMENT

Although the alternating bundle branch block is slightly more serious than an intermittent bundle branch block, it has a low potential to progress to a higher degree block. No specific treatment is indicated for the bundle branch block (Fig. 10-11).

FIG. 10–11. AN EXAMPLE OF ALTERNATING BUNDLE BRANCH BLOCK (MCL₁).

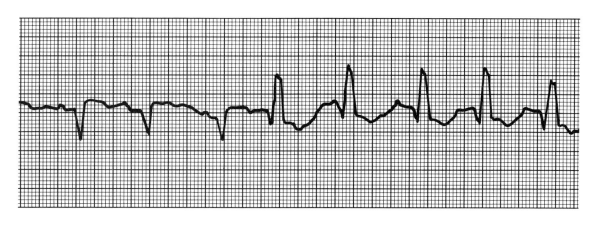

CRITERIA FOR ALTERNATING BUNDLE BRANCH BLOCK

Rhythm: Regular or irregular depending on the basic rhythm.

Rate: Dependent on the basic rhythm.

Atrial Conduction: P waves: may or may not be present depending on whether the basic rhythm has P waves.

AV Conduction: PR interval: may or may not be present depending on whether the basic rhythm has any P waves; may be normal or longer than normal.

Ventricular Conduction: QRS complexes: greater than 0.12 second; in an MCL₁ lead, some of the complexes are positive (upright) and some are negative (downward) (Fig. 10-12).

FIG. 10–12. AN EXAMPLE OF INTERMITTENT BUNDLE BRANCH BLOCK (MCL₁).

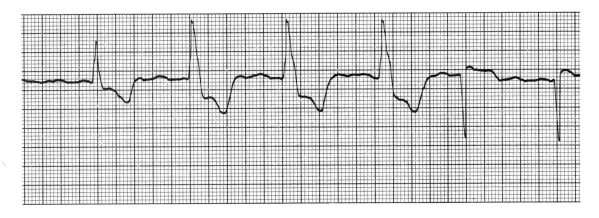

CRITERIA FOR INTERMITTENT BUNDLE BRANCH BLOCK

Rhythm: Regular or irregular depending on the basic rhythm.

Rate: Dependent on the basic rhythm.

Atrial Conduction: P waves: may or may not be present depending on whether the basic rhythm has P waves.

AV Conduction: PR interval: may or may not be present depending on whether the basic rhythm has any P waves. May be normal or longer than normal.

Ventricular Conduction: QRS complex: normal (0.06–0.10 second). QRS complexes are interspersed with wider than normal QRS complexes. These wide QRS complexes may be positive (upward) or negative (downward) in an MCL_1 lead depending on which bundle branch is blocked. The wide QRS complexes fall in cycle with the normal QRS complexes in regular rhythms.

PRACTICE ECG STRIPS FOR CHAPTER 10

Directions. On the following practice ECG strips, analyze each strip according to its rhythm, rate, atrial conduction, AV conduction, and ventricular conduction. Arrive at an interpretation of the strip based upon the analysis and criteria for the dysrhythmias due to abnormal conduction in the bundle branches as learned in this chapter. Remember that bundle branch blocks are not dysrhythmias in themselves but a condition imposed on another rhythm. Make sure also to analyze the underlying rhythm. All ECG strips in this section are in an MCL_1 lead unless indicated otherwise. (See Appendix II for interpretations.)

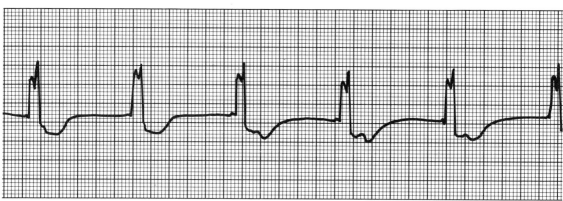

10–1

RHYTHM: _____

RATE: _____

ATRIAL CONDUCTION: _____

_____

AV CONDUCTION: _____

VENTRICULAR CONDUCTION: _____

INTERPRETATION: _____

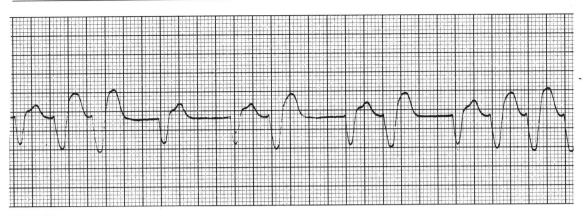

10–2

RHYTHM: _____

RATE: _____

ATRIAL CONDUCTION: _____

_____

AV CONDUCTION: _____

VENTRICULAR CONDUCTION: _____

INTERPRETATION: _____

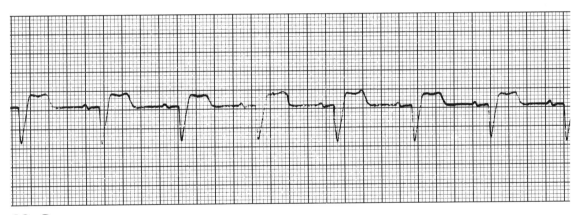

10–3

RHYTHM: _____

RATE: _____

ATRIAL CONDUCTION: _____

_____

AV CONDUCTION: _____

VENTRICULAR CONDUCTION: _____

INTERPRETATION: _____

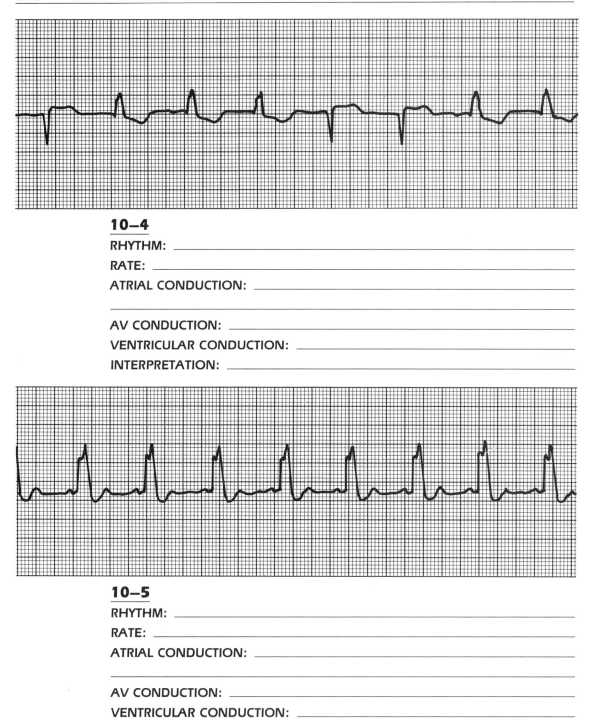

10–4

RHYTHM: _____

RATE: _____

ATRIAL CONDUCTION: _____

_____

AV CONDUCTION: _____

VENTRICULAR CONDUCTION: _____

INTERPRETATION: _____

10–5

RHYTHM: _____

RATE: _____

ATRIAL CONDUCTION: _____

_____

AV CONDUCTION: _____

VENTRICULAR CONDUCTION: _____

INTERPRETATION: _____

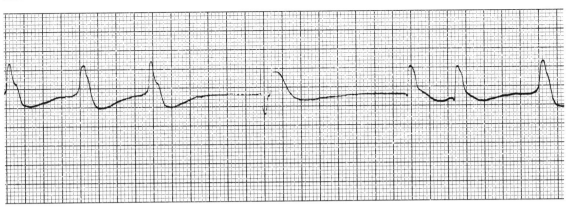

10–6

RHYTHM: _____

RATE: _____

ATRIAL CONDUCTION: _____

_____

AV CONDUCTION: _____

VENTRICULAR CONDUCTION: _____

INTERPRETATION: _____

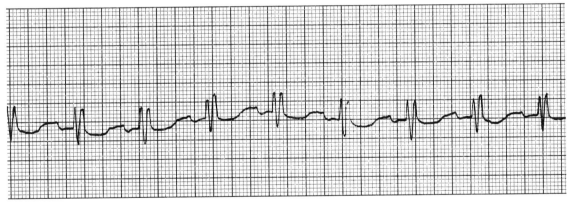

10–7

RHYTHM: _____

RATE: _____

ATRIAL CONDUCTION: _____

_____

AV CONDUCTION: _____

VENTRICULAR CONDUCTION: _____

INTERPRETATION: _____

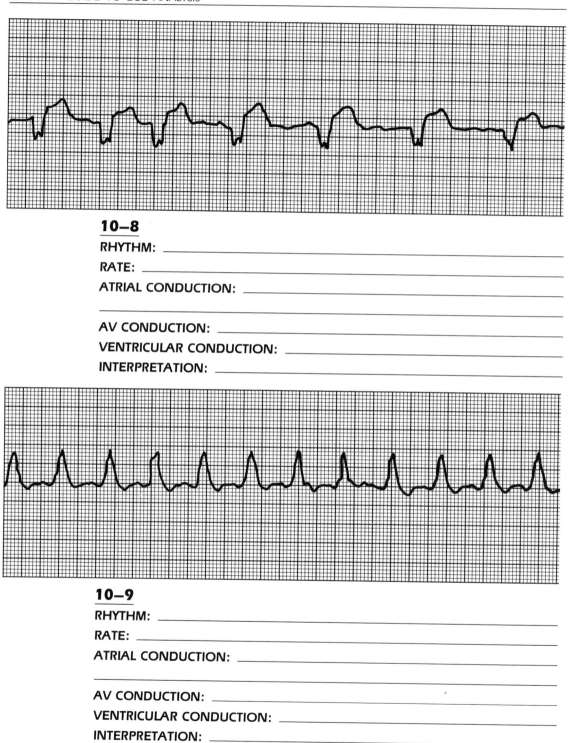

10–8

RHYTHM: _____

RATE: _____

ATRIAL CONDUCTION: _____

_____

AV CONDUCTION: _____

VENTRICULAR CONDUCTION: _____

INTERPRETATION: _____

10–9

RHYTHM: _____

RATE: _____

ATRIAL CONDUCTION: _____

_____

AV CONDUCTION: _____

VENTRICULAR CONDUCTION: _____

INTERPRETATION: _____

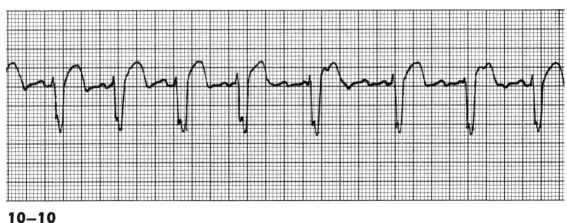

10–10

RHYTHM: _____

RATE: _____

ATRIAL CONDUCTION: _____

_____

AV CONDUCTION: _____

VENTRICULAR CONDUCTION: _____

INTERPRETATION: _____

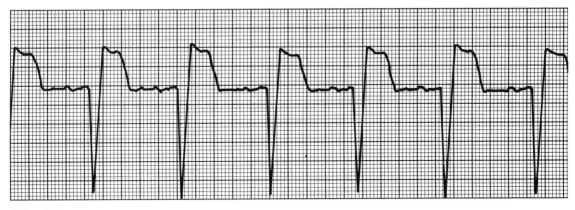

10–11

RHYTHM: _____

RATE: _____

ATRIAL CONDUCTION: _____

_____

AV CONDUCTION: _____

VENTRICULAR CONDUCTION: _____

INTERPRETATION: _____

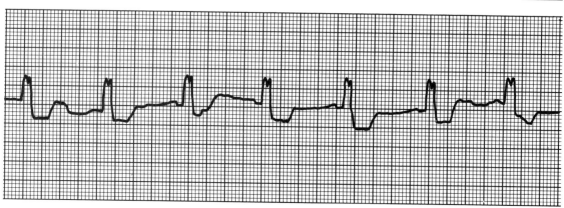

10–12

RHYTHM: _____

RATE: _____

ATRIAL CONDUCTION: _____

_____

AV CONDUCTION: _____

VENTRICULAR CONDUCTION: _____

INTERPRETATION: _____

11

DYSRHYTHMIAS ASSOCIATED WITH BYPASS MECHANISMS

LEARNING OBJECTIVES

After studying this section, the learner will be able to:

1. Identify the abnormal conduction mechanisms that produce the preexcitation syndromes.
2. Name the two most common dysrhythmia patterns produced by abnormal bypass mechanisms.
3. List the causes of the preexcitation syndromes.
4. Analyze and interpret ECG rhythm strips that contain preexcitation syndrome patterns.
5. List the treatments appropriate for preexcitation syndrome patterns.
6. Define preexcitation, preexcitation syndrome, and accessory pathways.

Changes in the PR interval reflect conduction abnormalities through the higher areas of the conduction system, especially in the atrioventricular (AV) node. Up to this point, the only abnormal PR intervals that have been discussed are ones that are longer than normal because of delays or blocks in the conduction to the Purkinje fibers. A *short* PR interval or a PR interval of less duration than normal can only be produced if the impulse travels more rapidly than expected from the sinoatrial (SA) node to the ventricles. Because the AV node delays all impulses from the SA node or atria for at least 0.1 second, the only way an impulse can travel to the ventricles more quickly than normal is through bypass mechanisms or what is commonly called *accessory pathways.*

Accessory pathways are abnormal tracts of extra cardiac muscular or conductive tissue between the atria and the ventricles. Basically, these accessory pathways bypass the AV node. The origin of these pathways can be traced to the normal embryologic development period of the heart. In the later stages of development of the embryonic heart or shortly after birth, these pathways normally become inactive and stop conducting impulses.

Because these accessory pathways are composed of tissue that is similar to that of the atria, they conduct impulses at a much faster rate than the AV node, although the refractory period is somewhat longer than the AV node. Also, because the main function of the AV node is to slow down impulses, when it is bypassed, the conduction is much faster. As a result of these impulses bypassing the AV node, part of the ventricular muscle tissue depolarizes earlier than it would be expected to depolarize if the impulse had traveled through the AV node. This early depolarization of the ventricular muscle tissue is called *preexcitation* and the dysrhythmias associated with the bypass mechanisms are referred to as *preexcitation syndromes.*

Although as many as seven different accessory pathways have been identified, Wolff-Parkinson-White syndrome and Lown-Ganong-Levine syndrome account for the majority of the cases of preexcitation syndrome. Overall, the preexcitation syndromes are a rare type of dysrhythmia, accounting for approximately 2% of all the dysrhythmias. When the AV node is bypassed and no delay occurs between atrial and ventricular contractions, there may be a small loss of ventricular filling from the atria and a small decrease in cardiac output. The loss of cardiac output increases as the rate of the dysrhythmia increases. Most individuals who have no other significant cardiac disease can compensate for this loss of cardiac output. Unless an individual develops symptoms from a secondary dysrhythmia associated with the preexcitation syndrome, there is no clinical way to determine its presence except to perform an electrocardiogram (ECG). Many individuals with preexcitation syndromes live normal lives with normal activity for many years without ever knowing they have the abnormal conduction pathways.

The most common dysrhythmia associated with the preexcitation syndromes is rapid supraventricular tachycardia. There are two mechanisms directly related to the production of supraventricular tachycardia in individuals who have accessory pathways.

RAPID 1:1 CONDUCTION

Because the AV node is being bypassed, it can no longer function as a gatekeeper to prevent too rapid or too frequent depolarization of the ventricles. The accessory pathways have very rapid conduction times compared to the AV node and will allow every impulse from the atria to be conducted to the ventricles. If the individual's basic rhythm is sinus rhythm or even sinus tachycardia, there is usually no difficulty, because the rate never exceeds what would be considered a realistic rate for the ventricles. If the individual should develop a dysrhythmia such as atrial flutter, atrial tachycardia, or atrial fibrillation, with a 1:1 conduction, every one of the atrial impulses will produce a ventricular contraction. The rate will soon exceed the maximal possible rate for the ventricles and severely compromise the cardiac output.

REENTRY TACHYCARDIA

Reentry tachycardia is also called retrograde atrial excitation, circus reentry tachycardia, and AV reciprocating tachycardia (Fig. 11-1).

Reentry-type tachycardias occur when there are two conduction pathways that

FIG. 11-1. REENTRY TACHYCARDIA.

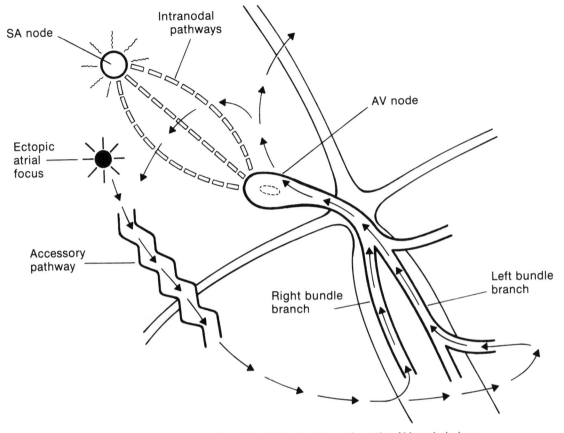

Reentry tachycardia occurs when an impulse falls at a time when the AV node is in a refractory period but the accessory pathway is not. The same impulse that depolarizes the ventricles returns through the AV node to depolarize the atria and then back to the ventricles via the accessory pathway.

have different conduction rates or different refractory periods. In the case of the preexcitation syndromes, the two pathways are the accessory pathway, which has a rapid conduction time but a somewhat longer refractory period, and the normal AV node and AV tracts, which have slower conduction times but somewhat shorter refractory periods. An impulse traveling from the SA node or the atria may be conducted either through the accessory pathway or through the AV node on its way to the ventricles. The impulse usually follows the accessory pathway because it has a more rapid conduction time than the AV node. Once the impulse reaches the ventricles and causes their depolarization, it is prevented from returning to the atria because the accessory pathway is still in its refractory period and the AV node has built-in mechanisms that usually prevent impulses from traveling backward through it from the ventricles to the atria.

If a beat should occur early in the cardiac cycle, such as a premature atrial contraction, and the accessory pathway is still in a refractory period from the previous impulse, then the impulse travels through the AV node and depolarizes the ventricles. That *same* impulse then travels backward through the accessory pathway, which has now recovered and is no longer in its refractory period, to the atria and causes them to contract. The impulse then is conducted to the ventricles through the AV node again (since the accessory pathway is in its refractory period from the previous contraction) and then backward through the accessory pathway to the atria, producing contractions in the respective chambers as it travels around the heart. This impulse traveling back and forth between the atria and ventricles unimpeded produces a self-sustaining, revolving, or circular dysrhythmia and rapidly increases in rate (see Fig. 11-1).

Less frequently, a similar type of reentry tachycardia can develop when the impulse travels through the accessory pathways to the ventricles, then back to the atria through the AV node. Termination of this type of dysrhythmia can occur spontaneously if the rate should become so fast that both pathways are in a refractory period at the same time, thus, preventing the passage of the impulse to the ventricles. A similar situation of simultaneous refractory periods can occur if a well-timed premature atrial contraction should happen at the moment that one or the other of the pathways was conducting the impulse. The main goal of treatment is aimed at lengthening the refractory period of the AV node. Vagal stimulation through such measures as the Valsalva's maneuver, carotid massage, or gagging increases the refractory period of the AV node. Cardiac medications, particularly the calcium-channel blocker, verapamil (Calan, Isoptin) also accomplishes this goal. Electric cardioversion produces total refractoriness of all the heart tissue and is effective in terminating reentry type tachycardias.

The preexcitation syndromes can be a dominant and permanent condition or they can be intermittent and transient, occurring at random intervals. Because the preexcitation syndromes sometimes alter the shape and duration of the QRS complex, particularly in rapid rhythms, supraventricular tachycardia may look like ventricular tachycardia.

WOLFF-PARKINSON-WHITE SYNDROME

Wolff-Parkinson-White syndrome is also called WPW, and accessory AV connections (Kent bundles) (Fig. 11-2).

Wolff-Parkinson-White syndrome is a type of preexcitation syndrome in which the accessory pathways that bypass the AV node are the bundles of Kent. The bundles of Kent are conduction pathways located along the sides of the heart and connect the atria directly to the ventricles. Normally present and functioning in the fetal heart and early newborn period, the bundles of Kent usually become nonfunctional within 24 hours after birth. Although there are two bundles of Kent, one on each side of the heart, in most individuals who have WPW, only one of the two pathways remains functional. On rare occasions, an individual may have both pathways functional, although, in these individuals, the rhythm tends to alternate from one side to the other.

Men comprise approximately 70% of all individuals who have WPW. Because there is only minimal decrease in cardiac output when the heart rate remains

FIG. 11–2. IN WPW, THE BUNDLES OF KENT (RIGHT AND LEFT) ARE THE ACCESSORY PATHWAYS. IMPULSES PASSING THROUGH THE BUNDLES OF KENT WILL BYPASS THE AV NODE, ALLOWING VERY RAPID CONDUCTION OF THE IMPULSE TO THE VENTRICLES. USUALLY ONE OR THE OTHER, BUT NOT BOTH BUNDLES OF KENT REMAIN ACTIVE. SINCE THE IMPULSE TERMINATES IN THE TOP OF THE VENTRICLES, IT DOES NOT FOLLOW THE NORMAL CONDUCTION PATHWAYS, MAKING THE QRS COMPLEX WIDER THAN NORMAL.

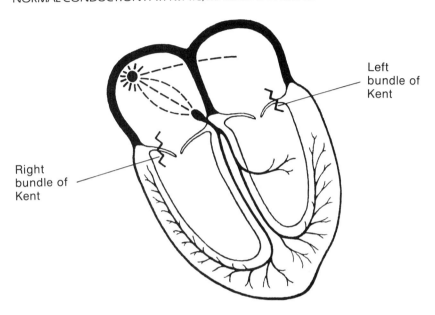

Left bundle of Kent

Right bundle of Kent

normal, the diagnosis of WPW may not be made until episodes of rapid supraventricular tachycardia produce symptoms.

There are some distinct ECG features produced when an individual has WPW that make its recognition fairly easy. Because the impulse from the SA node or atria is bypassing the AV node and going directly to the ventricles, there is an extremely short PR interval. The PR interval in WPW consists of only the width of the P wave located just before the QRS complex. There will *always* be one P wave for each QRS complex because of the obligatory 1:1 conduction ratio of the accessory pathways. The accessory pathways lack the ability to block out extra beats.

Another important identification feature of WPW is the shape of the QRS complex. Because the terminating end of the accessory pathway is in the top of the ventricles, the impulse from the atria does not follow the normal conduction pathways through the ventricles. This abnormal conduction produces a wider than normal QRS (0.12 second or greater) with a characteristic up-slope on the QRS complex. This up-slope is sometimes referred to as *slurred* and is called a *delta wave* because of its similarity in shape to the triangular-shaped Greek letter delta (Fig. 11-3). The delta wave can vary from a slight inclination after the P wave to a very large inclination, which may reach from the P wave to the top of the R wave (Fig. 11-4). The size of the delta wave has no relationship to the seriousness of the condition.

FIG. 11-3. FEATURES OF ECG PATTERN IN WPW.

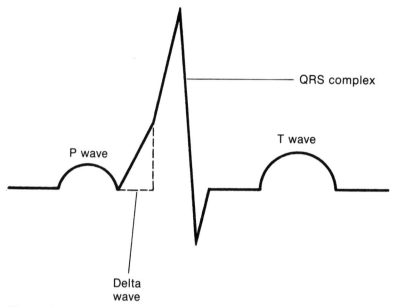

The ECG pattern produced when the impulses pass rapidly from the SA node to the ventricles through the bundles of Kent has some characteristic features. The PR interval is very short, consisting of only the P wave. A delta wave is present, which makes the QRS complex wider than normal.

FIG. 11-4. EXAMPLES OF VARIOUS DELTA WAVES IN ECG PATTERNS WITH WPW.

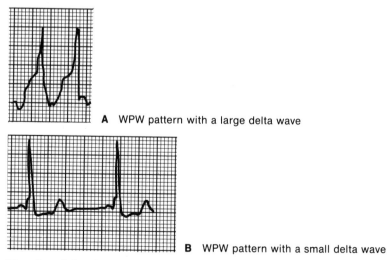

The size of the delta wave in a WPW pattern does not indicate the seriousness of the abnormality.

Because the two dominant bundles of Kent are located along the sides of the heart, WPW has classically been divided into type A and type B depending on the location of the functional bundle of Kent. It may be appropriate to develop a type C category for WPW to include the accessory pathway found in the area of the intraventricular septum. The difficulty with this third category is that it is difficult to identify on the ECG and its morphology often is identical to the LGL pattern.

TYPE A WPW

In type A WPW, the *left* bundle of Kent remains functional and connects the atria to the ventricles. Since the impulse first depolarizes the left ventricle and then travels across the intraventricular septum to depolarize the right ventricle, in a MCL_1 lead, the impulse travels toward the positive electrode. This electrical activity produces a QRS complex that is predominantly positive or upright (Fig. 11-5). Type A WPW is the most common and accounts for approximately 80% of all types of WPW.

FIG. 11–5. TYPE A WPW.

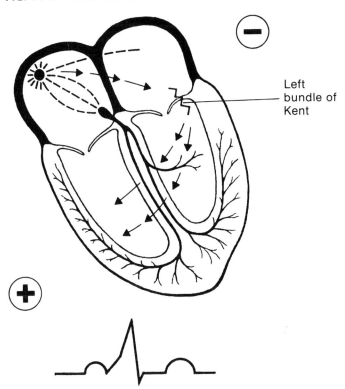

Left bundle of Kent

Type A WPW has a left bundle of Kent that is active. The impulses travel down the left side of the heart first and then across the interventricular septum to depolarize the right ventricle. The general current flow is toward the positive electrode in an MCL_1 so the QRS complex is generally positive.

TYPE B WPW

In type B WPW, the *right* bundle of Kent remains functional and connects the atria to the ventricles. Because the impulse first depolarizes the right ventricle and then travels across the intraventricular septum to depolarize the left ventricle, in a MCL$_1$ lead, the impulse travels away from the positive electrode. The QRS complex that this electrical activity produces is predominantly negative and appears downward on the ECG tracing (Fig. 11-6).

FIG. 11–6. TYPE B WPW.

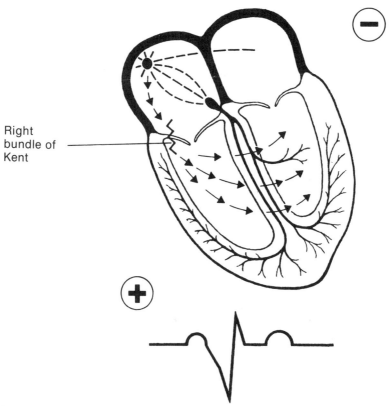

Right bundle of Kent

Type B WPW has a right bundle of Kent that is active. The impulses travel down the right side of the heart first and then across the interventricular septum to depolarize the left ventricle. The general current flow is away from the positive electrode in an MCL$_1$ so that the QRS complex will be predominantly negative.

CAUSES

There are no specific causes for WPW; acute or chronic cardiac disease states cannot cause it. Wolff-Parkinson-White syndrome is most often associated with congenital heart disease and is probably present from birth, although not detected until much later.

SYMPTOMS

The dysrhythmia itself does not decrease cardiac output enough to cause any symptoms. Patients become symptomatic when a supraventricular tachycardia is present because of rapid 1:1 conduction. With rapid rates, the signs and symptoms observed include those usually seen with all low cardiac output. Neurologically, the patient may display weakness, dizziness, and syncope. Cardiovascular symptoms include feelings of palpitations in the chest, chest pressure or pain, shortness of breath, low blood pressure, and weak, rapid pulses.

TREATMENT

The goal of treatment is to slow the cardiac rate to a point where the heart produces adequate cardiac output. If the underlying problem is due to a rapid atrial dysrhythmia with 1:1 conduction, that dysrhythmia must be terminated or slowed. If the tachycardia is due to a reentry problem, appropriate measures must be taken to terminate that dysrhythmia.

There is no definitive treatment for the WPW condition itself. The bundles of Kent, because of their dissimilarity to the tissues of the AV node, do not respond well to the usual cardiac medications such as digoxin, quinidine, and beta blockers. The calcium-channel blockers, particularly verapamil, have been more successful.

In WPW patients who have frequent prolonged episodes of supraventricular tachycardia that does not respond to medical treatment, heart surgery can be undertaken to ligate the bundles of Kent. One result of this type of surgery is that the patient is often left in a complete heart block, requiring the implantation of a permanent pacemaker (Fig. 11-7).

FIG. 11–7. AN EXAMPLE OF WPW PATTERN.

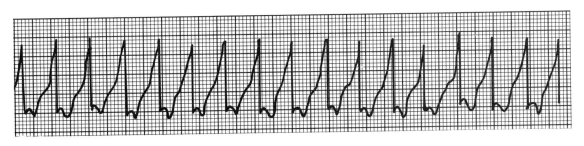

CRITERIA FOR WOLFF-PARKINSON-WHITE SYNDROME

Rhythm: Regular, although it may be irregular in the presence of atrial fibrillation or if alternating with another rhythm.

Rate: 60–100 beats/min if sinus in origin; may be much faster if the basic rhythm is atrial in origin or if in a SVT.

Atrial Conduction: P waves: usually normal, upright. Will always be one P wave before each QRS.

AV Conduction: PR interval: less than 0.11 second; will usually just be the width of the P wave; same across the whole strip.

Ventricular Conduction: QRS: greater than 0.10 second. Will have the characteristic delta wave. May be upright if type A or inverted if type B in MCL₁ lead.

LOWN-GANONG-LEVINE SYNDROME

Lown-Ganong-Levine syndrome is also called LGL, sinus rhythm with a short PR interval, and short PR normal QRS syndrome. Lown-Ganong-Levine syndrome is a type of preexcitation syndrome in which the AV node is bypassed by accessory pathways that terminate in or near the bundle of His. The accessory pathways of LGL are extensions of the normal intranodal conduction pathways of the atria and are sometimes referred to as *James fibers*.

The accessory pathways of LGL may totally bypass the AV node or may pass through the AV node. In either case, they terminate at the bundle of His (Figs. 11-8 and 11-9). A condition that can sometimes produce an ECG pattern identical

FIG. 11–8. ONE TYPE OF ACCESSORY PATHWAY IN LGL.

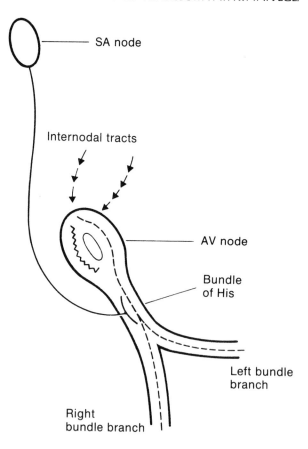

SA node

Internodal tracts

AV node

Bundle of His

Left bundle branch

Right bundle branch

The normal pathway through the AV node (dotted lines) is bypassed in LGL by one of the internodal tracts, which terminates in the bundle of His. The impulse then follows the normal conduction pathways through the ventricles, resulting in a normal QRS complex.

FIG. 11–9. A SECOND TYPE OF ACCESSORY PATHWAY IN LGL.

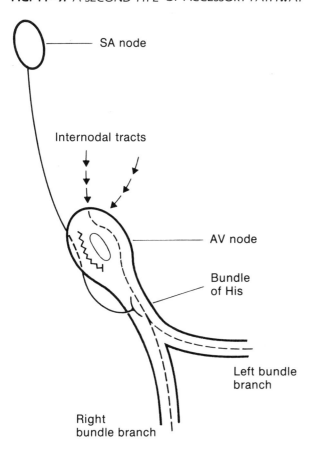

Although the internodal tract runs through the AV node, the impulses it carries bypass the normal conduction through the node. The impulse again terminates in the bundle of His. From there, the impulse follows the normal conduction pathways through the ventricles with a normal QRS complex.

to the pattern produced in LGL exists when the AV node is small, nonfunctional, and incapable of delaying atrial impulses. Strictly speaking, the LGL name should not be used in describing the small AV node syndrome. Because it produces a pattern identical to LGL, it is usually impossible to distinguish between the two on the ECG.

Females comprise approximately 70% of all cases of LGL. Cardiac output is decreased very little in LGL that remains at a normal rate and, like WPW, often not diagnosed until complications develop from other associated dysrhythmias. Lown-Ganong-Levine syndrome has the same potential for supraventricular tachycardia as WPW developing from rapid 1:1 conduction.

The key identifying features of LGL arise from the fact that the AV node is bypassed but the conduction through the ventricles follows the normal pathways. The bypass of the AV node appears on the ECG strip as a PR interval that is less than 0.11 second. As in the WPW, there really is no PR interval except the width of the P wave. The QRS complex in LGL is normal because the impulse that depolarizes the ventricles follows the normal conduction pathways in the ventricles. There is no delta wave. Lown-Ganong-Levine is sometimes misidentified as a junctional rhythm.

CAUSES

The origin of LGL is usually traceable to a congenital abnormality during the formation of the conduction system of the heart. There are no specific causes related to cardiac disease.

SYMPTOMS

The dysrhythmia does not produce any symptoms by itself. Symptoms appear in conjunction with LGL when supraventricular tachycardia is present. These include the usual low cardiac output symptoms.

TREATMENT

The goal of treatment is to keep the heart at a rate that produces adequate output and systemic circulation. Termination or control of rapid atrial dysrhythmias or SVT is fundamental.

Because the accessory pathways in LGL are identical in tissue structure to the normal intranodal pathways of the atria, LGL responds better to the cardiac medications used to control other rapid atrial dysrhythmias. Digoxin, quinidine, and the beta blockers control rapid tachycardias in LGL. The calcium channel-blockers are still the most effective. Surgical intervention for patients with LGL is dangerous and not often effective (Fig. 11-10).

FIG. 11–10. AN EXAMPLE OF LGL PATTERN.

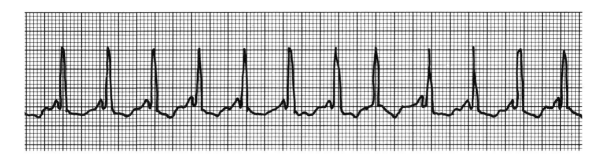

CRITERIA FOR LOWN-GANONG-LEVINE SYNDROME

Rhythm: Regular except when the underlying rhythm is atrial fibrillation or when alternating with other rhythms.

Rate: 60–100 beats/min if sinus in origin. Much faster if the underlying rhythm is atrial or if in a supraventricular tachycardia.

Atrial Conduction: P waves: usually normal, upright. Will always be one P wave before each QRS complex.

AV Conduction: PR Interval: less than 0.11 second; consists of the width of the P wave; same across the whole strip.

Ventricular Conduction: QRS: 0.06–0.10 second; same shape, *no* delta wave.

12

ECG PATTERNS PRODUCED BY PACEMAKERS

LEARNING OBJECTIVES

After studying this section, the learner will be able to:

1. Describe the parts of a pacemaker system.
2. List the most common reasons for the use of pacemakers.
3. Identify the type of pacemaker and its function based on the three letter ICHD code.
4. Recognize a normal single chamber pacemaker pattern on an ECG strip.
5. Analyze and interpret ECG rhythm strips that have abnormal pacemaker patterns.

An artificial pacemaker is an electronic device that delivers a depolarizing impulse to the myocardium when the heart's own internal pacemaker mechanisms fail. The topics of pacemakers and pacemaker rhythms are included here because of the frequency with which they are encountered by hospital personnel. While a comprehensive and indepth treatment of all types of pacemakers and the rhythms they can produce is beyond the scope of this book, basic information is included here that will serve as a building block for more detailed study in the future.

Although artificial pacemakers are common today, the first successful implantation of one in a human was accomplished a mere 30 years ago. Technologic advances in microcircuitry in recent years have revolutionized the capabilities of these devices. Although the basic pacemaker system is still composed of a pulse generator, which contains the pacemaker electronics and a power source, and a pacemaker catheter or lead electrode (or electrodes in multichamber pacemakers), there is little similarity to models of even a few years ago in both physical size and electronic capabilities (Fig. 12-1). Modern implantable pacemakers are much smaller, weigh less than one ounce, and have the potential for a variety of activities, ranging from simple demand pacing to multichamber termination of tachy-dysrhythmias.

FIG. 12–1. SINGLE CHAMBER PERMANENT PACEMAKER SYSTEM.

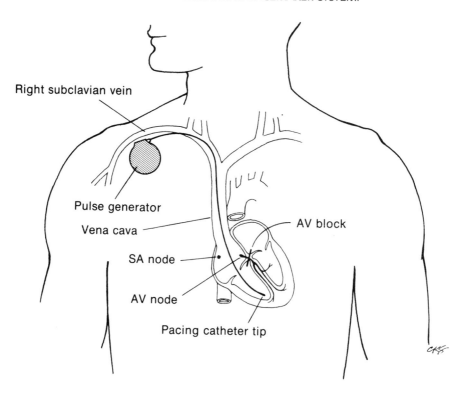

The most common type of pacemakers uses a transvenous pacing catheter with a bipolar tip, which is ideally lodged in or near the apex of the right ventricle. When an impulse is delivered from the pulse generator through the pacing catheter to the right ventricle, depolarization of the myocardium occurs. Because the depolarization originates from a ventricular focus, the QRS complex produced does not appear normal. The current travels in the heart from the right ventricle across the interventricular septum to the left ventricle. Because the current flow is away from the positive electrode in the MCL_1 lead, the QRS complex will appear wide and with a negative or downward deflection, much as the QRS complex of a left bundle branch block or a right ventricular PVC (Fig. 12-2). When the pacemaker "fires," the electrical activity produced by the pulse generator is recorded on the electrocardiogram (ECG) strip as an electrical artifact or pacing "spike" (discussed below), which should just precede the wide QRS complex.

INDICATIONS FOR PERMANENT (IMPLANTED) PACEMAKER USE

There are a variety of reasons why permanent or implantable pacemakers are used in patients. Generally, the underlying conditions are ones that cause low cardiac output because of malfunction or failure of the heart's internal pacemaker

FIG. 12–2. CURRENT FLOW WITH A SINGLE CHAMBER PACEMAKER WITH RESULTING ECG PATTERN.

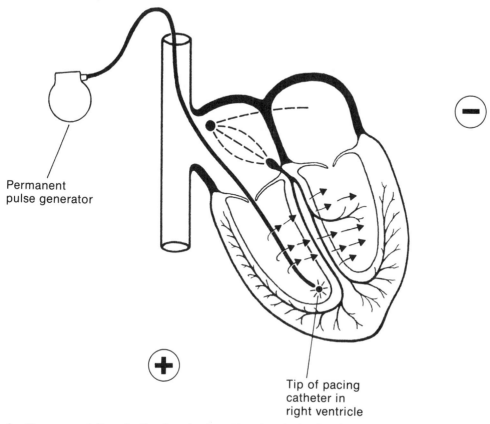

A   The current flow in the heart when the depolarization is initiated by a pacing catheter is away from the positive electrode in the MCL_1 lead.

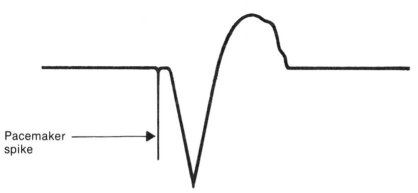

B   The wave form produced by a pacemaker is predominantly negative in the MCL_1 lead. A pacemaker "spike" precedes the wide QRS complex.

mechanisms. Some of the most common reasons permanent pacemakers are implanted include the following:

1. Sinus node dysfunction (including brady-tachy syndrome, sinus block and arrest, and slow sinus bradycardia)
2. Intermittent high grade atrioventricular (AV) block
3. Complete heart block (either AV block or trifascicular)
4. Atrial fibrillation with a ventricular rate below 50 beats/min
5. Wolff-Parkinson-White syndrome after surgery
6. Medication-induced bradycardia and sinus arrest

INDICATIONS OF TEMPORARY (EXTERNAL) PACEMAKER USE

The temporary pacemaker system is similar to the permanent pacemaker except that the pulse generator is external to the body (Fig. 12-3). Temporary pacemakers

FIG. 12–3. AN EXAMPLE OF A SINGLE CHAMBER TEMPORARY PACEMAKER SYSTEM.

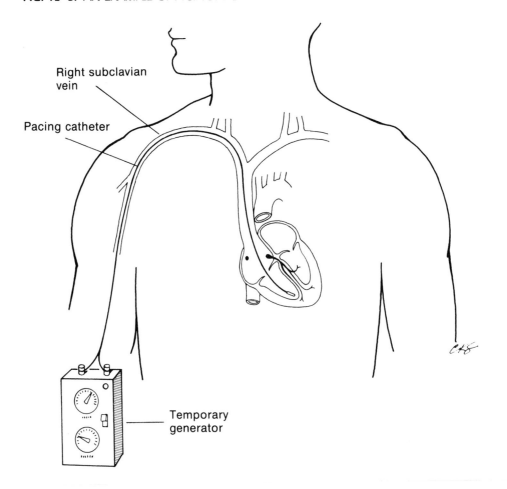

are used in emergency situations when there is not time to insert a permanent pacemaker or prophylactically for certain types of dysrhythmias that have the potential to progress to high grade blocks. The more common reasons for use of a temporary pacemaker include the following:

1. Right bundle branch block with left anterior hemiblock post myocardial infarction (MI)
2. Right bundle branch block with left posterior hemiblock post MI
3. Complete left bundle branch block post MI
4. An alternating bundle branch block post MI
5. Second or third degree AV block post MI
6. Failure of a permanent pacemaker
7. During a cardiac arrest in which cardiopulmonary resuscitation and medications have been ineffective in restoring a cardiac rhythm

As in the treatment of all dysrhythmias, the clinical condition of the patient and the underlying cardiac disease must be considered before any action is taken. To some extent, the determination of the type of pacemaker system used depends upon the underlying condition that requires treatment. Rather than "curing" the underlying dysrhythmia, the pacemaker merely increases the cardiac output to an adequate level, despite the defects in the heart's own conduction system. A pacemaker uses the heart's remaining capabilities and simulates the normal electrophysiologic functioning of the heart as closely as possible to produce the best cardiac output. A pacemaker inserted in a patient who has little functioning myocardium would be of no value to that patient and may even decrease the cardiac output because the normal depolarization of the heart has been altered.

CLASSIFICATIONS OF PACEMAKERS

At best, the classification of pacemakers is complicated and confusing. Pacemakers are classified by catheter type, method of insertion, and generator type.

The pacemaker catheter or electrode is the wire that connects the pulse generator to the myocardium of the heart. It is generally made of a metal alloy containing titanium and other metals and is surrounded with an inert silicon coating that acts as an insulator. The end of the catheter that makes contact with the myocardium is bare metal so the impulse is conducted to the muscle tissue of the heart.

CLASSIFICATION BY TYPE OF CATHETER

1. Unipolar catheter: This type of catheter contains just one wire and has one bare metal area at the end of it. Because two poles (positive and negative) are needed to create a current flow, the outside case of the pulse generator acts as the other pole. This type of catheter is infrequently used today.
2. Bipolar catheter: This type of catheter contains two wires. The end of the catheter has two bare metal areas separated by an insulated area. This type of catheter is the most common type used.

CLASSIFICATION BY METHOD OF CATHETER INSERTION

External (Skin Electrodes)

The pacemaker catheter is attached externally by needles, paddles, or skin electrodes to the skin on the chest wall over the heart. While this is a quick way to begin pacing a patient's heart, it requires much higher energy levels than internal catheters. Patients may experience a small electrical "twinge" as the pacemaker discharges. Portable pacing base units weighing up to 30 pounds are capable of delivering external stimulation of 50–200 mV by two wires connected to conducting pads. This method of pacing is used in emergency situations and has the advantage of being initiated quickly and effectively by a nurse without having to wait for a physician. Paramedics, emergency room personnel, and cardiac arrest teams could use this technology to save lives.

External pacing is used only for short periods of time; it is used only with temporary (external) pulse generators or base units.

Transthoracic

The pacemaker catheter is attached to long needles that pass through the chest wall and enter the myocardium of the heart. Again, it is a quick and effective way to begin pacing a patient's heart in an emergency situation but has some definite disadvantages. If the patient is awake, it can be a very painful procedure. It also has the potential to produce a pneumothorax or myocardial hemorrhage. Other complications include laceration of the coronary arteries, laceration of the conduction system of the heart, and cardiac tamponade. This method is used only with temporary (external) pulse generators.

Epicardial

The pacemaker catheter in epicardial pacing is attached to the epicardium through the pericardium after a thoracic incision has been made. This catheter may be connected to a temporary or permanent pulse generator. If the permanent pulse generator is used, it is implanted in the abdomen. This type of catheter placement is most often used when patients do not have adequate-sized subclavian veins for transvenous catheter insertion. It has the advantage of being able to pace the left ventricle directly but involves a much more complicated surgical procedure, with increased risks for complications.

Transvenous

In the transvenous method, the pacemaker catheter is passed through the venous side of the circulatory system into the right ventricle. The subclavian vein is the most commonly used site, but the brachial vein or even a femoral vein may be used. This type of catheter can be used with either permanent or temporary pulse generators of either the single or dual chamber types. It is a relatively simple procedure, usually does not require the use of general anesthesia, and can be done quickly in emergency situations. Transvenous pacemaker catheter placement is, by far, the most frequently used method of artificial cardiac pacing today.

Myocardial

In the myocardial method of catheter placement, a catheter is inserted directly into the myocardium of either the right or left ventricle. This procedure is similar to the procedure for the epicardial catheter placement. It is only used with a permanent pulse generator.

CLASSIFICATION BY PULSE GENERATOR TYPE

Temporary Pulse Generator

This type of pulse generator is external to the body and is connected to the heart by a catheter that must pass though the skin at some point. It is used for short-term emergency and prophylactic pacing. Temporary pulse generators may be (1) single chamber—only one pacing catheter from the pulse generator is inserted into the heart, generally into the right ventricle; or (2) dual chamber—two pacing catheters are inserted into the heart: one for the right atrium and one for the right ventricle. This procedure is more complicated and time-consuming and is not used as much as the single chamber pacing procedure.

Permanent Pulse Generator

This type of pulse generator is inserted under the skin into a pocket made in the chest wall or abdomen (in the case of epicardial pacemakers). It is connected to a pacing catheter that is, in turn, connected to the heart. Because of the potential complexity of permanent pacemakers, a special classification code has been developed by the Intersociety Commission for Heart Disease (ICHD). The original three position (letter) code (Table 12-1) was first developed in 1974. With the advent of more complex dual chamber pacemakers, the code was expanded to five positions in 1981. This expanded code is more comprehensive but is still

TABLE 12–1. THREE POSITION ICHD PACEMAKER CODE

Position	I	II	III
Classification of Letters	Chamber(s) Paced	Chamber(s) Sensed	Mode of Response
	V–Ventricle	V–Ventricle	I–Inhibited
	A–Atrium	A–Atrium	T–Triggered
	D–Dual (both)	D–Dual (both)	D–Dual (both)
	S–Single chamber	S–Single chamber	R–Reverse
		O–Neither chamber (none)	O–Neither mode (none or fixed rate)

inadequate to include all the possible types of pulse generators currently being developed. In this book, the three letter code is used in presenting the more common types of pulse generators used. Understanding the ICHD code requires knowledge of each of the three positions and the definition of each letter in the code. There is also some terminology used in the description of pacemaker function that is helpful in understanding the code.

KEY DEFINITIONS IN PACEMAKER LANGUAGE

SENSING

Sensing is the ability of the pacemaker to "see" electrically what the heart is doing. When a pulse generator senses, it is detecting the intrinsic electrical activity produced by the heart's own depolarizations through the pacemaker catheter. The pulse generator can actually ready the ECG and distinguish R waves from T waves or P waves based on amplitude, voltage, and width of the wave form the heart produces.

CAPTURE

Capture is the response by the heart to an impulse delivered through the pacemaker catheter that results in atrial or ventricular depolarization. A pacemaker that is functioning normally will have capture with each impulse delivered.

NONCAPTURE

A condition that exists when a pacemaker pulse generator is initiating impulses but the heart is not depolarizing in response to the impulses. Causes for noncapture pacemakers usually revolve around problems with the pacing catheter, such as increased resistance and broken or displaced catheters.

PACEMAKER SPIKE

A *pacemaker spike* is a type of electrical artifact that is produced on an ECG strip when a pacemaker pulse generator discharges an impulse. It appears as a dark line that should be just before the QRS complex produced by the pacemaker. The spike may be positive (upward) or negative (downward), depending on the monitoring equipment and how the leads are placed. Spikes without QRS complexes after them indicate noncapture.

Most monitoring equipment has built-in circuits to eliminate electrical interference. A pacemaker spike is often treated by the equipment as interference and may be suppressed unless the monitor is told that there is a pacemaker present. In a monitoring system that lacks a pacemaker selection, use of the "diagnostic" setting rather than the "monitoring" setting allows the pacemaker spike to be seen.

THRESHOLD

Threshold indicates the amount of electrical energy produced by the pulse generator that is required for capture. This setting is adjustable in all temporary pacemakers and most permanent pacemakers. The normal threshold for most permanent pacemakers ranges between 0.5 and 1.5 milliampheres (MA). Temporary pacemakers require a somewhat higher setting and may range up to 20 MA. The threshold may change after pacemaker insertion because of fibrin formation around the tip of the catheter that acts as an insulator.

ESCAPE INTERVAL (PACING INTERVAL)

In single chamber, demand pacemakers, the escape interval is the time interval measured from a sensed intrinsic QRS complex to the next paced beat (Fig. 12-4). The escape interval is the longest time the pacemaker allows the heart to remain in asystole. This setting is also adjustable and, in single chamber pacemakers, determines the rate of the pacing rhythm.

FIG. 12–4. AN EXAMPLE OF A PACING ESCAPE INTERVAL.

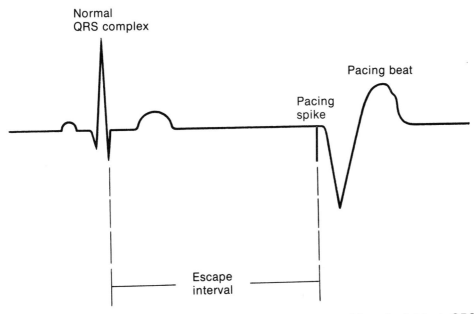

The escape interval in single chamber pacemakers is measured from the intrinsic QRS complex to the pacing spike. This interval is the longest time the pacemaker will allow the heart to go without contracting. Measured in milliseconds, the average escape interval for adults ranges between 1091 ms (55 beats/min) to 857 ms (70 beats/min).

DEMAND PACEMAKERS

A *demand pacemaker* is a type of artificial cardiac pacing that allows the heart to beat normally as long as it does not fall below a preset rate. For example, if the pulse generator was set to deliver 60 impulses per minute, it would not discharge pacing impulses until the patient's own rate fell below 60 beats/min.

FIXED RATE (ASYNCHRONOUS) PACEMAKERS

A *fixed rate pacemaker* is a type of artificial cardiac pacing in which the pacemaker delivers pacing impulses at a preset rate no matter what the heart is doing on its own. For example, a fixed rate pacemaker set to deliver 60 impulses per minute would discharge impulses even if the patient's own intrinsic rate was above 60. This type of activity leads to what is called *competition* between the pacemaker and the intrinsic rhythm of the heart. The major potential problem associated with fixed rate pacing is the occurrence of a pacing impulse during the relative refractory period of the normal cardiac cycle (a type of R on T effect) that could put the patient into ventricular tachycardia or ventricular fibrillation. Fixed rate pacemakers are seldom used.

THREE LETTER ICHD CODE

The letters in the code usually refer to transvenous pacemakers inserted into the right side of the heart where most pacemakers are inserted. Left-sided and epicardial pacemakers use the same designations in the majority of situations but may also differ.

The first position or letter in the ICHD code indicates the chamber that is *paced*. There are four choices possible for pacing chambers: (1) the atrium may be paced, indicated by the letter A; (2) the ventricle may be paced, indicated by the letter V; (3) both chambers may be paced, indicated by the letter D (stands for dual); and (4) some manufacturers use the S (single chamber) designation because their pacemakers may be used for either atrial or ventricular pacing. Upon implantation, an additional letter is added (such as S-V) to indicate which of the single chambers is being paced.

The second position or letter in the ICHD code indicates the chamber that is being *sensed*. There are five choices possible here. If the atrium is the chamber that is being sensed, the letter is A. If it is the ventricle that is being sensed, the letter is V. When both chambers are sensed, the designation is D. When neither chamber is sensed, it is designated by O. Again, some manufacturers like to remain noncommittal until the pacemaker has been implanted and use the letter S as a designation.

The third letter position in the ICHD code, *mode of response*, indicates how the pacemaker generator is programmed to respond to the information it has received through the pacing catheter concerning the heart's own intrinsic activity. Depending on how it is programmed, the pulse generator responds by increasing the cardiac output to an optimal level. There are basically five designations that may be used in this third position. The most common mode of response is the inhibited mode designated by the letter I. In the inhibited mode, the pulse generator constantly monitors the heart's intrinsic beats (from either the atrium or the ventricle or both). If the pulse generator senses intrinsic beats occurring at intervals shorter than the escape interval, it is "inhibited" and does not fire. When the escape interval of the intrinsic heart beats becomes longer than the programmed escape interval (*i.e.*, when the heart rate falls below the preset rate in the pulse generator), it will start initiating impulses. This mode of inhibition is commonly referred to as the *demand mode*.

The T or *triggered* mode of response actually provides the pulse generator with the capability or option of two activities in response to intrinsic cardiac activity. First, in the triggered mode, the pulse generator is able to sense and respond to abnormal fast dysrhythmias such as supraventricular tachycardia or ventricular tachycardia. The pulse generator programmed to respond in the T mode will produce impulses at a rate faster than that of the tachy-dysrhythmia until capture occurs, then will gradually reduce the rate of the heart. The second way the pulse generator may respond in the triggered mode is by sensing normal currents in the atrium (produced by atrial depolarization). These currents, after a preset interval, then trigger the pacemaker to provide an impulse to the ventricle. This mode of response is particularly useful when the patient has a normally functioning sinus node but a complete block in the AV conduction system. The pacemaker maintains the normal sequence of cardiac activity. This type of pacemaker also responds to increased cardiac output demands caused by increased physical activity, or disease states when the sinus node increases its inherent rate. The triggered mode generally requires the use of two pacing catheters: one for the atrium and one for the ventricle.

In the dual (D) mode of response, the pulse generator has the capability to both trigger or inhibit the impulse produced. Functionally, cardiac output is maximized when the pulse generator is programmed in the atrial triggered, ventricular inhibited configuration, again requiring two pacing catheters.

In the none (O) mode, the pulse generator produces impulses at a predetermined or fixed rate, regardless of intrinsic cardiac activity. The O mode in the third position usually follows an O in the second position. For example, VOO is the designation for the fixed rate single chamber pacemaker discussed above.

The reverse (R) designation of the third position of the ICHD code indicates that the pulse generator responds to fast rhythms. The R mode is actually a type of triggered mode that responds to bursts of supraventricular tachycardia or ventricular tachycardia. This mode requires a higher energy level than most of the commonly used pacemakers are able to produce.

COMMON TYPES OF PACEMAKERS AND THEIR ICHD DESIGNATION

While a theoretical total of some 2400 variations and combinations of pacemaker pulse generators are possible with the five positions and 23 letters of the ICHD code, there are only 15 types of pulse generators currently available. Of these 15 pulse generators, there are three that are commonly used. These are described and identified below.

SINGLE CHAMBER PACEMAKERS: VVI

The single chamber pacemaker VVI is also called ventricular demand pacemaker, ventricular inhibited pacemaker, stimulus blocking pacemaker, and standby pacemaker (Fig. 12-5). The VVI (ventricle paced, ventricle sensed, inhibited mode of response) pacemaker is, by far, the most common type used. Impulses are only delivered when the patient's intrinsic heart rate falls below the rate that is programmed into the pacemaker. The inhibited mode prevents competition between the pacemaker and the patient's own rhythm.

    This type of pacemaker is used for a variety of cardiac conditions, including sinus node dysfunction, blocks of the atrial conduction system, and high-grade AV blocks (Fig. 12-6).

FIG. 12–5. VVI PACEMAKER SYSTEM.

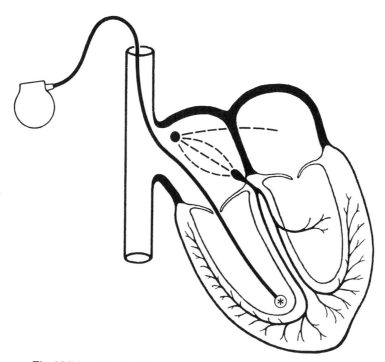

The VVI (ventricular demand) pacemaker is the most common type used. It both senses and paces the right ventricle through a transvenous catheter when the heart's intrinsic rate falls below the pacemaker's programmed rate. ⊛ = both sensing and pacing.

FIG. 12–6. AN EXAMPLE OF VVI ECG PACEMAKER PATTERN.

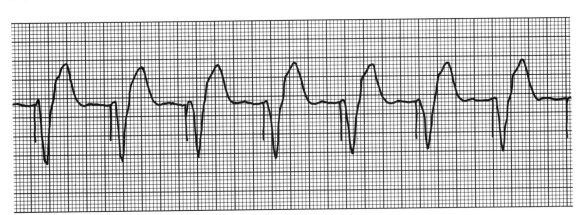

In the VVI pacemaker pattern, the pacing spike falls just before the wide QRS complex. P waves may or may not be present on the strip.

CRITERIA FOR VVI PACEMAKER

Rhythm: Regular while in the pacing rhythm. May have ectopics or fusion beats mixed with the pacing rhythm. Underlying rhythm may be irregular.

Rate: Should be for what the pacemaker is set. Generally, adult rates range between 50 and 80 beats/min. Children usually are set between 80 and 100 beats/min, depending on the size and age of the child.

Atrial Conduction: P waves may or may not be present. There should be one pacemaker spike (either positive or negative) before each QRS complex.

AV Conduction: PR interval may be present but is incidental in pacing rhythms. The pacemaker spike should precede the QRS complex by 0.04 second or less.

Ventricular Conduction: QRS complexes in the pacing rhythm are greater than 0.10 second, negative (downward) in lead MCL_1, and appear similar to the QRS complexes of a left bundle branch block pattern.

SINGLE CHAMBER PACEMAKERS: AAI

The single chamber pacemaker AAI is also called atrial demand pacemaker, atrial standby pacemaker, and atrial inhibited pacemaker (Fig. 12-7).

The AAI (atrium paced, atrium sensed, inhibited mode of response) is a type of single chamber pacemaker that controls only the atrium. For this type of pacemaker to function, the AV node and conduction system of the ventricles must be intact and functional. Impulses from the pulse generator are only delivered to the atrium when the intrinsic rate of the sinus node falls below the preset rate of the pulse generator. The inhibited mode prevents competition with normal atrial contractions.

The AAI pacemaker is used when the only problem in the conduction system

FIG. 12–7. *AAI PACEMAKER SYSTEM.*

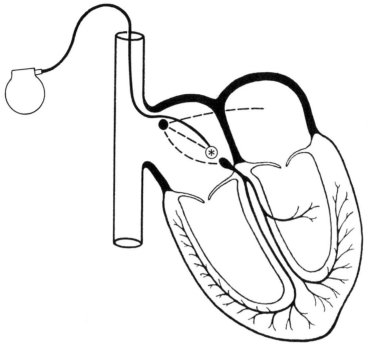

The AAI (atrial demand) pacemaker is used when there is damage to the SA node but the AV and ventricular conduction systems remain intact. It both senses and paces the right atrium through a transvenous catheter when the rate of the SA node falls below the preset rate of the pulse generator. ⊛ = both sensing and pacing.

FIG. 12–8. *AN EXAMPLE OF AAI ECG PACEMAKER PATTERN.*

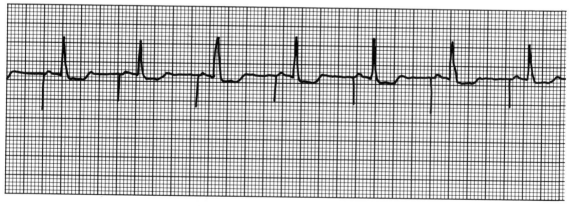

In the AAI pacemaker pattern, the pacing spike falls just before the P wave. The PR interval and QRS complexes should be normal because the impulse follows the normal conduction pathways through the AV node and ventricular conduction system.

of the heart is a nonfunctional or poorly functioning sinus node. Any abnormalities in the AV conduction system would render this pacemaker useless (Fig. 12-8).

CRITERIA FOR AAI PACEMAKER

Rhythm: Regular while in the pacing rhythm.

Rate: Rate of the pacemaker.

Atrial Conduction: Intrinsic P waves may be present when the pacemaker is in the inhibited mode. There should be one pacemaker spike just before each P wave and one P wave for each QRS complex. The P waves following the pacemaker spike may be normal in shape and size but may also be larger than normal, negative, or more peaked.

AV Conduction: PR interval: 0.12–0.20 second after the paced P wave. Consistent across the whole strip.

Ventricular Conduction: QRS complex: 0.06–0.10 second; uniform in shape across the strip.

DUAL CHAMBER PACEMAKERS: DDD

The dual chamber pacemaker DDD is also called dual chamber pacemaker fully automatic and atrial/ventricular synchronous pacemaker (Fig. 12-9).

The DDD (both atrium and ventricle paced, both atrium and ventricle sensed, both inhibited and triggered mode of response, or combinations thereof) is a type of dual chamber pacemaker that attempts to maintain the atrial-ventricular synchronous contractions of the chambers of the heart, despite a variety of potential conduction problems. The DDD pacemaker generator uses advanced electronic technology to maintain optimal cardiac output.

This type of pacemaker requires two pacing catheters. The atrial catheter may be difficult to insert and remain in the atrium due to the normal tendency of the blood flow from the atria into the ventricles. The DDD has the capability of switching modes to meet the needs of the heart. The modes of function range from the simple VVI pacemaker, where only the ventricle is sensed and paced, to the more complex DVI pacemaker, where both the atrium and ventricle are sensed and paced, producing spikes before both the P waves and the QRS complexes. Other possible modes that the DDD pacemaker may function in include the following: VVI, AOO, VOO, DOO, DAD, VAT, AAI, AAT, VVT, VAT, and VDD.

Although the DDD pacemaker may be used for almost any conduction problem, it is usually reserved for the more severe conditions because of its increased cost and difficulty of insertion. A DDD pulse generator may cost as much as ten times more than a VVI. The DDD pacemaker may not be appropriate for slow atrial fibrillation or atrial flutter type rhythms.

It is difficult to identify just one pattern for a DDD pacemaker generator because it can easily and quickly switch modes as the conduction problems in the heart change. The pattern included here is the one found if the DDD pulse

FIG. 12–9. DDD PACEMAKER SYSTEM.

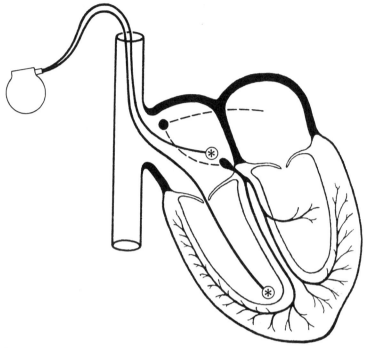

The DDD (fully automatic) pacemaker is the most advanced of all the pacemaker systems. It requires two pacing catheters: one for the atrium and one for the ventricles. It can function as a variety of other types of pacemakers, but its main goal is to maintain the atrial-ventricular sequence of cardiac contraction. When functioning as a fully DDD pacemaker, there will be pacing spikes before both the P waves and QRS complexes. ⊛ = both sensing and pacing.

FIG. 12–10. AN EXAMPLE OF DDD ECG PACEMAKER PATTERN.

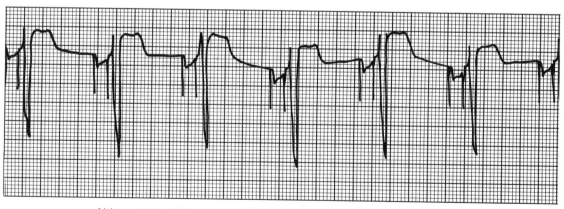

Although the DDD pacmaker may also produce other types of ECG patterns, the most common pattern is that of the dual pacemaker spikes produced by both the atrial and the ventricular catheters.

generator is functioning in its most advanced mode, with both chambers being sensed and paced (Fig. 12-10).

CRITERIA FOR DDD PACEMAKER

Rhythm: Regular when in the pacing mode.

Rate: Should be the same as the predetermined rate of the pacemaker. One difficulty in determining the rate of this type of pacemaker is that DDD pulse generators may permit a rate slower than what it is programmed for if the pattern producing the rate is normal, that is, has a normal P wave followed by a normal PR interval and normal QRS complex. This capability of DDD pulse generators is called *hysteresis* and may lead to the conclusion that the generator is not functioning properly. There is an absolute lower rate limit for DDD pulse generators below which it will not permit a rate to go, no matter what the configuration of the cardiac cycle.

Atrial Conduction: Each P wave should have a pacemaker spike in front of it. May be normal or abnormal in shape.

AV Conduction: PR interval should be what is programmed into the pacemaker. The PR interval in a dual chamber pacemaker is called the *AV interval* and is the distance between the atrial pacemaker spike and the ventricular spike. The AV interval ranges between 0.12 and 0.25 second with an average of 0.16 second.

Ventricular Conduction: QRS complex is greater than 0.10 second, negatively deflected in lead MCL$_1$, and appears similar to a left bundle branch block pattern. It should follow the pacing spike.

CAUSES FOR PACEMAKER FAILURE

There are three major causes for pacemaker failure, arising from the malfunction of the three major components of the pacemaker system. Probably the most common cause for pacemakers to malfunction is dislocation of the pacing catheter from its normal position in the apex of the right ventricle. Normally, patients who have just had a permanent pacemaker implanted are kept on bedrest for 12–24 hours after the procedure to allow the pacing catheter to lodge itself securely in the right ventricle. Pacing catheters may also become loosened or detached from the pulse generator or may actually fracture internally. These malfunctions of the pacemaker catheter lead to conditions of noncapture or nonpacing.

Malfunctions of the pacemaker generator may involve the electronic circuits or the batteries. If the electronic circuits fail, they usually do so within the first 24 hours after implantation, although this is by no means an absolute rule. The conditions produced by circuit failure may range from a simple nonpacing state to a condition called *runaway pacemaker* where the pacemaker begins firing at a very rapid rate. Battery failure can also occur at any point in the pacemaker generator's life. The modern pacemaker batteries are designed to last some 10 to 15 years, depending on how much actual pacing the generator does. If the generator functions mostly in the standby mode, the batteries last longer. Many of the modern pacemakers are programmed to begin fixed rate pacing of 100 beats/min when the batteries start to weaken. If the generator is not replaced with a new one, battery failure eventually leads to total pacemaker failure.

SIGNS AND SYMPTOMS OF PACEMAKER FAILURE

Although there are a few unique symptoms associated with pacemaker failure, generally, the signs and symptoms observed are the symptoms of low cardiac output that follow slow rhythms. These include the dizziness, weakness, and syncope from poor circulation to the brain, as well as the cardiac symptoms of shortness of breath, chest pain and pressure, low blood pressure, and a slow, irregular pulse.

The pulse is a particularly sensitive indicator of pacemaker problems, especially with single chamber pacemakers. Patients need to be taught how to take their pulses, and the rate setting of their pacemakers. A pulse rate consistently 5–10 beats or more below what the pulse generator is set for indicates problems with the generator. A slow irregular pulse is also an indication of problems.

One symptom that is unique and associated with problematic pacemakers is hiccups. Hiccups in nonpacemaker patients are often caused by spasms of the diaphragm caused by irritation from the gastrointestinal system. In patients who have pacemakers, occasionally the pacing catheter burrows its way through the myocardium and pericardium and comes in contact with the diaphragm. If a pacing impulse is delivered while the pacemaker wire is in contact with the diaphragm, a hiccup will occur. Pacemaker patients who have very frequent hiccups or hiccups at regular intervals and rates that are the same as the pacemaker rate require further evaluation for this problem.

TREATMENT FOR PACEMAKER FAILURE

Because pacemaker failure allows the symptomatology and reduced cardiac output from the underlying condition to reoccur, the goal of treatment is to reverse the underlying condition. Most pacemakers are inserted because of slow dysrhythmias such as sinus bradycardia, sinus arrest, and complete heart block. The specific treatments for these dysrhythmias are appropriate for pacemaker failure. Generally, the use of atropine sulfate or other medications to maintain the heart rate is effective for short time periods. The permanent pacemaker may need to be turned off. This task can be accomplished by placing a very strong magnet over the chest wall of the patient in the area of the permanent generator. A temporary pacemaker may need to be inserted and maintained for a short time until a new permanent generator and/or catheter can be inserted.

ABNORMAL PACEMAKER PATTERNS (PACEMAKER DYSRHYTHMIAS)

The following abnormal pacemaker patterns are limited to malfunctions of the single chamber, ventricular pacemaker systems (VVI). This limited presentation is necessary because of the complexity and many potential arrangements of pacemaker spikes and wave forms that dual chamber pacemaker systems are capable of producing.

FIG. 12–11. AN EXAMPLE OF PACEMAKER FUSION BEATS.

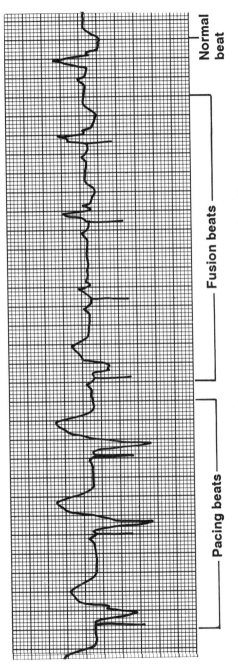

Pacemaker fusion beats occur when an intrinsic beat occurs at the same time the pacemaker is delivering an impulse. Fusion beats have pacemaker spikes in front of them but look like neither the pacing beats nor the patient's normal beats. Often, they are smaller than either.

PACEMAKER FUSION BEAT

A pacemaker fusion beat (Fig. 12-11) occurs when an intrinsic impulse begins to depolarize the ventricle at the same time the pacemaker initiates an impulse. This type of electrical activity produces a QRS complex that looks neither like the patient's normal nonpacing beats nor like the pacing beats. There is a pacing spike in front of the fusion beat and it is often much smaller in size than the other beats. Although there is little circulation produced by fusion beats, a rare or isolated fusion beat is common in pacemaker rhythms and does not indicate a major problem. If the intrinsic heart rate of the patient is close to the rate of the pacemaker, then there may be frequent fusion beats. Because this type of pattern may reduce cardiac output greatly and has an increased risk for a R on T situation, the rate of the pacemaker needs to be reduced to a point where the fusion beats stop.

NONCAPTURE PACING PATTERN

Noncapture pacing patterns (Fig. 12-12) occur when the impulse produced by the pulse generator fails to produce a paced QRS complex. The noncapture pacemaker pattern is the second most common type of abnormal pacing pattern,

FIG. 12–12. AN EXAMPLE OF NONCAPTURE PACEMAKER.

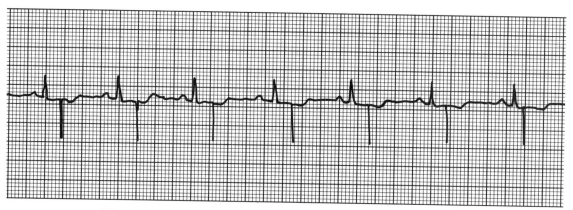

When a pacemaker is in a state of noncapture, the pacemaker spikes will fall randomly across the strip without regard to the patient's own intrinsic beats. A state of non-sensing always accompanies a noncapture pacemaker although it is possible to have a non-sensing pacemaker that still captures.

after fusion beats. The causes for noncapture include dislodgment of the pacing catheter from the ventricular myocardium, a threshold setting that is too low, or increased fibrin formation on the catheter tip. The noncapture pacemaker is recognized on the ECG strip as pacing spikes that have no QRS complexes after them. Treatment for noncapture pacing may be as simple as increasing the MA output of the pacemaker or as complicated as repositioning the catheter or replacing the generator.

An occasional noncapture occurrence is called *intermittent capture* or *intermittent pacing*. This condition is less serious than a permanent state of noncapture, and may require no treatment other than bedrest for a short time.

NON-SENSING PACEMAKER PATTERN

A non-sensing pacemaker pattern (undersensing pacemaker pattern) (Fig. 12-13) occurs when the pacemaker fails to sense the heart's intrinsic beats. This pattern appears as pacemaker spikes, and paced QRS complexes that are close to the patient's intrinsic QRS complexes, that is, less than the established escape interval. The primary problem with this pattern is its potential for competition and R on T situations.

FIG. 12–13. *AN EXAMPLE OF NON-SENSING PACEMAKER.*

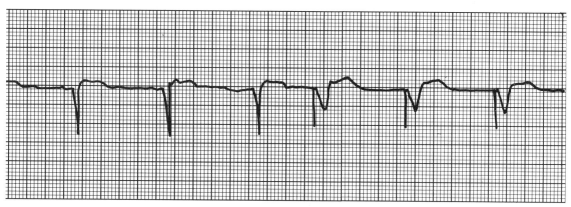

In the non-sensing pacemaker, the pacemaker fails to "see" the previous intrinsic beat and fires before its present escape interval.

Common causes for non-sensing or undersensing include pacemaker catheter dislodgment; poor catheter connection with the pulse generator; improper catheter placement; and a malfunctioning generator. In some types of pulse generators, the sensitivity setting is adjustable and may need to be increased. Otherwise, treatment requires either catheter manipulation or replacement, or generator replacement.

Oversensing is an abnormal condition that occurs when the pacemaker senses and misidentifies repolarization of the ventricles (the T wave of the intrinsic QRS complex) as the QRS complex. Oversensing appears as pacing spikes and paced QRS complexes that come after the preset escape interval of the pacemaker. In pacemakers with an adjustable sensitivity, decreasing this setting treats the problem effectively.

TOTAL PACEMAKER FAILURE

Total pacemaker failure (Fig. 12-14) occurs when the pacemaker completely stops initiating impulses to depolarize the ventricles. Total pacemaker failure is observed as a pattern where there are no pacemaker spikes and no paced QRS complexes. The underlying condition for which the pacemaker was initially inserted reappears and may be seen as asystole, slow bradycardia, complete heart block, and so on. Pacemaker failure may be permanent or intermittent. Intermittent pacemaker failure may lead to transient episodes of syncope. Total pacemaker failure is usually treated as an emergency situation, depending on the symptomatology the patient is showing.

FIG. 12–14. AN EXAMPLE OF TOTAL PACEMAKER FAILURE.

Lead MCL₆

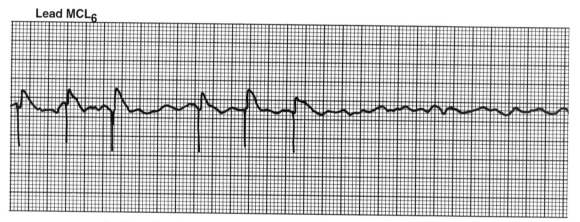

In this strip, the complexes after the spikes are in a positive direction because it is a lead MCL₆. When a pacemaker fails completely, the patient's rhythm returns to what it was before the pacemaker was inserted—in this case, ventricular fibrillation.

PRACTICE ECG STRIPS FOR CHAPTER 12

Directions. On the following practice ECG strips, analyze each strip according to its rhythm, rate, atrial conduction, AV conduction, and ventricular conduction. Arrive at an interpretation of the strip based upon the analysis and criteria for abnormal pacemaker patterns as learned in this chapter. (See Appendix II for interpretations.)

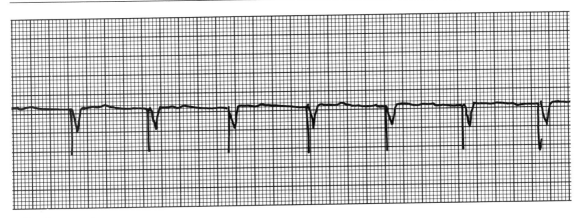

12–1

RHYTHM: _____

RATE: _____

ATRIAL CONDUCTION: _____

_____

AV CONDUCTION: _____

VENTRICULAR CONDUCTION: _____

INTERPRETATION: _____

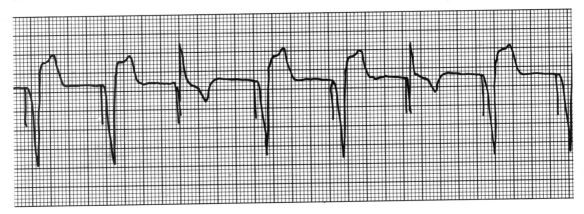

12–2

RHYTHM: _____

RATE: _____

ATRIAL CONDUCTION: _____

_____

AV CONDUCTION: _____

VENTRICULAR CONDUCTION: _____

INTERPRETATION: _____

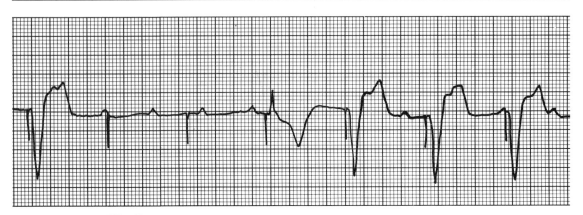

12–3

RHYTHM: _____

RATE: _____

ATRIAL CONDUCTION: _____

_____

AV CONDUCTION: _____

VENTRICULAR CONDUCTION: _____

INTERPRETATION: _____

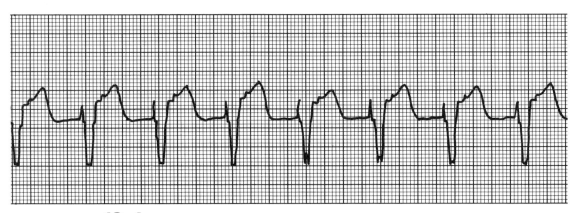

12–4

RHYTHM: _____

RATE: _____

ATRIAL CONDUCTION: _____

_____

AV CONDUCTION: _____

VENTRICULAR CONDUCTION: _____

INTERPRETATION: _____

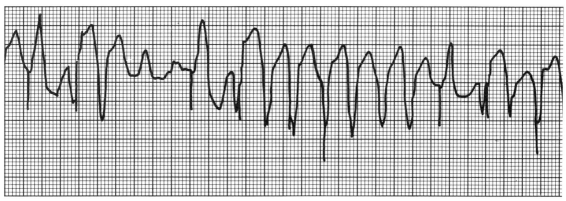

12–5
RHYTHM: _____

RATE: _____

ATRIAL CONDUCTION: _____

_____

AV CONDUCTION: _____

VENTRICULAR CONDUCTION: _____

INTERPRETATION: _____

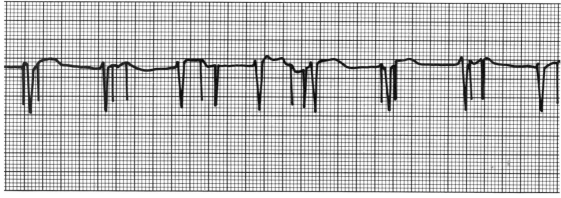

12–6
RHYTHM: _____

RATE: _____

ATRIAL CONDUCTION: _____

_____

AV CONDUCTION: _____

VENTRICULAR CONDUCTION: _____

INTERPRETATION: _____

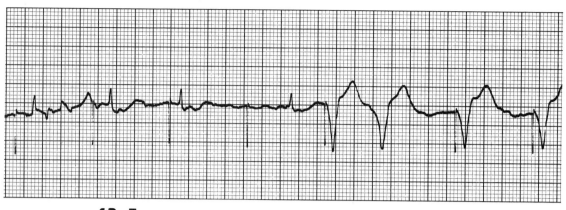

12–7

RHYTHM: _____

RATE: _____

ATRIAL CONDUCTION: _____

_____

AV CONDUCTION: _____

VENTRICULAR CONDUCTION: _____

INTERPRETATION: _____

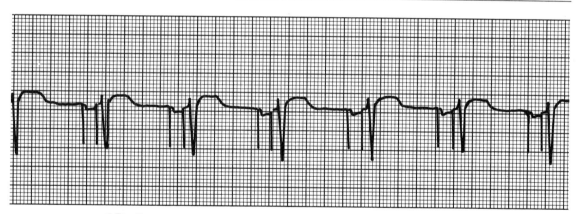

12–8

RHYTHM: _____

RATE: _____

ATRIAL CONDUCTION: _____

_____

AV CONDUCTION: _____

VENTRICULAR CONDUCTION: _____

INTERPRETATION: _____

GENERAL PRACTICE STRIPS

DIRECTIONS

This appendix is composed completely of ECG practice strips. Analyze each ECG strip and then arrive at an interpretation of that strip based on the criteria learned throughout the rest of the book. Many of these strips contain multiple dysrhythmias; make sure to note each dysrhythmia in the interpretation. There may be some room for variations in interpretation on some of the ECG strips. (See interpretations at end of Appendix I.)

App. 1–1

RHYTHM: _____

RATE: _____

ATRIAL CONDUCTION: _____

_____

AV CONDUCTION: _____

VENTRICULAR CONDUCTION: _____

INTERPRETATION: _____

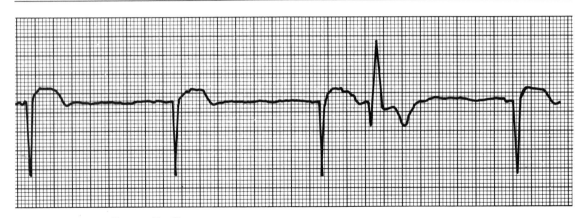

App. 1–2

RHYTHM: _____

RATE: _____

ATRIAL CONDUCTION: _____

_____

AV CONDUCTION: _____

VENTRICULAR CONDUCTION: _____

INTERPRETATION: _____

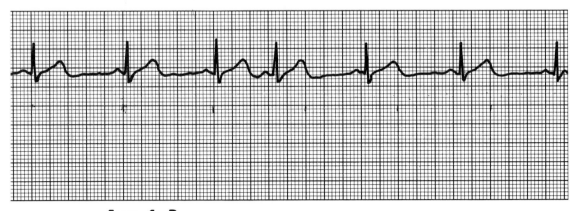

App. 1–3

RHYTHM: _____

RATE: _____

ATRIAL CONDUCTION: _____

_____

AV CONDUCTION: _____

VENTRICULAR CONDUCTION: _____

INTERPRETATION: _____

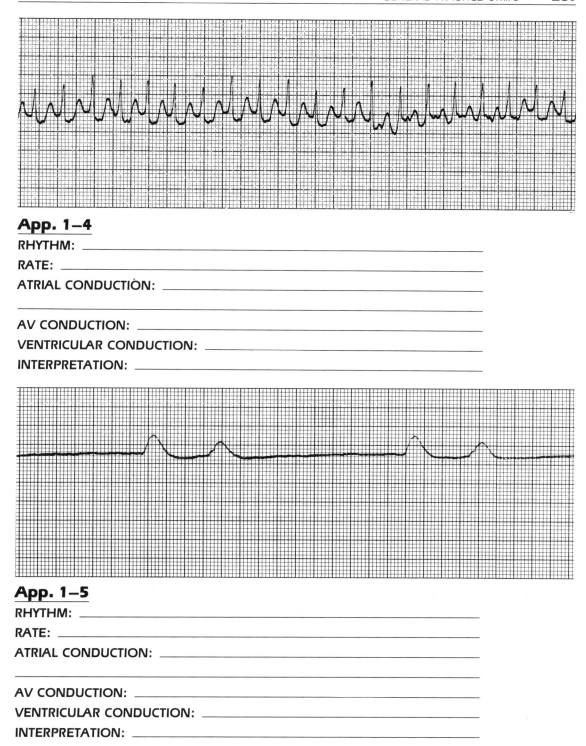

App. 1–4

RHYTHM: _____

RATE: _____

ATRIAL CONDUCTIÓN: _____

_____

AV CONDUCTION: _____

VENTRICULAR CONDUCTION: _____

INTERPRETATION: _____

App. 1–5

RHYTHM: _____

RATE: _____

ATRIAL CONDUCTION: _____

_____

AV CONDUCTION: _____

VENTRICULAR CONDUCTION: _____

INTERPRETATION: _____

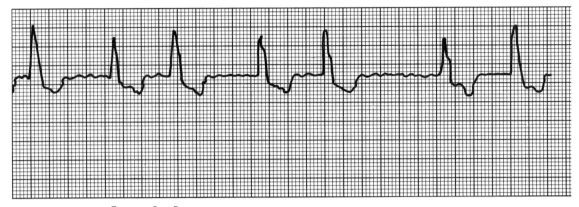

App. 1–6

RHYTHM: _____

RATE: _____

ATRIAL CONDUCTION: _____

_____

AV CONDUCTION: _____

VENTRICULAR CONDUCTION: _____

INTERPRETATION: _____

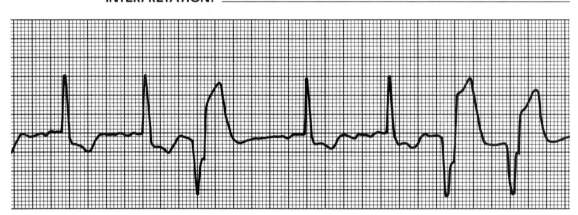

App. 1–7

RHYTHM: _____

RATE: _____

ATRIAL CONDUCTION: _____

_____

AV CONDUCTION: _____

VENTRICULAR CONDUCTION: _____

INTERPRETATION: _____

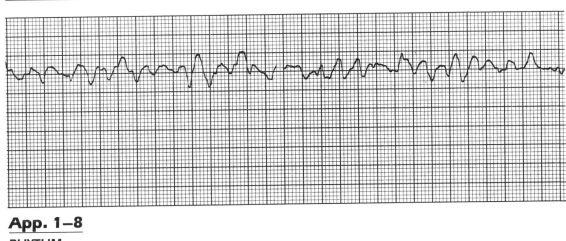

App. 1–8

RHYTHM: _____

RATE: _____

ATRIAL CONDUCTION: _____

_____

AV CONDUCTION: _____

VENTRICULAR CONDUCTION: _____

INTERPRETATION: _____

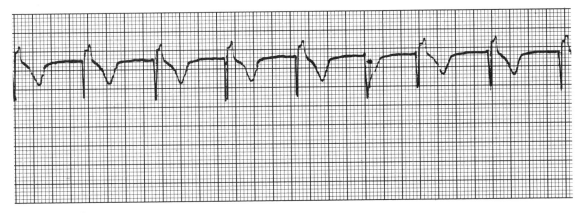

App. 1–9

RHYTHM: _____

RATE: _____

ATRIAL CONDUCTION: _____

_____

AV CONDUCTION: _____

VENTRICULAR CONDUCTION: _____

INTERPRETATION: _____

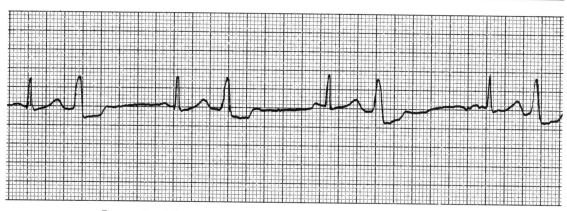

App. 1–10

RHYTHM: _____

RATE: _____

ATRIAL CONDUCTION: _____

_____

AV CONDUCTION: _____

VENTRICULAR CONDUCTION: _____

INTERPRETATION: _____

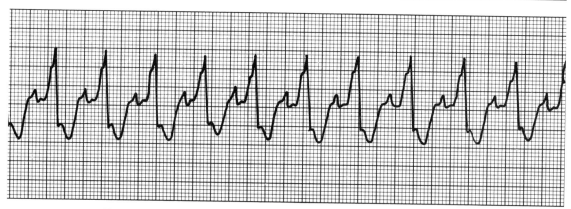

App. 1–11

RHYTHM: _____

RATE: _____

ATRIAL CONDUCTION: _____

_____

AV CONDUCTION: _____

VENTRICULAR CONDUCTION: _____

INTERPRETATION: _____

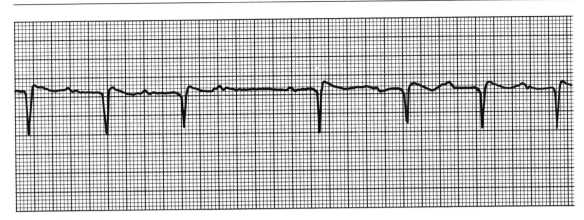

App. 1–12

RHYTHM: _____

RATE: _____

ATRIAL CONDUCTION: _____

_____

AV CONDUCTION: _____

VENTRICULAR CONDUCTION: _____

INTERPRETATION: _____

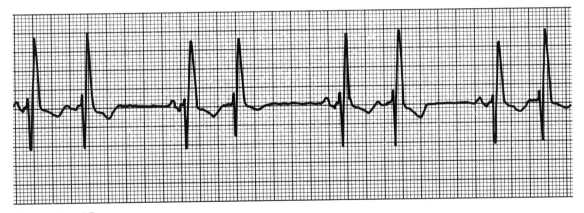

App. 1–13

RHYTHM: _____

RATE: _____

ATRIAL CONDUCTION: _____

_____

AV CONDUCTION: _____

VENTRICULAR CONDUCTION: _____

INTERPRETATION: _____

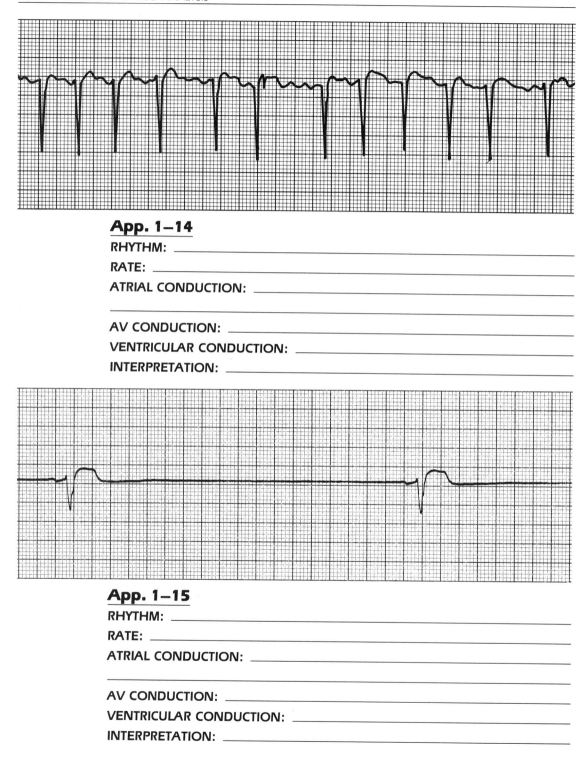

App. 1–14

RHYTHM: _____

RATE: _____

ATRIAL CONDUCTION: _____

_____

AV CONDUCTION: _____

VENTRICULAR CONDUCTION: _____

INTERPRETATION: _____

App. 1–15

RHYTHM: _____

RATE: _____

ATRIAL CONDUCTION: _____

_____

AV CONDUCTION: _____

VENTRICULAR CONDUCTION: _____

INTERPRETATION: _____

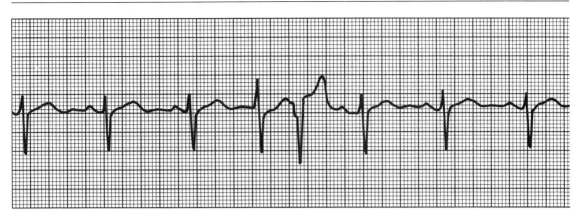

App. 1–16

RHYTHM: _____

RATE: _____

ATRIAL CONDUCTION: _____

_____

AV CONDUCTION: _____

VENTRICULAR CONDUCTION: _____

INTERPRETATION: _____

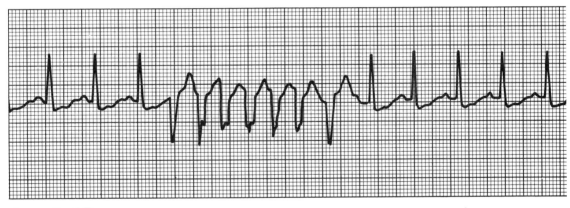

App. 1–17

RHYTHM: _____

RATE: _____

ATRIAL CONDUCTION: _____

_____

AV CONDUCTION: _____

VENTRICULAR CONDUCTION: _____

INTERPRETATION: _____

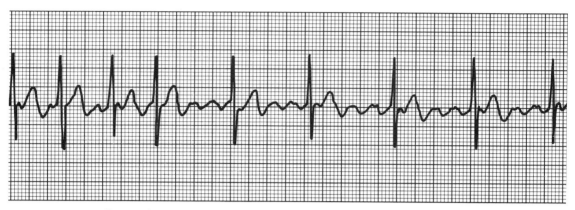

App. 1–18

RHYTHM: _____

RATE: _____

ATRIAL CONDUCTION: _____

_____

AV CONDUCTION: _____

VENTRICULAR CONDUCTION: _____

INTERPRETATION: _____

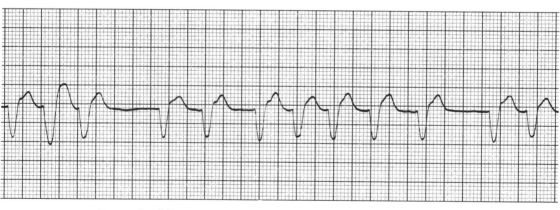

App. 1–19

RHYTHM: _____

RATE: _____

ATRIAL CONDUCTION: _____

_____

AV CONDUCTION: _____

VENTRICULAR CONDUCTION: _____

INTERPRETATION: _____

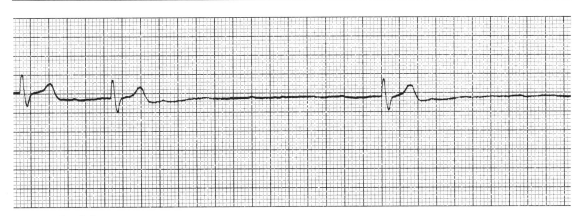

App. 1–20

RHYTHM: _____

RATE: _____

ATRIAL CONDUCTION: _____

_____

AV CONDUCTION: _____

VENTRICULAR CONDUCTION: _____

INTERPRETATION: _____

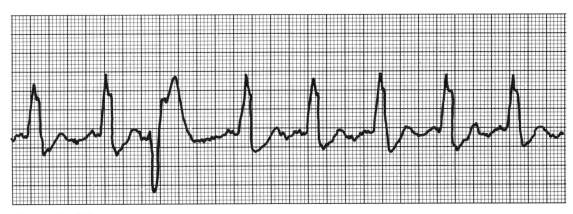

App. 1–21

RHYTHM: _____

RATE: _____

ATRIAL CONDUCTION: _____

_____

AV CONDUCTION: _____

VENTRICULAR CONDUCTION: _____

INTERPRETATION: _____

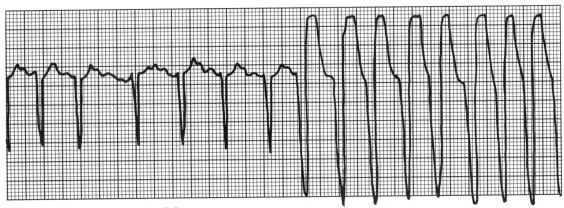

App. 1–22

RHYTHM: _____

RATE: _____

ATRIAL CONDUCTION: _____

_____

AV CONDUCTION: _____

VENTRICULAR CONDUCTION: _____

INTERPRETATION: _____

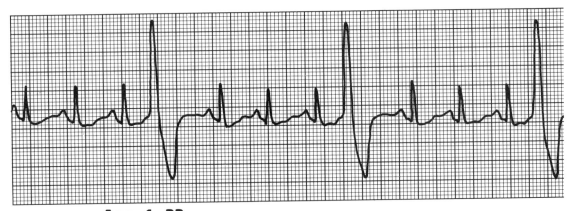

App. 1–23

RHYTHM: _____

RATE: _____

ATRIAL CONDUCTION: _____

_____

AV CONDUCTION: _____

VENTRICULAR CONDUCTION: _____

INTERPRETATION: _____

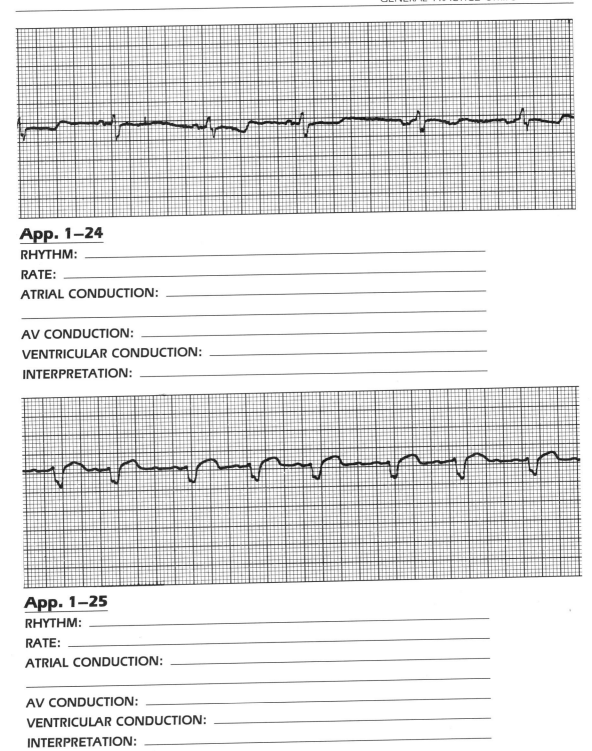

App. 1–24

RHYTHM: ⸻

RATE: ⸻

ATRIAL CONDUCTION: ⸻
⸻

AV CONDUCTION: ⸻

VENTRICULAR CONDUCTION: ⸻

INTERPRETATION: ⸻

App. 1–25

RHYTHM: ⸻

RATE: ⸻

ATRIAL CONDUCTION: ⸻
⸻

AV CONDUCTION: ⸻

VENTRICULAR CONDUCTION: ⸻

INTERPRETATION: ⸻

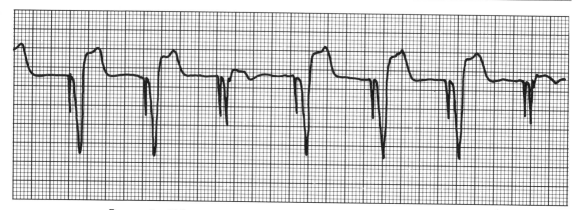

App. 1–26

RHYTHM: _____

RATE: _____

ATRIAL CONDUCTION: _____

_____

AV CONDUCTION: _____

VENTRICULAR CONDUCTION: _____

INTERPRETATION: _____

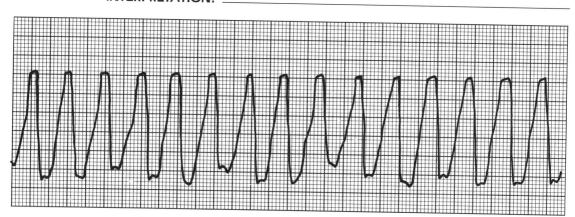

App. 1–27

RHYTHM: _____

RATE: _____

ATRIAL CONDUCTION: _____

_____

AV CONDUCTION: _____

VENTRICULAR CONDUCTION: _____

INTERPRETATION: _____

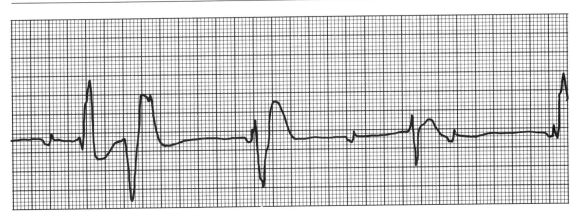

App. 1–28

RHYTHM: _____

RATE: _____

ATRIAL CONDUCTION: _____

_____

AV CONDUCTION: _____

VENTRICULAR CONDUCTION: _____

INTERPRETATION: _____

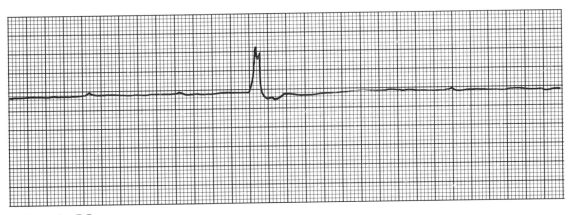

App. 1–29

RHYTHM: _____

RATE: _____

ATRIAL CONDUCTION: _____

_____

AV CONDUCTION: _____

VENTRICULAR CONDUCTION: _____

INTERPRETATION: _____

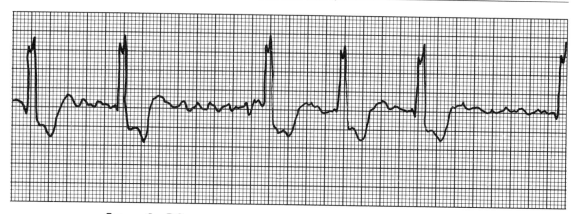

App. 1–30

RHYTHM: _____

RATE: _____

ATRIAL CONDUCTION: _____

_____

AV CONDUCTION: _____

VENTRICULAR CONDUCTION: _____

INTERPRETATION: _____

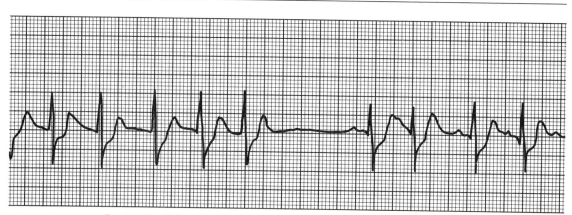

App. 1–31

RHYTHM: _____

RATE: _____

ATRIAL CONDUCTION: _____

_____

AV CONDUCTION: _____

VENTRICULAR CONDUCTION: _____

INTERPRETATION: _____

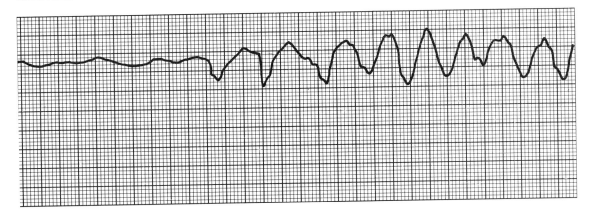

App. 1–32

RHYTHM: _____

RATE: _____

ATRIAL CONDUCTION: _____

_____

AV CONDUCTION: _____

VENTRICULAR CONDUCTION: _____

INTERPRETATION: _____

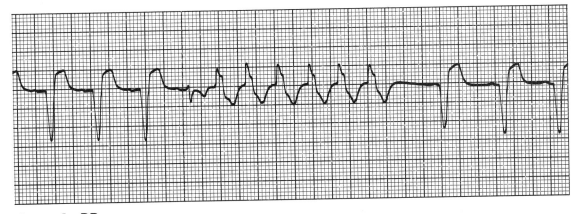

App. 1–33

RHYTHM: _____

RATE: _____

ATRIAL CONDUCTION: _____

_____

AV CONDUCTION: _____

VENTRICULAR CONDUCTION: _____

INTERPRETATION: _____

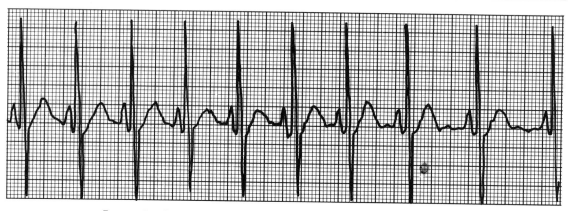

App. 1–34

RHYTHM: _____

RATE: _____

ATRIAL CONDUCTION: _____

_____

AV CONDUCTION: _____

VENTRICULAR CONDUCTION: _____

INTERPRETATION: _____

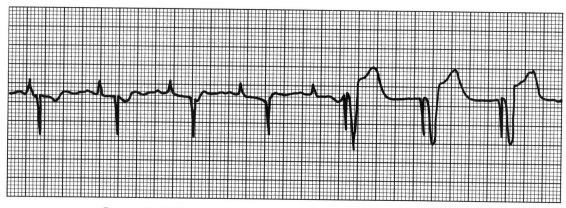

App. 1–35

RHYTHM: _____

RATE: _____

ATRIAL CONDUCTION: _____

_____

AV CONDUCTION: _____

VENTRICULAR CONDUCTION: _____

INTERPRETATION: _____

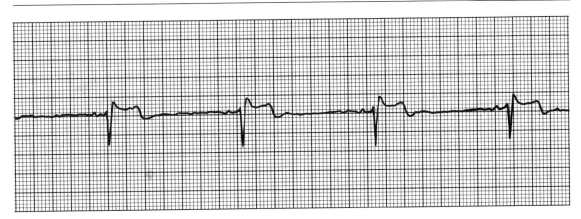

App. 1–36

RHYTHM: _____

RATE: _____

ATRIAL CONDUCTION: _____
_____

AV CONDUCTION: _____

VENTRICULAR CONDUCTION: _____

INTERPRETATION: _____

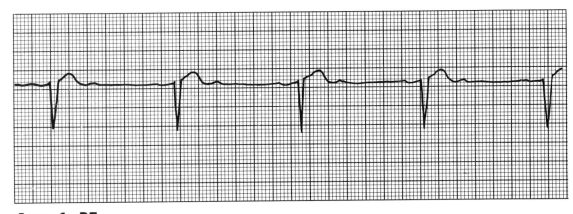

App. 1–37

RHYTHM: _____

RATE: _____

ATRIAL CONDUCTION: _____
_____

AV CONDUCTION: _____

VENTRICULAR CONDUCTION: _____

INTERPRETATION: _____

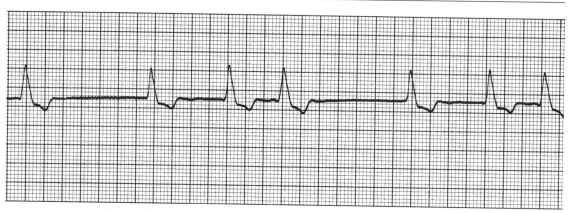

App. 1–38

RHYTHM: _____

RATE: _____

ATRIAL CONDUCTION: _____

_____

AV CONDUCTION: _____

VENTRICULAR CONDUCTION: _____

INTERPRETATION: _____

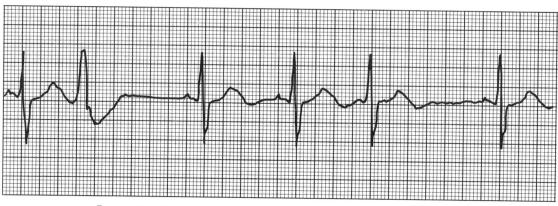

App. 1–39

RHYTHM: _____

RATE: _____

ATRIAL CONDUCTION: _____

_____

AV CONDUCTION: _____

VENTRICULAR CONDUCTION: _____

INTERPRETATION: _____

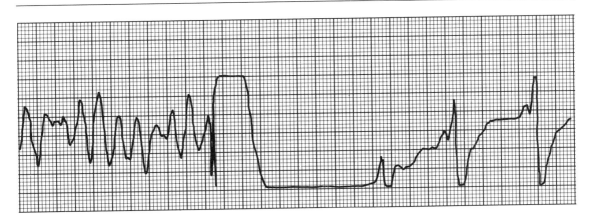

App. 1–40

RHYTHM: _____

RATE: _____

ATRIAL CONDUCTION: _____

_____

AV CONDUCTION: _____

VENTRICULAR CONDUCTION: _____

INTERPRETATION: _____

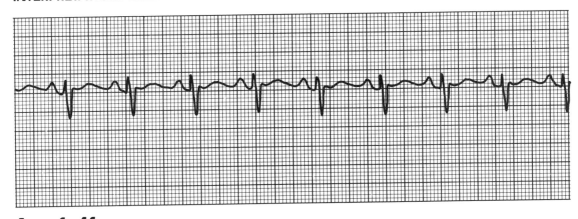

App. 1–41

RHYTHM: _____

RATE: _____

ATRIAL CONDUCTION: _____

_____

AV CONDUCTION: _____

VENTRICULAR CONDUCTION: _____

INTERPRETATION: _____

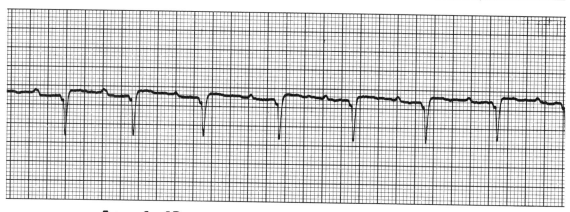

App. 1–42

RHYTHM: _____

RATE: _____

ATRIAL CONDUCTION: _____

_____

AV CONDUCTION: _____

VENTRICULAR CONDUCTION: _____

INTERPRETATION: _____

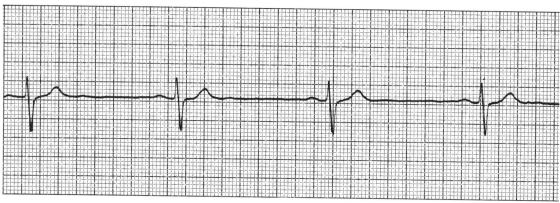

App. 1–43

RHYTHM: _____

RATE: _____

ATRIAL CONDUCTION: _____

_____

AV CONDUCTION: _____

VENTRICULAR CONDUCTION: _____

INTERPRETATION: _____

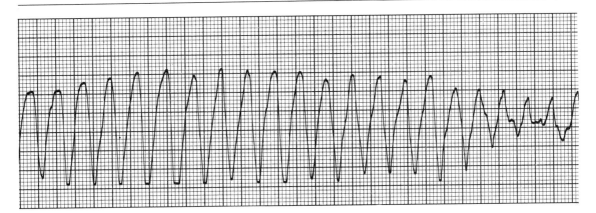

App. 1–44

RHYTHM: _____

RATE: _____

ATRIAL CONDUCTION: _____

_____

AV CONDUCTION: _____

VENTRICULAR CONDUCTION: _____

INTERPRETATION: _____

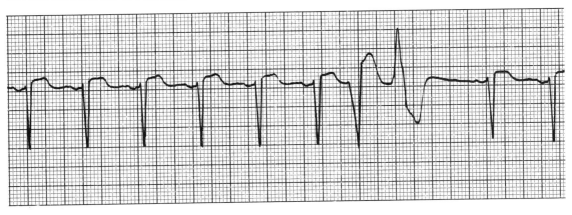

App. 1–45

RHYTHM: _____

RATE: _____

ATRIAL CONDUCTION: _____

_____

AV CONDUCTION: _____

VENTRICULAR CONDUCTION: _____

INTERPRETATION: _____

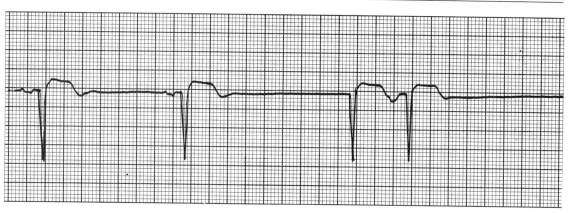

App. 1–46

RHYTHM: _____

RATE: _____

ATRIAL CONDUCTION: _____

_____

AV CONDUCTION: _____

VENTRICULAR CONDUCTION: _____

INTERPRETATION: _____

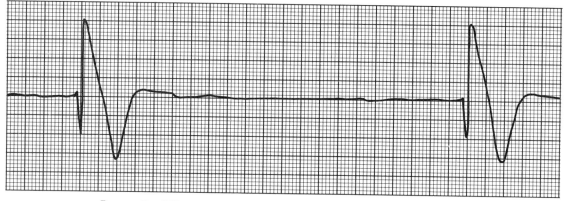

App. 1–47

RHYTHM: _____

RATE: _____

ATRIAL CONDUCTION: _____

_____

AV CONDUCTION: _____

VENTRICULAR CONDUCTION: _____

INTERPRETATION: _____

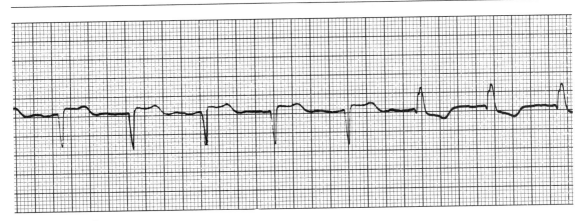

App. 1–48

RHYTHM: _____

RATE: _____

ATRIAL CONDUCTION: _____

_____

AV CONDUCTION: _____

VENTRICULAR CONDUCTION: _____

INTERPRETATION: _____

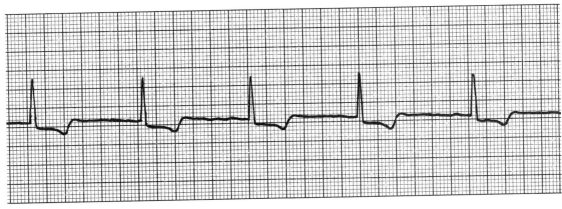

App. 1–49

RHYTHM: _____

RATE: _____

ATRIAL CONDUCTION: _____

_____

AV CONDUCTION: _____

VENTRICULAR CONDUCTION: _____

INTERPRETATION: _____

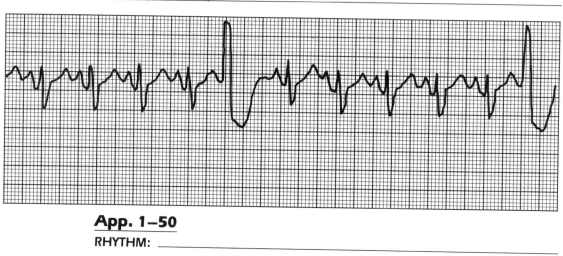

App. 1–50

RHYTHM: _____

RATE: _____

ATRIAL CONDUCTION: _____

_____

AV CONDUCTION: _____

VENTRICULAR CONDUCTION: _____

INTERPRETATION: _____

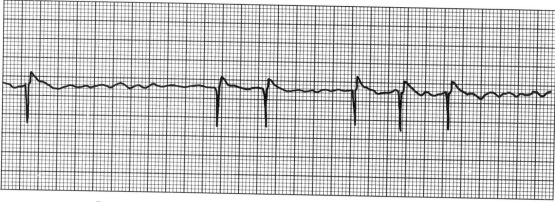

App. 1–51

RHYTHM: _____

RATE: _____

ATRIAL CONDUCTION: _____

_____

AV CONDUCTION: _____

VENTRICULAR CONDUCTION: _____

INTERPRETATION: _____

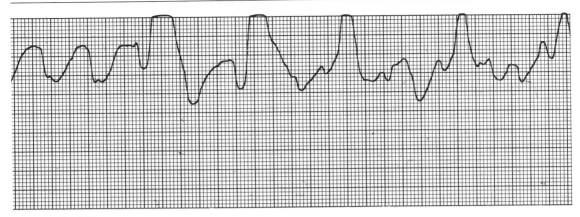

App. 1–52

RHYTHM: _____

RATE: _____

ATRIAL CONDUCTION: _____

_____

AV CONDUCTION: _____

VENTRICULAR CONDUCTION: _____

INTERPRETATION: _____

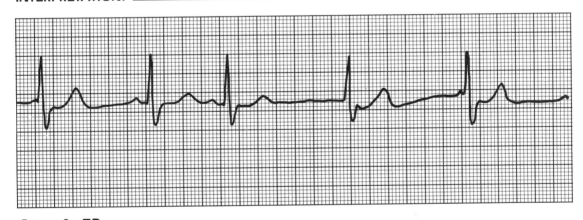

App. 1–53

RHYTHM: _____

RATE: _____

ATRIAL CONDUCTION: _____

_____

AV CONDUCTION: _____

VENTRICULAR CONDUCTION: _____

INTERPRETATION: _____

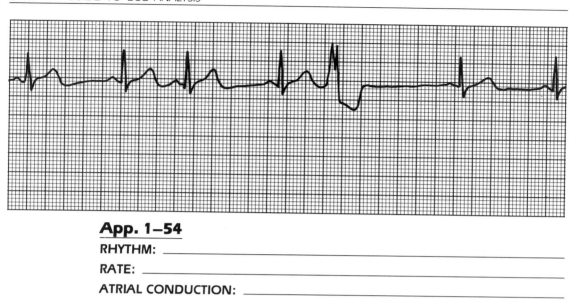

App. 1–54

RHYTHM: _____

RATE: _____

ATRIAL CONDUCTION: _____

_____

AV CONDUCTION: _____

VENTRICULAR CONDUCTION: _____

INTERPRETATION: _____

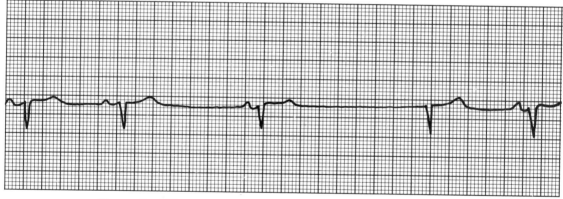

App. 1–55

RHYTHM: _____

RATE: _____

ATRIAL CONDUCTION: _____

_____

AV CONDUCTION: _____

VENTRICULAR CONDUCTION: _____

INTERPRETATION: _____

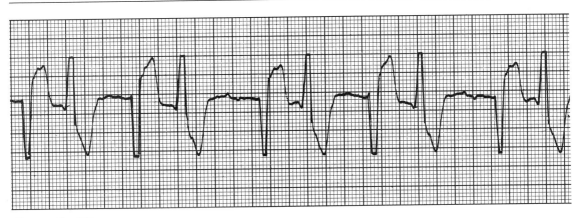

App. 1–56

RHYTHM: _____

RATE: _____

ATRIAL CONDUCTION: _____

_____

AV CONDUCTION: _____

VENTRICULAR CONDUCTION: _____

INTERPRETATION: _____

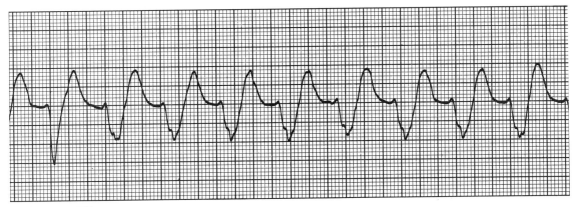

App. 1–57

RHYTHM: _____

RATE: _____

ATRIAL CONDUCTION: _____

_____

AV CONDUCTION: _____

VENTRICULAR CONDUCTION: _____

INTERPRETATION: _____

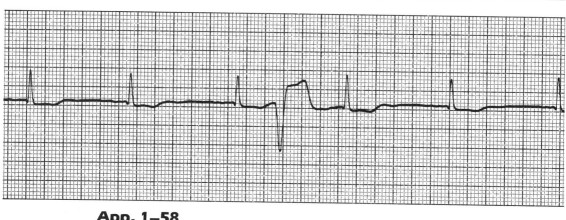

App. 1–58

RHYTHM: _____

RATE: _____

ATRIAL CONDUCTION: _____

_____

AV CONDUCTION: _____

VENTRICULAR CONDUCTION: _____

INTERPRETATION: _____

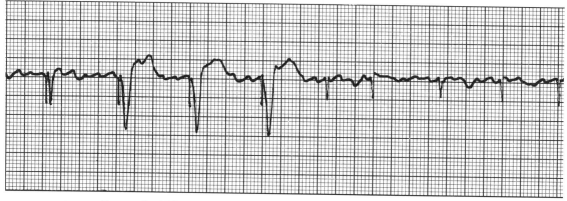

App. 1–59

RHYTHM: _____

RATE: _____

ATRIAL CONDUCTION: _____

_____

AV CONDUCTION: _____

VENTRICULAR CONDUCTION: _____

INTERPRETATION: _____

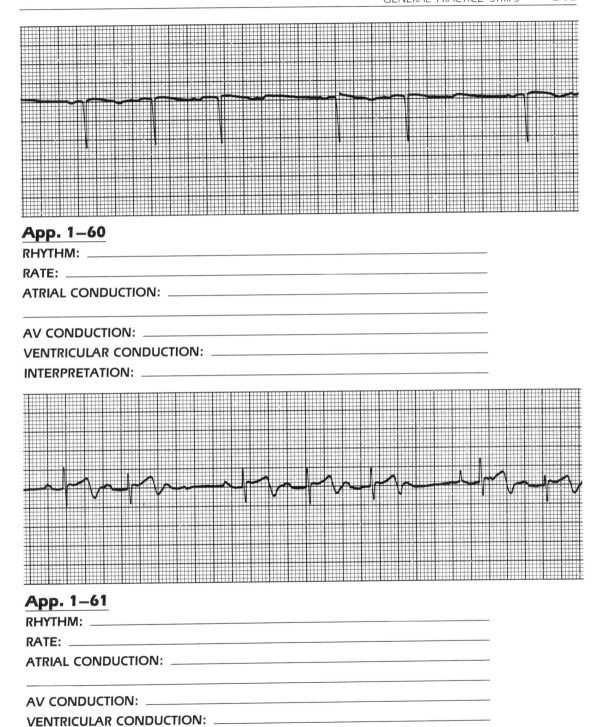

App. 1–60

RHYTHM: _____

RATE: _____

ATRIAL CONDUCTION: _____

AV CONDUCTION: _____

VENTRICULAR CONDUCTION: _____

INTERPRETATION: _____

App. 1–61

RHYTHM: _____

RATE: _____

ATRIAL CONDUCTION: _____

AV CONDUCTION: _____

VENTRICULAR CONDUCTION: _____

INTERPRETATION: _____

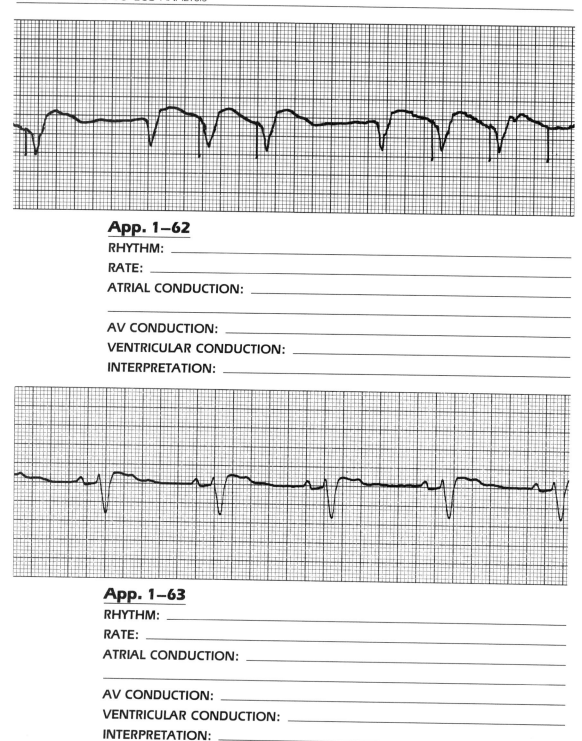

App. 1–62

RHYTHM: _____

RATE: _____

ATRIAL CONDUCTION: _____

_____

AV CONDUCTION: _____

VENTRICULAR CONDUCTION: _____

INTERPRETATION: _____

App. 1–63

RHYTHM: _____

RATE: _____

ATRIAL CONDUCTION: _____

_____

AV CONDUCTION: _____

VENTRICULAR CONDUCTION: _____

INTERPRETATION: _____

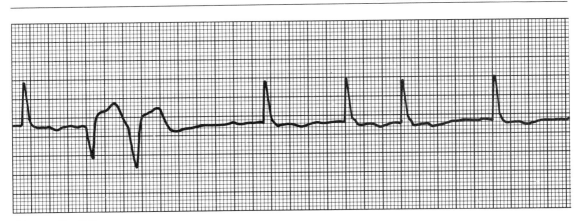

App. 1–64

RHYTHM: _____

RATE: _____

ATRIAL CONDUCTION: _____
_____

AV CONDUCTION: _____

VENTRICULAR CONDUCTION: _____

INTERPRETATION: _____

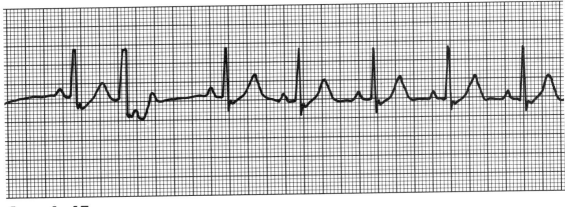

App. 1–65

RHYTHM: _____

RATE: _____

ATRIAL CONDUCTION: _____
_____

AV CONDUCTION: _____

VENTRICULAR CONDUCTION: _____

INTERPRETATION: _____

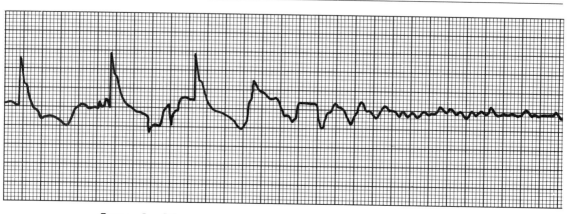

App. 1–66

RHYTHM: _____

RATE: _____

ATRIAL CONDUCTION: _____

_____

AV CONDUCTION: _____

VENTRICULAR CONDUCTION: _____

INTERPRETATION: _____

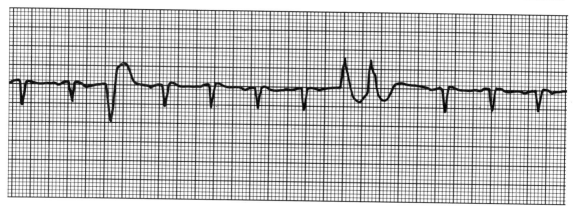

App. 1–67

RHYTHM: _____

RATE: _____

ATRIAL CONDUCTION: _____

_____

AV CONDUCTION: _____

VENTRICULAR CONDUCTION: _____

INTERPRETATION: _____

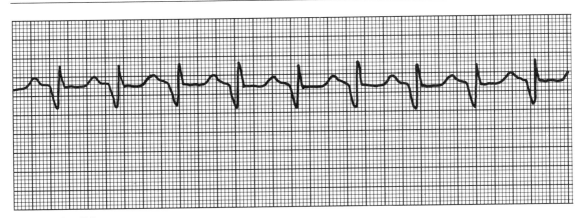

App. 1–68

RHYTHM: _____

RATE: _____

ATRIAL CONDUCTION: _____

_____

AV CONDUCTION: _____

VENTRICULAR CONDUCTION: _____

INTERPRETATION: _____

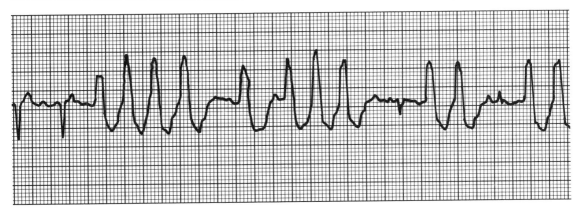

App. 1–69

RHYTHM: _____

RATE: _____

ATRIAL CONDUCTION: _____

_____

AV CONDUCTION: _____

VENTRICULAR CONDUCTION: _____

INTERPRETATION: _____

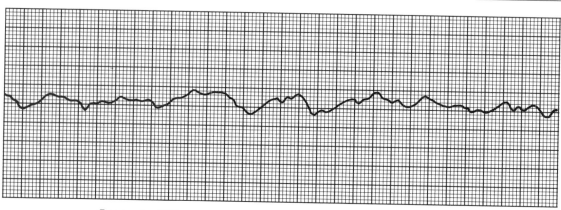

App. 1–70

RHYTHM: _____

RATE: _____

ATRIAL CONDUCTION: _____

_____

AV CONDUCTION: _____

VENTRICULAR CONDUCTION: _____

INTERPRETATION: _____

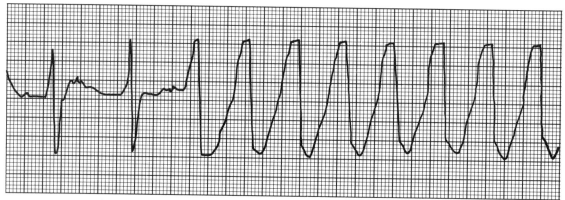

App. 1–71

RHYTHM: _____

RATE: _____

ATRIAL CONDUCTION: _____

_____

AV CONDUCTION: _____

VENTRICULAR CONDUCTION: _____

INTERPRETATION: _____

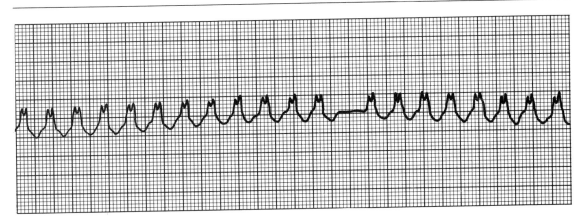

App. 1–72

RHYTHM: _____

RATE: _____

ATRIAL CONDUCTION: _____

_____

AV CONDUCTION: _____

VENTRICULAR CONDUCTION: _____

INTERPRETATION: _____

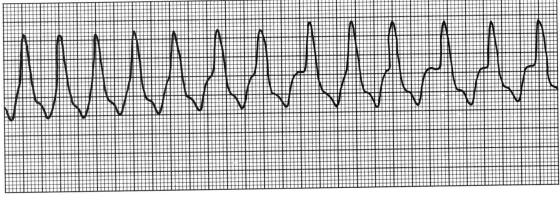

App. 1–73

RHYTHM: _____

RATE: _____

ATRIAL CONDUCTION: _____

_____

AV CONDUCTION: _____

VENTRICULAR CONDUCTION: _____

INTERPRETATION: _____

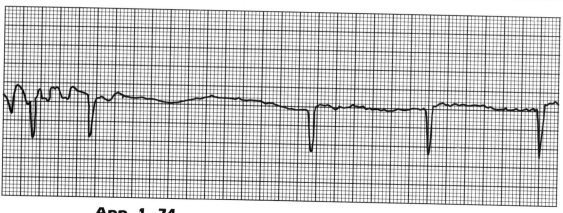

App. 1–74

RHYTHM: _____

RATE: _____

ATRIAL CONDUCTION: _____
_____

AV CONDUCTION: _____

VENTRICULAR CONDUCTION: _____

INTERPRETATION: _____

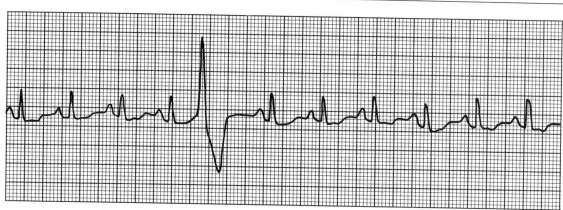

App. 1–75

RHYTHM: _____

RATE: _____

ATRIAL CONDUCTION: _____
_____

AV CONDUCTION: _____

VENTRICULAR CONDUCTION: _____

INTERPRETATION: _____

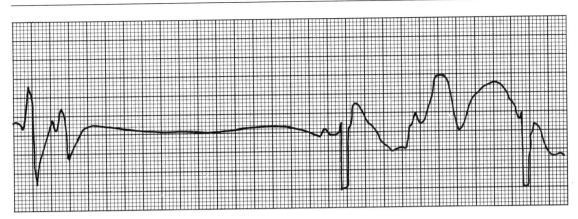

App. 1–76

RHYTHM: _____

RATE: _____

ATRIAL CONDUCTION: _____

_____

AV CONDUCTION: _____

VENTRICULAR CONDUCTION: _____

INTERPRETATION: _____

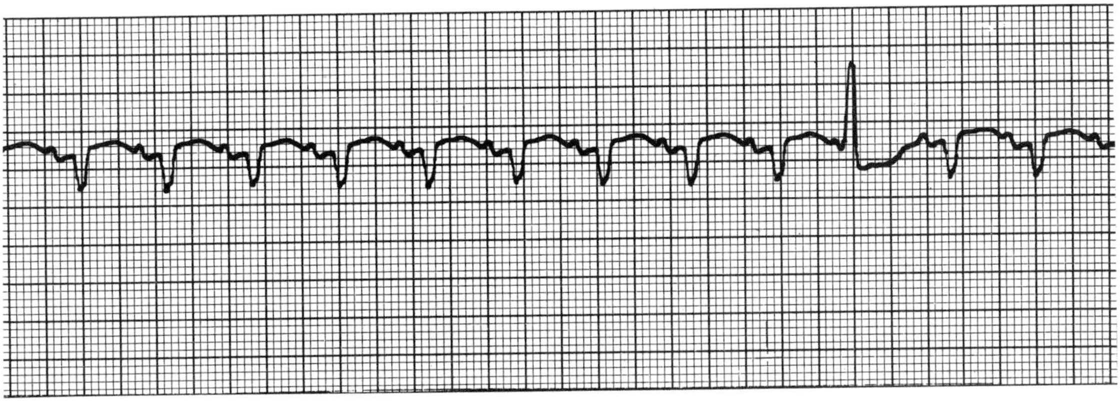

App. 1–77

RHYTHM: _____

RATE: _____

ATRIAL CONDUCTION: _____

_____

AV CONDUCTION: _____

VENTRICULAR CONDUCTION: _____

INTERPRETATION: _____

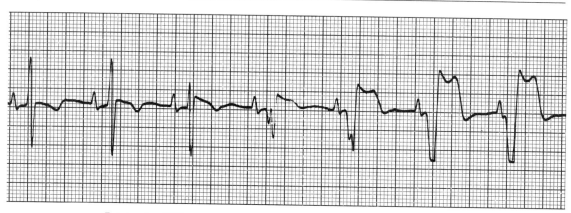

App. 1–78

RHYTHM: _____

RATE: _____

ATRIAL CONDUCTION: _____

_____

AV CONDUCTION: _____

VENTRICULAR CONDUCTION: _____

INTERPRETATION: _____

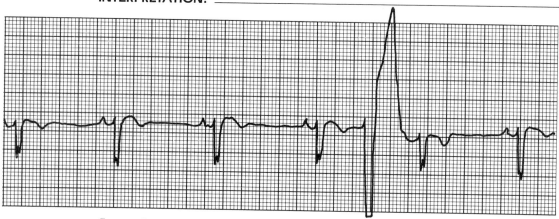

App. 1–79

RHYTHM: _____

RATE: _____

ATRIAL CONDUCTION: _____

_____

AV CONDUCTION: _____

VENTRICULAR CONDUCTION: _____

INTERPRETATION: _____

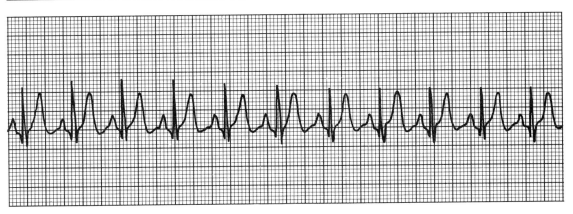

App. 1–80

RHYTHM: _____

RATE: _____

ATRIAL CONDUCTION: _____

_____

AV CONDUCTION: _____

VENTRICULAR CONDUCTION: _____

INTERPRETATION: _____

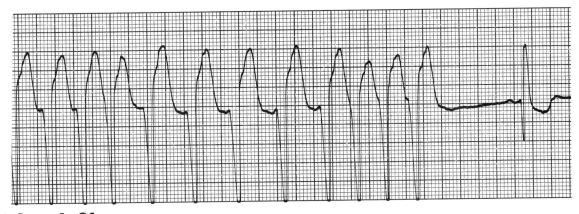

App. 1–81

RHYTHM: _____

RATE: _____

ATRIAL CONDUCTION: _____

_____

AV CONDUCTION: _____

VENTRICULAR CONDUCTION: _____

INTERPRETATION: _____

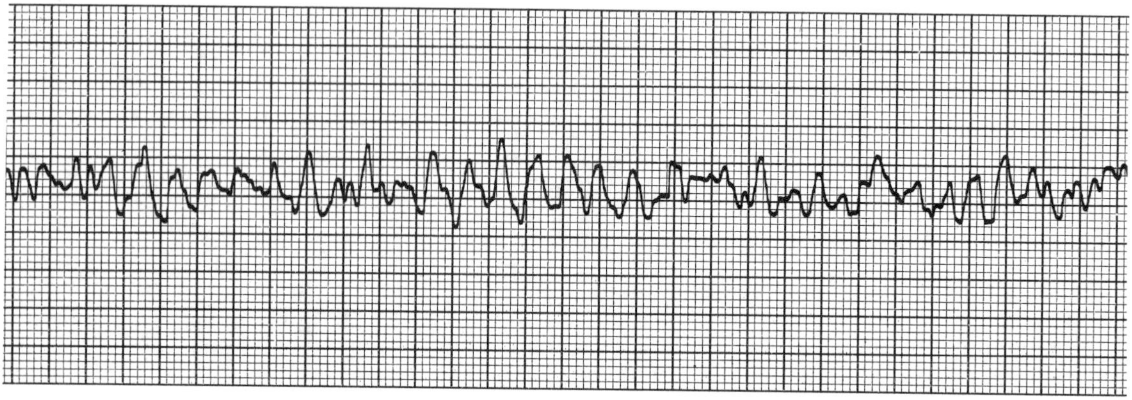

App. 1–82

RHYTHM: _____

RATE: _____

ATRIAL CONDUCTION: _____
_____

AV CONDUCTION: _____

VENTRICULAR CONDUCTION: _____

INTERPRETATION: _____

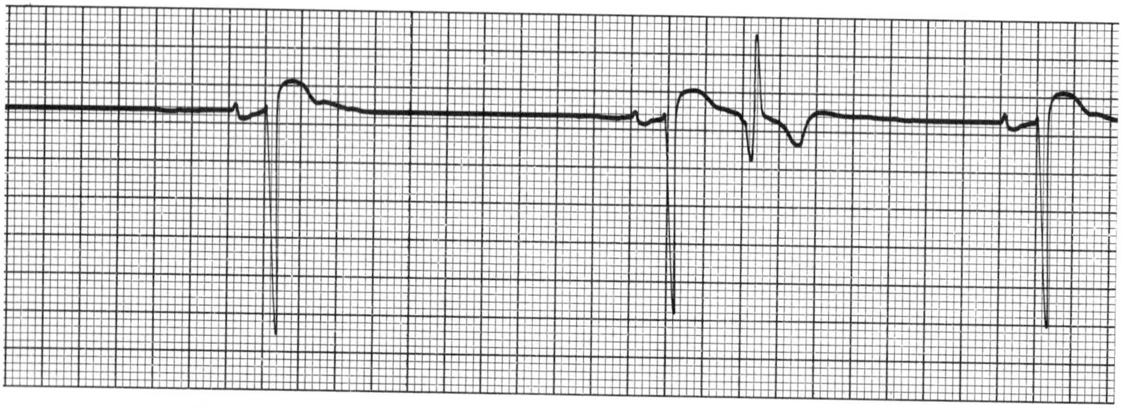

App. 1–83

RHYTHM: _____

RATE: _____

ATRIAL CONDUCTION: _____
_____

AV CONDUCTION: _____

VENTRICULAR CONDUCTION: _____

INTERPRETATION: _____

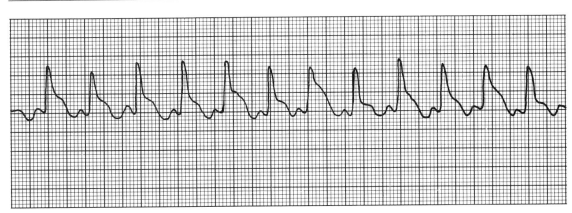

App. 1–84
RHYTHM: _____

RATE: _____

ATRIAL CONDUCTION: _____

_____

AV CONDUCTION: _____

VENTRICULAR CONDUCTION: _____

INTERPRETATION: _____

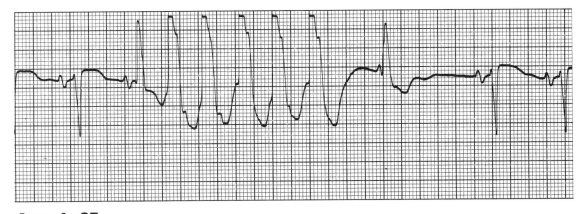

App. 1–85
RHYTHM: _____

RATE: _____

ATRIAL CONDUCTION: _____

_____

AV CONDUCTION: _____

VENTRICULAR CONDUCTION: _____

INTERPRETATION: _____

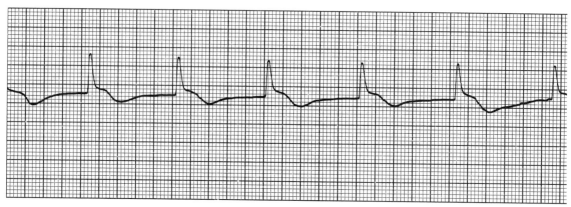

App. 1–86

RHYTHM: _____

RATE: _____

ATRIAL CONDUCTION: _____

_____

AV CONDUCTION: _____

VENTRICULAR CONDUCTION: _____

INTERPRETATION: _____

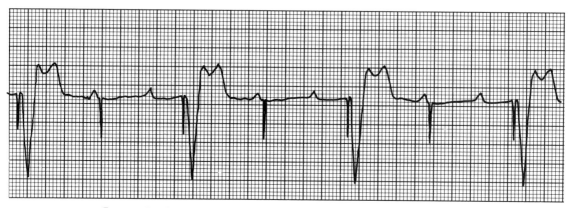

App. 1–87

RHYTHM: _____

RATE: _____

ATRIAL CONDUCTION: _____

_____

AV CONDUCTION: _____

VENTRICULAR CONDUCTION: _____

INTERPRETATION: _____

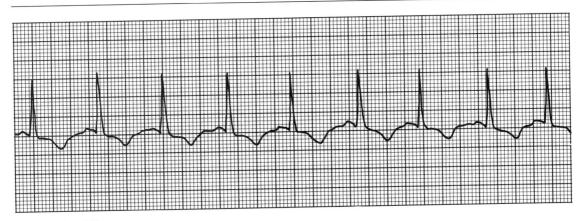

App. 1–88

RHYTHM: _____

RATE: _____

ATRIAL CONDUCTION: _____

_____

AV CONDUCTION: _____

VENTRICULAR CONDUCTION: _____

INTERPRETATION: _____

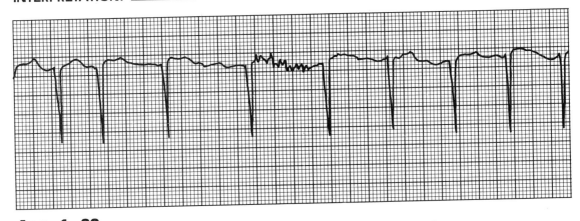

App. 1–89

RHYTHM: _____

RATE: _____

ATRIAL CONDUCTION: _____

_____

AV CONDUCTION: _____

VENTRICULAR CONDUCTION: _____

INTERPRETATION: _____

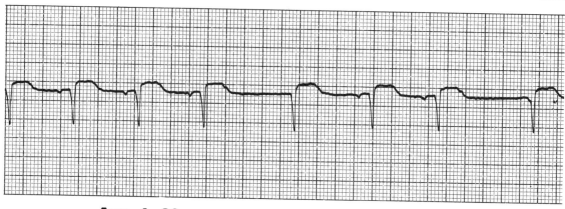

App. 1–90

RHYTHM: _____

RATE: _____

ATRIAL CONDUCTION: _____
_____

AV CONDUCTION: _____

VENTRICULAR CONDUCTION: _____

INTERPRETATION: _____

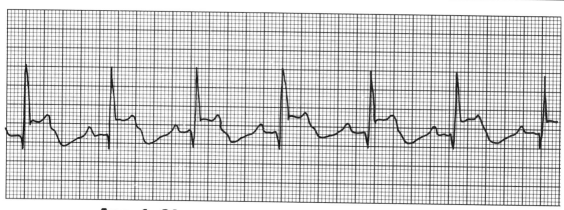

App. 1–91

RHYTHM: _____

RATE: _____

ATRIAL CONDUCTION: _____
_____

AV CONDUCTION: _____

VENTRICULAR CONDUCTION: _____

INTERPRETATION: _____

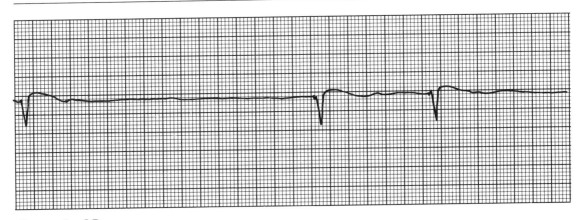

App. 1–92

RHYTHM: _____

RATE: _____

ATRIAL CONDUCTION: _____

AV CONDUCTION: _____

VENTRICULAR CONDUCTION: _____

INTERPRETATION: _____

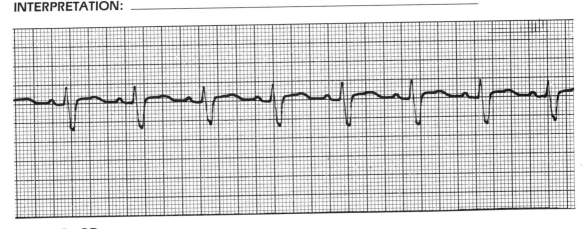

App. 1–93

RHYTHM: _____

RATE: _____

ATRIAL CONDUCTION: _____

AV CONDUCTION: _____

VENTRICULAR CONDUCTION: _____

INTERPRETATION: _____

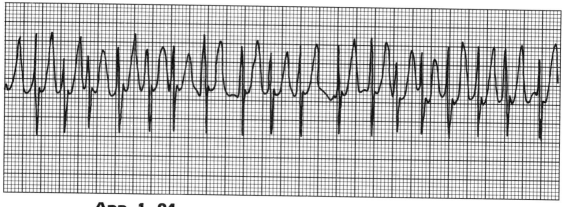

App. 1–94

RHYTHM: _____

RATE: _____

ATRIAL CONDUCTION: _____
_____

AV CONDUCTION: _____

VENTRICULAR CONDUCTION: _____

INTERPRETATION: _____

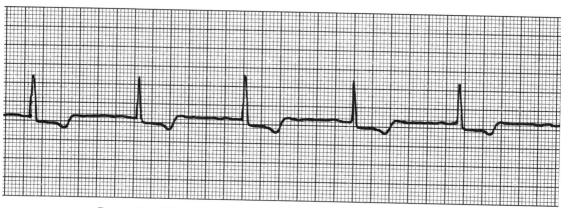

App. 1–95

RHYTHM: _____

RATE: _____

ATRIAL CONDUCTION: _____
_____

AV CONDUCTION: _____

VENTRICULAR CONDUCTION: _____

INTERPRETATION: _____

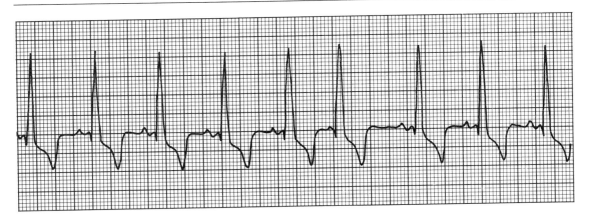

App. 1–96

RHYTHM: _____

RATE: _____

ATRIAL CONDUCTION: _____

_____

AV CONDUCTION: _____

VENTRICULAR CONDUCTION: _____

INTERPRETATION: _____

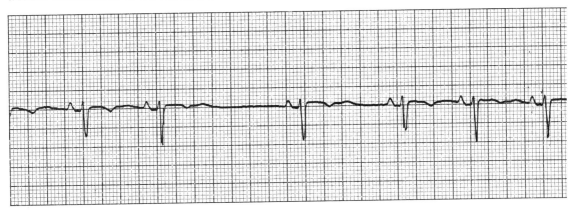

App. 1–97

RHYTHM: _____

RATE: _____

ATRIAL CONDUCTION: _____

_____

AV CONDUCTION: _____

VENTRICULAR CONDUCTION: _____

INTERPRETATION: _____

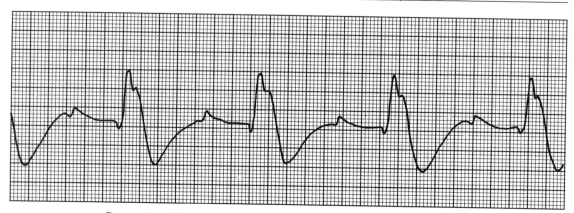

App. 1–98

RHYTHM: _____

RATE: _____

ATRIAL CONDUCTION: _____

_____

AV CONDUCTION: _____

VENTRICULAR CONDUCTION: _____

INTERPRETATION: _____

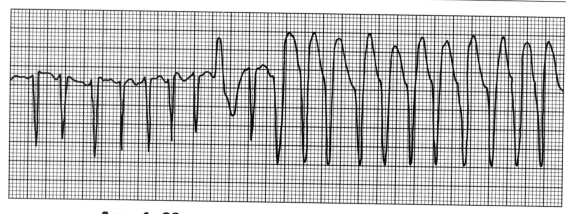

App. 1–99

RHYTHM: _____

RATE: _____

ATRIAL CONDUCTION: _____

_____

AV CONDUCTION: _____

VENTRICULAR CONDUCTION: _____

INTERPRETATION: _____

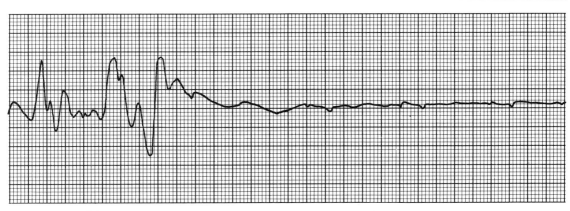

App. 1–100

RHYTHM: _____

RATE: _____

ATRIAL CONDUCTION: _____

_____

AV CONDUCTION: _____

VENTRICULAR CONDUCTION: _____

INTERPRETATION: _____

INTERPRETATIONS

App. 1–1

Rhythm: Regular
Rate: 79
Atrial: P waves: one P wave for each QRS complex; normal
AV Cond: PRI: 0.22 second; consistent
Vent: QRS: 0.08 second; same shape across strip
Interp: Sinus rhythm with first degree AV block

App. 1–2

Rhythm: Basically regular, interrupted by one premature ectopic
Rate: 38
Atrial: P waves: small P wave after each QRS complex in T waves
AV Cond: PRI: not measured
Vent: QRS: 0.08 second in nonectopic; ectopic = 0.20+ second
Interp: Junctional escape rhythm with one PVC

App. 1–3

Rhythm: Basically regular with one premature ectopic
Rate: 60
Atrial: P waves: one P wave for each QRS complex; P wave before ectopic is different shape
AV Cond: PRI: 0.14 second; consistent; ectopic PRI = 0.18 second
Vent: QRS: 0.06 second; same shape including ectopic QRS complex
Interp: Sinus rhythm with one PAC

App. 1–4

Rhythm: Regular P to P; regular R to R
Rate: 250 atrial; 125 ventricular
Atrial: P waves: 2 P waves for each QRS complex
AV Cond: PRI: 0.016 second; difficult to measure
Vent: QRS: 0.06 second; same shape across strip
Interp: Atrial flutter in 2 : 1 ratio (or atrial tachycardia in a 2 : 1 ratio)

App. 1–5

Rhythm: Totally irregular
Rate: Approximately 40
Atrial: P waves: not visible
AV Cond: PRI: not measured
Vent: QRS: 0.24 second; low amplitude
Interp: Agonal rhythm

App. 1–6

Rhythm: Totally irregular
Rate: Approximately 70
Atrial: P waves: chaotic, irregular base line; no clear P waves
AV Cond: PRI: not measured
Vent: QRS: 0.16 second; all positive; shape varies slightly
Interp: Controlled atrial fibrillation with RBBB

App. 1–7

Rhythm: Basically regular interrupted by premature ectopics
Rate: Approximately 70
Atrial: P waves: one P wave for each nonectopic QRS complex; none before the ectopics
AV Cond: PRI: 0.20 second; consistent; none before ectopics
Vent: QRS: 0.10 second for nonectopics; 0.20 + second for ectopics in ventricular configuration
Interp: Sinus rhythm with one PVC and a set of coupled PVCs

App. 1–8

Rhythm: Totally chaotic
Rate: Rapid; unable to count
Atrial: P waves: none visible
AV Cond: PRI: not measured
Vent: QRS: irregular shaped; small; variable rate
Interp: Fine ventricular fibrillation

App. 1–9

Rhythm: Regular
Rate: 75
Atrial: P waves: after the QRS complex before T waves
AV Cond: PRI: not measured
Vent: 0.06 second; same shape
Interp: Accelerated idiojunctional rhythm

App. 1–10

Rhythm: Regularly irregular; repetitive pattern of a normal QRS complex followed by a premature ectopic
Rate: 80
Atrial: P waves: before nonectopic QRS complexes; none before ectopic beats
AV Cond: PRI: 0.14 second; consistent where present
Vent: QRS: 0.08 second for nonectopic; 0.16 second in ectopics
Interp: Sinus rhythm with bigeminal PVCs

App. 1–11

Rhythm: Regular P to P; regular R to R
Rate: Atrial = 214; ventricular = 107
Atrial: P waves: two P waves for each QRS complex (one is in the bottom of the T wave)
AV Cond: PRI: 0.18 second; consistent where present
Vent: QRS: 0.16 second; positive in rR_1 configuration
Interp: Atrial tachycardia in 2:1 ratio with RBBB

App. 1–12

Rhythm: Regular P to P; irregular R to R
Rate: Atrial = 79; ventricular = approximately 70
Atrial: P waves: one more P wave than QRS complexes
AV Cond: PRI: 0.32–0.40 second; gets progressively longer until a P wave without a QRS complex
Vent: QRS: 0.08 second; same shape
Interp: Wenckebach pattern

App. 1–13

Rhythm: Regularly irregular; repetitive pattern of nonectopic followed by premature ectopic
Rate: 80
Atrial: P waves: one for each QRS complex; ectopic beats have different shaped P waves
AV Cond: PRI: 0.16 second for nonectopics; 0.14 second for ectopic beats
Vent: 0.10 second; same shape across strip
Interp: Sinus rhythm with bigeminal PACs

App. 1–14

Rhythm: Totally irregular
Rate: Approximately 120
Atrial: P waves: no clear P waves; irregular, chaotic base line
AV Cond: PRI: not measured
Vent: QRS: 0.08 second; same shape across strip
Interp: Uncontrolled atrial fibrillation

App. 1–15

Rhythm: Regular?
Rate: 16
Atrial: P waves: one small diphasic P wave for each QRS complex
AV Cond: PRI: 0.20 second; consistent
Vent: QRS: 0.14 second; negative deflection
Interp: Slow sinus bradycardia with a LBBB

App. 1–16

Rhythm: Basically regular interrupted by two premature ectopics
Rate: 65
Atrial: P waves: one P wave before each QRS complex; flattened P wave before first ectopic
AV Cond: PRI: 0.20 second nonectopic; 0.22 second for ectopic
Vent: QRS: 0.08 second; same for first ectopic; second ectopic QRS complex = 0.14+ second
Interp: Sinus rhythm with one PAC and one PVC

App. 1–17

Rhythm: Basically regular with a run of seven premature ectopics
Rate: 125; ectopic run 215
Atrial: P waves: one P wave before each nonectopic QRS complex; no P waves with ectopics
AV Cond: PRI: 0.12 second; consistent where present
Vent: QRS: 0.08 second for nonectopics; 0.14+ second in ventricular configuration for ectopics
Interp: Sinus tachycardia with a seven beat run of ventricular tachycardia

App. 1–18

Rhythm: Totally irregular
Rate: Approximately 80
Atrial: P waves: in sawtooth pattern; more P waves than QRS complexes
AV Cond: PRI: not measured
Vent: QRS: 0.08 second; same shape across strip
Interp: Controlled atrial flutter with variable ratio

App. 1–19

Rhythm: Totally irregular
Rate: Approximately 120
Atrial: P waves: no clear P waves; undulating, almost straight base line
AV Cond: PRI: not measured
Vent: QRS: 0.16 second; negative deflection; same shape
Interp: Uncontrolled atrial fibrillation with LBBB

App. 1–20

Rhythm: Totally irregular; long pauses between beats
Rate: Approximately 30
Atrial: P waves: not visible
AV Cond: PRI: not measured
Vent: QRS: 0.10 second; same shape across strip
Interp: Irregular junctional escape beats

App. 1–21

Rhythm: Basically regular with one premature ectopic
Rate: 83
Atrial: P waves: one before each nonectopic QRS complex; no P wave before ectopic
AV Cond: PRI: 0.18 second; consistent where present
Vent: QRS: 0.20 second; positive with Rr_1 configuration for nonectopic beats; ectopic = 0.18+ second with negative deflection
Interp: Sinus rhythm with RBBB and one PVC

App. 1–22

Rhythm: Totally irregular basic rhythm with run of nine premature ectopics which are regular
Rate: Approximately 140 for nonectopic part; 214 for ectopic rhythm
Atrial: P waves: no clear P waves; chaotic, uneven baseline; no P waves with ectopic QRS complexes
AV Cond: PRI: not measured
Vent: QRS: 0.08 second for nonectopics; 0.20+ second for ectopics in ventricular configuration
Interp: Uncontrolled atrial fibrillation changing to run of ventricular tachycardia

App. 1–23

Rhythm: Regularly irregular; repetitive pattern of three normal beats followed by premature ectopic
Rate: 115
Atrial: P waves: one for each nonectopic QRS complex; none with ectopic beats
AV Cond: PRI: 0.16 second; consistent where present
Vent: QRS: 0.08 second for nonectopics; 0.20 + second for ectopics in ventricular configuration
Interp: Sinus tachycardia with quadrigeminal PVCs

App. 1–24

Rhythm: Slightly irregular
Rate: 55
Atrial: P waves: one for each QRS complex; change shape—some positive, some negative
AV Cond: PRI: 0.16 second; consistent
Vent: QRS: 0.10 second; same shape
Interp: Wandering pacemaker pattern

App. 1–25

Rhythm: Totally irregular
Rate: Approximately 80
Atrial: P waves; no clear P waves; chaotic, uneven base line
AV Cond: PRI: not measured
Vent: QRS: 0.16 second; negative in sS_1 configuration
Interp: Controlled atrial fibrillation with LBBB

App. 1–26

Rhythm: Regular spike to spike; regular R to R
Rate: 71
Atrial: P waves: none; one spike for each QRS complex
AV Cond: PRI: not measured; spike falls >0.04 second before QRS complex
Vent: QRS: 0.16 second; two are smaller at 0.10 second but all are negatively deflected
Interp: Single chamber pacemaker pattern with two fusion beats

App. 1–27

Rhythm: Regular
Rate: 150
Atrial: P waves: one before each QRS complex (at the bottom of the complexes)
AV Cond: PRI: 0.10 second; consistent
Vent: QRS: 0.22 second with large delta wave at beginning of each complex
Interp: Sinus tachycardia in WPW pattern

App. 1–28

Rhythm: Regular P to P; totally irregular R to R
Rate: Atrial = 55; Ventricular = approximately 40
Atrial: P waves: more diphasic P waves than QRS complexes; unrelated to QRS complexes
AV Cond: PRI: variable and inconsistent
Vent: QRS: 0.20 second; some positive, some negative
Interp: Complete heart block with ventricular escape rhythm and PVCs (probably be considered a high grade block)

App. 1–29

Rhythm: Regular P to P; regular(?) R to R.
Rate: Atrial = 63; ventricular = 10(?)
Atrial: P waves: small P waves across entire strip without QRS complexes
AV Cond: PRI: not measured
Vent: QRS: 0.12 second
Interp: Ventricular standstill with one junctional escape beat

App. 1–30

Rhythm: Totally irregular
Rate: Approximately 60
Atrial: P waves: uneven, chaotic base line
AV Cond: PRI: not measured
Vent: QRS: 0.16 second; upright in rsR_1 configuration
Interp: Controlled atrial fibrillation with RBBB

App. 1–31

Rhythm: Totally irregular with one-second pause in middle
Rate: Approximately 90
Atrial: P waves: no clear P waves for first half of strip; one P wave for each QRS complex for second half
AV Cond: PRI: 0.16 second; consistent where present
Vent: QRS: 0.08 second; same shape across strip
Interp: Atrial fibrillation converting to sinus dysrhythmia

App. 1–32

Rhythm: Pause followed by totally irregular
Rate: Approximately 100 where complexes are present
Atrial: P waves: none visible
AV Cond: PRI: not measured
Vent: QRS: 0.20 second where present; irregular shaped
Interp: Asystole going into fast agonal rhythm

App. 1–33

Rhythm: Basically regular with a run of six premature ectopics
Rate: 115 nonectopics; 188 for ectopics
Atrial: P waves: one for each nonectopic QRS complex; none with ectopics
AV Cond: PRI: 0.16 second; consistent where present
Vent: QRS: 0.10 second for nonectopics; 0.16+ second for ectopics; one small QRS complex starting run of ectopics
Interp: Sinus tachycardia with a fusion beat and run of ventricular tachycardia

App. 1–34

Rhythm: Regular
Rate: 94
Atrial: P waves: one before each QRS complex; tall; peaked
AV Cond: PRI: 0.14 second; consistent
Vent: QRS: 0.10 second; same shape across strip
Interp: Normal sinus rhythm

App. 1–35

Rhythm: Regular spike to spike; regular R to R
Rate: Pacemaker rate 71
Atrial: P waves: none; spikes fall randomly for first four beats, last three beats, QRS complex follows spike
AV Cond: PRI: not measured; spike >0.04 second before QRS complex in captured beats
Vent: QRS: 0.08 second in first five beats; 0.16 second with negative deflection in captured beats
Interp: Intermittent capture pacemaker (underlying rhythm probably junctional escaped rhythm)

App. 1–36

Rhythm: Regular
Rate: 43
Atrial: P waves: one before each QRS complex
AV Cond: PRI: 0.16 second; consistent
Vent: QRS: 0.08 second; same shape across strip
Interp: Sinus bradycardia (note elevated S-T segment)

App. 1–37

Rhythm: Regular P to P; regular R to R
Rate: Atrial = 88; ventricular = 44
Atrial: P waves: small; two P waves for each QRS complex
AV Cond: PRI: 0.26 second; constant where present
Vent: QRS: 0.08 second; same shape across strip
Interp: Classic second degree AV block (type II) in a 2:1 ratio with a long PR interval

App. 1–38

Rhythm: Totally irregular
Rate: Approximately 70
Atrial: P waves: none seen; straight line between QRS complexes
AV Cond: PRI: not measured
Vent: QRS: 0.14 second; positive monophasic R wave; same shape across strip
Interp: Controlled atrial fibrillation with RBBB

App. 1–39

Rhythm: Basically regular with two premature ectopics
Rate: 60
Atrial: P waves: one before each nonectopic QRS complex; P wave before narrow ectopic is different shaped; no P wave before wide ectopic QRS complex
AV Cond: PRI: 0.18 second; consistent where present
Vent: QRS: 0.10 second for nonectopic and narrow ectopic; 0.16+ second for wide ectopic
Interp: Sinus rhythm with one PVC and one PAC

App. 1–40

Rhythm: Totally irregular—pause—slightly irregular
Rate: Approximately 68 for last half of strip
Atrial: P waves: none for first half of strip; one P wave for each QRS complex for second half of strip
AV Cond: PRI: 0.12 second; consistent where present
Vent: QRS: irregular and chaotic for first half of strip; 0.12 second for second half of strip after pause
Interp: Coarse ventricular fibrillation electrocardioverted to sinus rhythm

App. 1–41

Rhythm: Regular
Rate: 88
Atrial: P waves: one P before each QRS complex; normal shape
AV Cond: PRI: 0.20 second; consistent
Vent: QRS: 0.08 second; same shape
Interp: Normal sinus rhythm

App. 1–42

Rhythm: Regular
Rate: 83
Atrial: P waves: one P before each QRS complex; normal shape
AV Cond: PRI: 0.28 second; consistent
Vent: QRS: 0.10 second; same shape
Interp: Sinus rhythm with first degree AV block

App. 1–43

Rhythm: Slightly irregular
Rate: 36
Atrial: P waves: one flattened P wave before each QRS complex
AV Cond: PRI: 0.22 second; consistent
Vent: QRS: 0.08 second; same shape
Interp: Sinus bradycardia with first degree AV block

App. 1–44

Rhythm: Slightly irregular
Rate: 200
Atrial: P waves: none visible
AV Cond: PRI: not measured
Vent: QRS: 0.20+ second; shape changes some at end
Interp: Ventricular tachycardia

App. 1–45

Rhythm: Basically regular interrupted by two premature ectopic beats in a row
Rate: 94
Atrial: P waves: one P wave before each nonectopic beat; none before the ectopic beats
AV Cond: PRI: 0.20 second; none with ectopic beats
Vent: QRS: 0.08 second for nonectopic beats; ectopic beats 0.18+ second; R waves in different directions
Interp: Sinus rhythm with a set of coupled multifocal PVCs

App. 1–46

Rhythm: Basically regular with one ectopic that comes late in the cycle
Rate: Approximately 40
Atrial: P waves: diphasic P waves before the first two and last QRS complexes
AV Cond: PRI: 0.20 second where present
Vent: QRS: 0.08 second; same shape for all beats
Interp: Sinus bradycardia with a junctional escape beat

App. 1–47

Rhythm: Regular(?)
Rate: 20(?)
Atrial: P waves: not visible
AV Cond: PRI: not measured
Vent: QRS: 0.40+ second; same shape
Interp: Slow ventricular escape rhythm (or agonal rhythm)

App. 1–48

Rhythm: Regular
Rate: 75
Atrial: P waves: not visible; hidden in QRS complexes
AV Cond: PRI: not measured
Vent: QRS: 0.08 second for first five beats, then changing to 0.16 second with a positive deflection for last three beats
Interp: Accelerated junctional rhythm with intermittent RBBB

App. 1–49

Rhythm: Regular
Rate: 52
Atrial: P waves: not visible; hidden in QRS complexes
AV Cond: PRI: not measured
Vent: QRS: 0.08 second; same shape
Interp: Junctional escape rhythm

App. 1–50

Rhythm: Basically regular interrupted by two premature ectopic beats
Rate: 107
Atrial: P waves: one P wave before each nonectopic QRS complex; none before the ectopic beats
AV Cond: PRI: 0.14 second; consistent where present
Vent: QRS: 0.06 second for nonectopic beats; ectopic beats 0.16+ second; same shape
Interp: Sinus tachycardia with two PVCs (unifocal)

App. 1–51

Rhythm: Totally irregular
Rate: Undetermined
Atrial: P waves: uneven, irregular undulations; pacemaker spikes at irregular intervals
AV Cond: PRI: not measured
Vent: QRS: no distinct QRS complexes; uneven small undulations
Interp: Fine ventricular fibrillation with noncapture malfunctioning pacemaker

App. 1–52

Rhythm: Totally irregular
Rate: 50–70
Atrial: P waves: none present
AV Cond: PRI: not measured
Vent: QRS: 0.40–0.60+ second; irregular shaped
Interp: Agonal rhythm

App. 1–53

Rhythm: Totally irregular
Rate: Approximately 60
Atrial: P waves: irregular P to P intervals; vary in shape; some QRS complexes without P waves before them
AV Cond: PRI: 0.18 second where present
Vent: QRS: 0.08 second; same shape
Interp: Sinus dysrhythmia with junctional escape beats

App. 1–54

Rhythm: Totally irregular with one wide premature ectopic
Rate: Approximately 70
Atrial: P waves: one P wave before each nonectopic QRS complex; none before ectopic beat
AV Cond: PRI: 0.16 second; consistent where present
Vent: QRS: 0.10 second for nonectopics; ectopic = 0.20+ second
Interp: Sinus dysrhythmia with one PVC

App. 1–55

Rhythm: Totally irregular with one ectopic after a long pause
Rate: Approximately 50
Atrial: P waves: one P wave before each nonectopic QRS complex; none before ectopic beat
AV Cond: PRI: 0.20; consistent where present
Vent: QRS: 0.06 second; all same shape
Interp: Sinus dysrhythmia with a sinus arrest and junctional escape beat

App. 1–56

Rhythm: Totally irregular in a pattern of grouped beats
Rate: Approximately 100
Atrial: P waves: no distinct P waves; irregular base line
AV Cond: PRI: not measured
Vent: QRS: 0.12 second; both positive and negative deflections
Interp: Atrial fibrillation with RBBB and bigeminal PVCs

App. 1–57

Rhythm: Regular
Rate: 100
Atrial: P waves: none visible
AV Cond: PRI: not measured
Vent: QRS: 0.20+ second; same shape
Interp: Slow ventricular tachycardia

App. 1–58

Rhythm: Slightly irregular with one premature ectopic that does not interrupt the underlying rhythm
Rate: 60
Atrial: P waves: hidden in the QRS complexes
AV Cond: PRI: not measured
Vent: QRS: 0.08 second for nonectopic beats; ectopic is 0.16+ second
Interp: Junctional rhythm with an interpolated PVC

App. 1–59

Rhythm: Regular becoming totally irregular
Rate: Overall approximately 90
Atrial: P waves: no clear P waves; uneven base line: pacemaker spikes present for first four beats rate of 75
AV Cond: PRI: not measured; pacemaker spikes just before QRS
Vent: QRS: 0.14 second for pacing beats with one at 0.08 second; nonpacing beats measure 0.06 second
Interp: Pacing fusion beat followed by three capture ventricular demand pacemaker beats changing to atrial fibrillation

App. 1–60

Rhythm: Regular P to P intervals; irregular R to R intervals
Rate: Atrial = 88; ventricular = approximately 60
Atrial: P waves: small, diphasic P waves; more P waves than QRS complexes
AV Cond: PRI: varies 0.20–0.28 second; gets progressively longer until there is a P wave without a QRS complex; pattern repeats
Vent: QRS: 0.06 second; same shape
Interp: Wenckebach pattern (second degree AV block)

App. 1–61

Rhythm: Regular P to P intervals; irregular R to R intervals
Rate: Atrial = 100; ventricular = approximately 70
Atrial: P waves: more P waves than QRS complexes; some are difficult to see
AV Cond: PRI: varies 0.20–0.32 second; gets progressively longer until there is a P wave without a QRS complex; pattern repeats itself
Vent: QRS: 0.06 second; same shape
Interp: Wenckebach pattern (second degree AV block)

App. 1–62

Rhythm: Totally irregular with irregular pacemaker spikes
Rate: Approximately 70
Atrial: P waves: none visible; pacemaker spikes present at irregular intervals, some without QRS complexes after them
AV Cond: PRI: not measured
Vent: QRS: 0.20 second; negative deflection; same shape
Interp: Malfunctioning pacemaker with intermittent capture

App. 1–63

Rhythm: Regular
Rate: 47
Atrial: P waves: one P before each QRS complex; normal shape
AV Cond: PRI: 0.22 second; consistent
Vent: QRS: 0.16 second; negative deflection; same shape
Interp: Sinus bradycardia with first degree AV block and LBBB

App. 1–64

Rhythm: Totally irregular with two premature ectopics in a row
Rate: Approximately 70
Atrial: P waves: no clear P waves; irregular base line
AV Cond: PRI: not measured
Vent: QRS: 0.14 second with positive deflection in nonectopic QRS complexes; ectopics = 0.18+ second in a negative direction
Interp: Controlled atrial fibrillation with a RBBB and a set of coupled PVC

App. 1–65

Rhythm: Basically regular interrupted by one premature ectopic
Rate: 71
Atrial: P waves: one P wave before each QRS complex; P wave after ectopic beat which falls in cycle with other P waves
AV Cond: PRI: 0.20 second: consistent where present
Vent: QRS: 0.10 second; ectopic is same width but different shape
Interp: Sinus rhythm with one PJC

App. 1–66

Rhythm: Totally irregular
Rate: 30(?) - undetermined
Atrial: P waves: not visible
AV Cond: PRI: not measured
Vent: QRS: first three = 0.20+ second then becomes irregular; chaotic base line in small undulations
Interp: Agonal rhythm changing to fine ventricular fibrillation

App. 1–67

Rhythm: Basically regular interrupted by three premature ectopic beats
Rate: 120
Atrial: P waves: small inverted P waves before nonectopic QRS complexes; no P waves before ectopic beats
AV Cond: PRI: 0.14 second where present
Vent: QRS: 0.08 second for nonectopic beats; ectopics all about 0.16+ second with one negative and two positive in a row
Interp: Sinus tachycardia with multifocal PVCs (one set of coupled PVCs)

App. 1–68

Rhythm: Regular
Rate: 88
Atrial: P waves: hidden in the QRS complexes
AV Cond: PRI: not measured
Vent: QRS: 0.10 second; same shape
Interp: Accelerated junctional rhythm

App. 1–69

Rhythm: Overall, totally irregular; many ectopic beats
Rate: Approximately 130
Atrial: P waves: P waves before first two nonectopic QRS complexes; none before ectopic beats
AV Cond: PRI: 0.20 second where present
Vent: QRS: 0.08 second for nonectopic beats; ectopics 0.20+ second; few small, irregular shaped QRS complexes mixed in
Interp: Sinus rhythm changing to ventricular tachycardia and salvos of PVCs with fusion beats mixed in

App. 1–70

Rhythm: Totally chaotic base line
Rate: Undetermined
Atrial: P waves: none present
AV Cond: PRI: not measured
Vent: QRS: totally chaotic baseline in small undulations
Interp: Fine ventricular fibrillation

App. 1–71

Rhythm: Overall, irregular although regular in parts
Rate: Approximately 110
Atrial: P waves: small P waves before first two QRS complexes; none before ectopic beats
AV Cond: PRI: 0.22 second where present
Vent: QRS: 0.18 second for nonectopic beats; 0.20+ second for ectopic beats
Interp: Sinus rhythm with first degree AV block and RBBB changing to ventricular tachycardia

App. 1–72

Rhythm: Irregular
Rate: Approximately 190
Atrial: P waves: irregular base line
AV Cond: PRI: not measured
Vent: QRS: 0.14 second; positive deflection with rabbit ear pattern
Interp: Uncontrolled atrial fibrillation with RBBB

App. 1–73

Rhythm: Slightly irregular—pattern gradually slows
Rate: 150 to 83
Atrial: P waves: none visible
AV Cond: PRI: not measured
Vent: QRS: 0.20+ second; same shape
Interp: Ventricular tachycardia slowing to an accelerated idioventricular rhythm

App. 1–74

Rhythm: Overall, totally irregular
Rate: Approximately 60 overall, slows after first three beats
Atrial: P waves: no clear P waves; irregular base line
AV Cond: PRI: not measured
Vent: QRS: 0.08 second; same shape
Interp: Uncontrolled atrial fibrillation changing to slow atrial fibrillation

App. 1–75

Rhythm: Basically regular interrupted by one premature ectopic
Rate: 115
Atrial: P waves: one P wave before each QRS; none with ectopic
AV Cond: PRI: 0.16 second; consistent where present
Vent: QRS: 0.08 second for nonectopic beats; ectopic beat is 0.20+ second in ventricular configuration
Interp: Sinus tachycardia with one PVC

App. 1–76

Rhythm: Totally irregular
Rate: Approximately 40
Atrial: P waves: none visible
AV Cond: PRI: not measured
Vent: QRS: wide, irregular shaped first two QRS complexes, followed by a pause, then two QRS complexes at 0.10 second
Interp: Ventricular fibrillation with asystole changing to a junctional rhythm

App. 1–77

Rhythm: Basically regular with one premature ectopic beat
Rate: 125
Atrial: P waves: one P wave before each QRS complex; sinus P wave before the ectopic beat
AV Cond: PRI: 0.16 second; consistent where present
Vent: QRS: 0.08 second for nonectopic QRS complexes; 0.10 second for ectopic beat; has different configuration from other beats
Interp: Sinus tachycardia with one PJC with abnormal conduction

App. 1–78

Rhythm: Regular P to P interval; R to R interval gets shorter
Rate: Approximately 70 (68)
Atrial: P waves: one P wave before each QRS complex; normal shape
AV Cond: PRI: 0.18 second before first three beats, then gradually shortens to 0.10 second as the QRS complexes get wider
Vent: QRS: 0.10 second for first three beats; gradually widens to 0.18+ second in a ventricular configuration
Interp: Sinus rhythm changing to third degree AV block with a ventricular escape rhythm

App. 1–79

Rhythm: Basically regular with one premature ectopic that does not interrupt the underlying rhythm
Rate: 53
Atrial: P waves: one P wave before each QRS complex; none before ectopic beat
AV Cond: PRI: 0.16 second; consistent where present
Vent: QRS: 0.12 second for nonectopics; 0.16+ second for ectopic beat in ventricular configuration
Interp: Sinus bradycardia with one interpolated PVC

App. 1–80

Rhythm: Regular
Rate: 115
Atrial: P waves: one P wave before each QRS complex; normal shape
AV Cond: PRI: 0.16 second; consistent
Vent: QRS: 0.08 second; same shape (large T wave)
Interp: Sinus tachycardia

App. 1–81

Rhythm: Slightly irregular
Rate: Approximately 150
Atrial: P waves: one P wave before last QRS complex; none before ectopic QRS complexes
AV Cond: PRI: 0.16 second where present
Vent: QRS: 0.10 second for nonectopic QRS complex; ectopic QRS complexes = 0.16+ second in ventricular configuration
Interp: Ventricular tachycardia changing to sinus rhythm (beat)

App. 1–82

Rhythm: Totally chaotic
Rate: Undetermined
Atrial: P waves: none visible
AV Cond: PRI: not measured
Vent: QRS: totally chaotic small undulations
Interp: Fine ventricular fibrillation

App. 1–83

Rhythm: Slightly irregular interrupted by one premature ectopic
Rate: Approximately 40
Atrial: P waves: one P wave before each nonectopic QRS complex; none before ectopic beat
AV Cond: PRI: 0.20 second where present
Vent: QRS: 0.08 second for nonectopic beats; 0.14 second for ectopic beat with a different configuration
Interp: Sinus bradycardia with one PVC

App. 1–84

Rhythm: Regular
Rate: 115
Atrial: P waves: one P wave before each QRS complex; normal
AV Cond: PRI: 0.14 second; consistent
Vent: QRS: 0.10 second; same shape but appear wider due to elevated ST segment
Interp: Sinus tachycardia with elevated ST segment

App. 1–85

Rhythm: Basically regular with a run of seven ectopic beats in a row
Rate: Basic rhythm = 86; run of ectopics = 167
Atrial: P waves: one P wave before each nonectopic QRS complex
AV Cond: PRI: 0.20 second where present
Vent: QRS: 0.08 second for nonectopic beats; 0.22+ second for ectopic beats with two smaller beats in different direction from nonectopic QRS complexes
Interp: Sinus rhythm followed by a ventricular fusion beat followed by a run of ventricular tachycardia followed by a fusion beat changing back to sinus rhythm

App. 1–86

Rhythm: Slightly irregular
Rate: 60
Atrial: P waves: hidden in QRS complexes
AV Cond: PRI: not measured
Vent: QRS: 0.10 second; appear wider due to elevated ST segment
Interp: Junctional rhythm with elevated ST segment

App. 1–87

Rhythm: Regular P to P intervals; regular R to R intervals; regular pacemaker spike to spike intervals; all different
Rate: Atrial = 100; ventricular = 33; pacemaker = 65
Atrial: P waves: at regular intervals but not followed by QRS complexes; every other pacemaker spike followed by QRS complex
AV Cond: PRI: not measured; capture pacemaker spikes followed closely by QRS complexes
Vent: QRS: 0.16 second; same shape in negative deflection
Interp: Intermittent capture pacemaker (underlying rhythm probably complete heart block high grade)

App. 1–88

Rhythm: Regular
Rate: 86
Atrial: P waves: one small P wave before each QRS complex
AV Cond: PRI: 0.20 second; consistent
Vent: QRS: 0.06 second; same shape
Interp: Normal sinus rhythm

App. 1–89

Rhythm: Totally irregular
Rate: Approximately 100
Atrial: P waves: none, chaotic uneven base line
AV Cond: PRI: not measured
Vent: QRS: 0.08 second; same shape
Interp: Controlled atrial fibrillation

App. 1–90

Rhythm: Basically regular interrupted by two ectopic beats that come late in the cycle
Rate: 83
Atrial: P waves: one P wave before each nonectopic beat; P waves for ectopic beats hidden in QRS complexes
AV Cond: PRI: 0.14 second where present
Vent: QRS: 0.08 second; same shape for all beats
Interp: Sinus rhythm with two junctional escape beats

App. 1–91

Rhythm: Regular P to P intervals; regular R to R intervals
Rate: Atrial = 126; ventricular = 63
Atrial: P waves: two P waves for each QRS complex
AV Cond: PRI: 0.22 second; consistent where conducted
Vent: QRS: 0.08 second; elevated ST segment
Interp: Classic (type II) second degree AV block with a long PRI in a 2 : 1 ratio and with an elevated ST segment

App. 1–92

Rhythm: Totally irregular
Rate: Approximately 30
Atrial: P waves: no distinct P waves; irregular base line
AV Cond: PRI: not measured
Vent: QRS: 0.01 second; same shape
Interp: Very slow atrial fibrillation

App. 1–93

Rhythm: Regular
Rate: 81
Atrial: P waves: one P wave before each QRS complex
AV Cond: PRI: 0.18 second; consistent
Vent: QRS: 0.14 second; same shape in RS configuration
Interp: Sinus rhythm with RBBB

App. 1–94

Rhythm: Slightly irregular
Rate: 190
Atrial: P waves: not visible due to fast rate
AV Cond: PRI: not measured
Vent: QRS: 0.08 second
Interp: Supraventricular tachycardia, probably a fast atrial fibrillation due to irregularity

App. 1–95

Rhythm: Regular
Rate: 50
Atrial: P waves; not visible; hidden in QRS complexes
AV Cond: PRI: not measured
Vent: QRS: 0.08 second
Interp: Junctional escape rhythm

App. 1–96

Rhythm: Basically regular interrupted by one premature ectopic beat
Rate: 83
Atrial: P waves: one P wave before each QRS complex; P wave before ectopic beat is different shape than rest
AV Cond: PRI: 0.16 second for nonectopic beats; 0.12 second for ectopic
Vent: QRS: 0.12 second; same shape for all beats
Interp: Sinus rhythm with one PAC

App. 1–97

Rhythm: Totally irregular
Rate: Approximately 70
Atrial: P waves: one P wave before each QRS complex
AV Cond: PRI: 0.16 second; consistent
Vent: QRS: 0.10 second; same shape
Interp: Sinus dysrhythmia

App. 1–98

Rhythm: Regular
Rate: 41
Atrial: P waves: none present
AV Cond: PRI: not measured
Vent: QRS: 0.40 second; wide and bizarre shaped
Interp: Agonal rhythm

App. 1–99

Rhythm: Regular
Rate: 215
Atrial: P waves: no distinct P waves; chaotic base line present for first of strip
AV Cond: PRI: not measured
Vent: QRS: 0.08 second for first part of strip; 0.14+ second for second part of strip
Interp: Uncontrolled atrial fibrillation changing to ventricular tachycardia

App. 1–100

Rhythm: Chaotic, irregular
Rate: Undetermined
Atrial: P waves: none present
AV Cond: PRI: not measured
Vent: QRS: large undulations changing to straight line
Interp: Coarse ventricular fibrillation changing to asystole

INTERPRETATIONS FOR CHAPTER PRACTICE STRIPS

CHAPTER 3

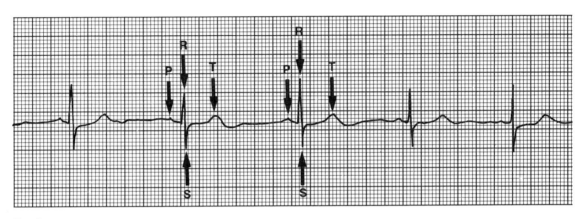

3–1

Rhythm: Slightly irregular
Rate: Approx. 50 (48) (abnormal = slower than normal)
Atrial: One P wave before each QRS; normal in shape
AV Cond: PRI: 0.14 second and consistent
Vent: QRS: 0.08 second and uniform in shape

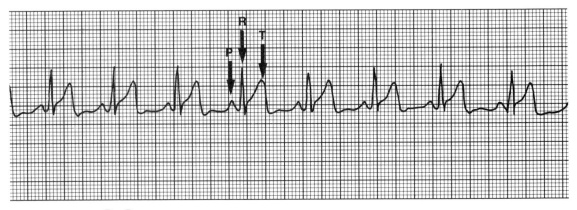

3–2

Rhythm: Regular
Rate: Approx. 90 (88)
Atrial: One P wave before each QRS; normal in shape
AV Cond: PRI: 0.12 second and consistent
Vent: QRS: 0.08 second and uniform in shape

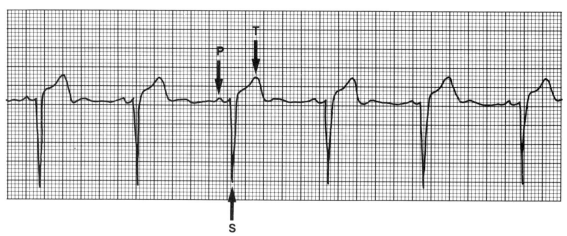

3–3

Rhythm: Regular
Rate: Approx. 60 (58)
Atrial: One P wave before each QRS; normal in shape
AV Cond: PRI: 0.16 second and consistent
Vent: QRS: 0.10 second and uniform in shape

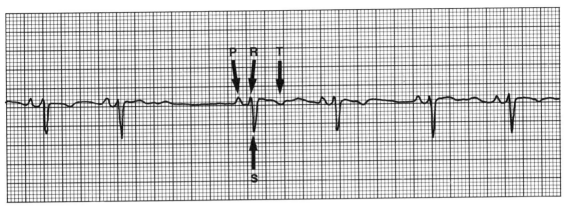

3—4

Rhythm: Totally irregular (abnormal)
Rate: Approx. 60
Atrial: One P wave before each QRS; normal in shape
AV Cond: PRI: 0.16 second and consistent
Vent: QRS: 0.10 second and uniform in shape

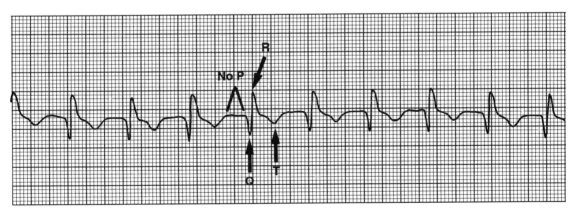

3—5

Rhythm: Regular
Rate: Approx. 90 (94)
Atrial: No visible P waves in this strip (abnormal)
AV Cond: Unable to measure a PR interval (abnormal)
Vent: QRS: 0.16 second and uniform in shape (abnormal)

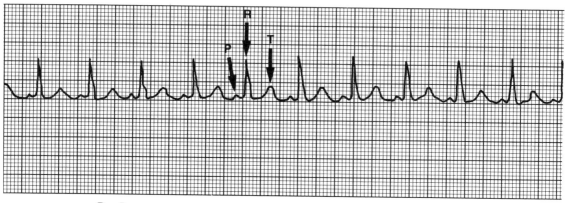

3-6

Rhythm: Regular
Rate: Approx. 100 (100)
Atrial: One P wave before each QRS: normal in shape
AV Cond: PRI: 0.12 second and consistent
Vent: QRS: 0.08 second and uniform in shape

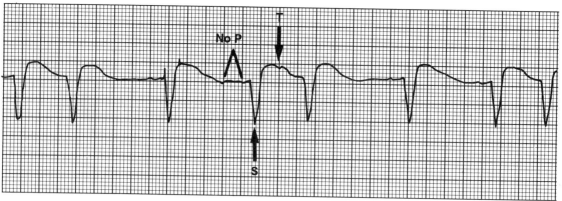

3-7

Rhythm: Totally irregular (abnormal)
Rate: Approx. 80
Atrial: No distinct P waves, undulating, wavy base line (abnormal)
AV Cond: Unable to measure a PRI (abnormal)
Vent: QRS: 0.16 second and uniform in shape (abnormal width)

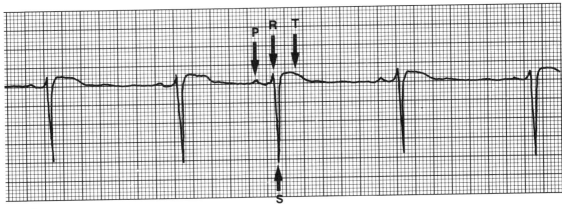

3—8

Rhythm: Totally irregular (abnormal)
Rate: Approx. 50 (abnormal—too slow)
Atrial: One P wave before each QRS: normal in shape
AV Cond: PRI: 0.20 second and consistent
Vent: QRS: 0.08 second and uniform in shape

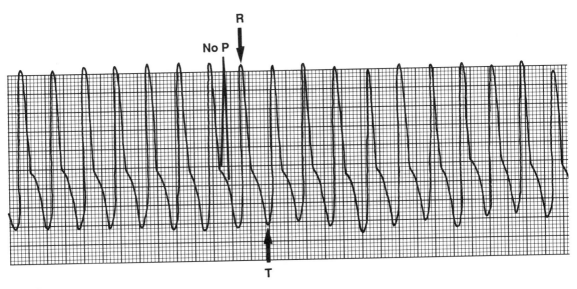

3—9

Rhythm: Regular
Rate: Approx. 170 (167) (abnormal—too fast)
Atrial: No P waves visible in this pattern (abnormal)
AV Cond: Unable to measure the PRI (abnormal)
Vent: QRS: 0.20 second and uniform in shape (abnormal)

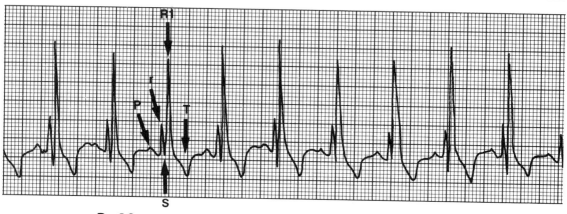

3–10

Rhythm: Regular
Rate: Approx. 100 (100)
Atrial: One P wave before each QRS: normal in shape
AV Cond: PRI: 0.14 second and consistent
Vent: QRS: 0.14 second and uniform in shape (abnormal)

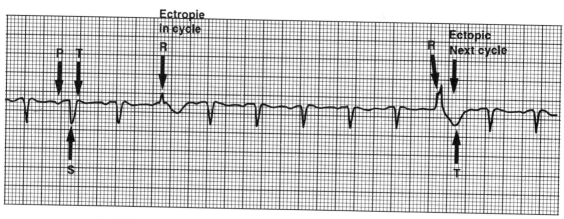

3–11

Rhythm: Basically regular interrupted by a premature ectopic complex (abnormal)
Rate: Approx. 120 (115)
Atrial: One P wave before each nonectopic QRS complex: inverted, no P wave before the premature ectopic
AV Cond: PRI: 0.18 second and consistent; no PRI with ectopic (abnormal)
Vent: QRS: nonectopic 0.08 and uniform in shape/first ectopic QRS is 0.04 second/second ectopic is 0.14 second (abnormal)

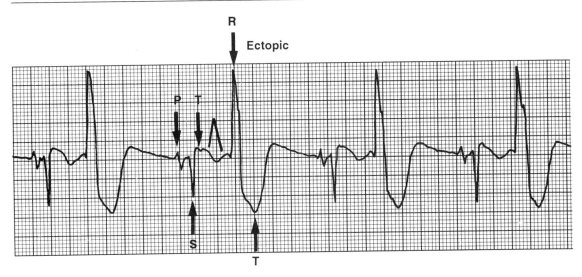

3—12

Rhythm: Regularly irregular (pattern of grouped beats) (abnormal)
Rate: Approx. 80
Atrial: One P wave for each nonectopic QRS complex: is diphasic in shape; no P waves before premature ectopic QRS complexes
AV Cond: PRI: 0.14 second for nonectopic: consistent; none for ectopics
Vent: QRS: nonectopic = 0.10 and consistent; ectopic = 0.18 second and consistent (abnormal)

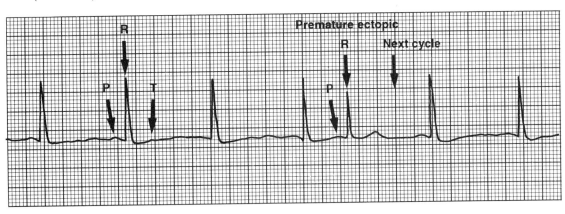

3—13

Rhythm: Slightly irregular interrupted by a premature ectopic (abnormal)
Rate: Approx. 70 (65)
Atrial: One P wave before each QRS complex: shape is flattened and uniform; P wave before ectopic is different shape
AV Cond: PRI: 0.16 and consistent nonectopics/PRI ectopic = 0.12
Vent: QRS: 0.08 second and consistent; same for ectopic

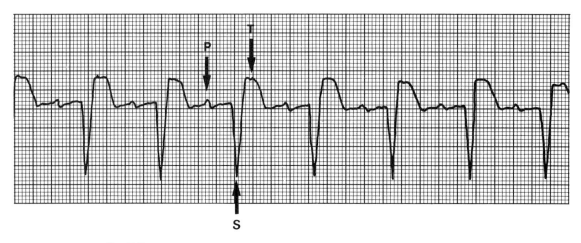

3–14

Rhythm: Regular
Rate: Approx. 70 (71)
Atrial: One P wave for each QRS complex: shape normal
AV Cond: PRI: 0.24 second and consistent (abnormal—too long)
Vent: QRS: 0.16 second and uniform in shape

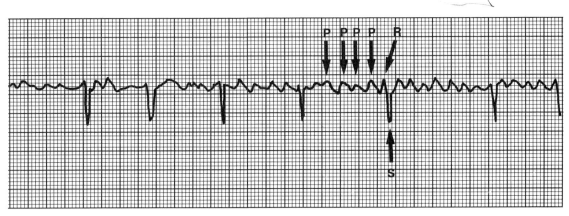

3–15

Rhythm: R to R totally irregular; P to P some regular; some irregular (abnormal)
Rate: Ventricular = approx. 70/atrial = 300
More P waves than QRS complexes (about 4 Ps for 1 QRS)
Atrial: P waves in a sawtooth pattern (abnormal)
AV Cond: PRI: not measured when P waves are in this pattern
Vent: QRS: 0.08 second and uniform in shape

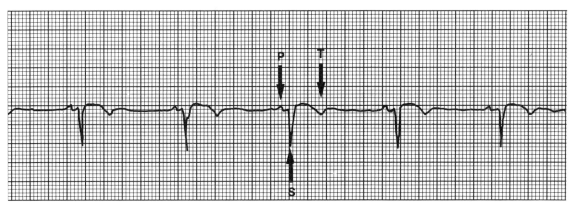

3–16

Rhythm: Regular
Rate: Approx. 50 (54) (abnormal—too slow)
Atrial: One P wave for each QRS complex; normal in shape
AV Cond: PRI: 0.12 second and consistent
Vent: QRS: 0.08 second and uniform in shape

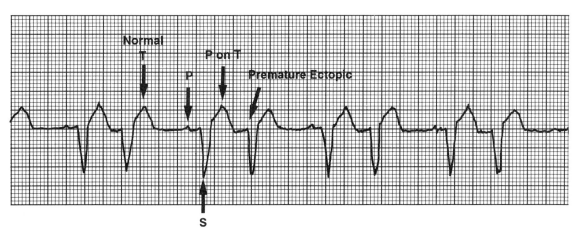

3–17

Rhythm: Regularly irregular (pattern of grouped beats)
Rate: Approx. 90
Atrial: One P wave before each QRS: normal shape before nonectopic; peaked
P wave on top of T wave before ectopics
AV Cond: PRI: nonectopic = 0.16; ectopics = 0.24 (abnormal)
Vent: QRS: 0.10 second for both nonectopics and ectopics

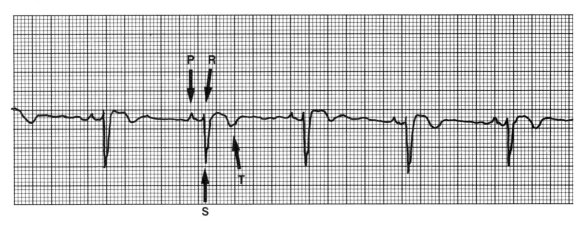

3–18

Rhythm: Regular
Rate: Approx. 50 (53) (abnormal—too slow)
Atrial: One P wave for each QRS complex; normal shape
AV Cond: PRI: 0.16 second and consistent
Vent: QRS: 0.12 second and uniform in shape

CHAPTER 4

4–1

Rhythm: Regular
Rate: 90
Atrial: P waves: one P before each QRS; normal shape; consistent
AV Cond: PRI: 0.14 second; same for whole strip
Vent: QRS: 0.08 second; same shape
Interp: Normal sinus rhythm

4–2

Rhythm: Regular
Rate: 100
Atrial: P waves: one P before each QRS; normal shape; consistent
AV Cond: PRI: 0.14 second; same for whole strip
Vent: QRS: 0.12 second; same shape
Interp: Sinus tachycardia

4–3

Rhythm: Irregular
Rate: Approx. 90
Atrial: P waves: one P before each QRS; normal shape; consistent
AV Cond: PRI: 0.12 second; same for whole strip
Vent: QRS: 0.08 second; same shape
Interp: Normal sinus rhythm

4–4

Rhythm: Regular
Rate: 50
Atrial: P waves: one P before each QRS; normal shape; consistent
AV Cond: PRI: 0.16 second; same for whole strip
Vent: QRS: 0.06 second; same shape
Interp: Sinus bradycardia

4–5

Rhythm: Regular
Rate: 107
Atrial: P waves: one before each QRS; normal shape; consistent
AV Cond: PRI: 0.16 second; same for whole strip
Vent: QRS: 0.16 second; same shape
Interp: Sinus tachycardia

4–6

Rhythm: Regular
Rate: 75
Atrial: P waves: one P before each QRS; normal; consistent
AV Cond: PRI: 0.20 second; same for whole strip
Vent: QRS: 0.06 second; same shape
Interp: Normal sinus rhythm

4–7

Rhythm: Regular
Rate: 136
Atrial: P waves: one P before each QRS; normal; consistent
AV Cond: PRI: 0.12 second; same for whole strip
Vent: QRS: 0.10 second; same for whole strip
Interp: Sinus tachycardia

4–8

Rhythm: Regular
Rate: 79
Atrial: P waves: one P before each QRS; normal; consistent
AV Cond: PRI: 0.20 second; same for whole strip
Vent: QRS: 0.10 second; same shape
Interp: Normal sinus rhythm

4–9

Rhythm: Totally irregular with missed beat out of cycle
Rate: Approx. 70 (67)
Atrial: P waves: one P before each QRS; normal; consistent
AV Cond: PRI: 0.16 second; same for whole strip
Vent: QRS: 0.08 second; same shape
Interp: Sinus rhythm with a sinus arrest (possibly sinus dysrhythmia)

4–10

Rhythm: Regular
Rate: 106
Atrial: P waves: one P before each QRS; tall, but probably normal; same shape for all
AV Cond: PRI: 0.20 second; same for whole strip
Vent: QRS: 0.08 second; same shape
Interp: Sinus tachycardia

4–11

Rhythm: Regular
Rate: 180
Atrial: P waves: one P before each QRS; some are partially buried in the preceding T wave; same shape
AV Cond: PRI: 0.16 second; same for whole strip
Vent: QRS: 0.08 second; same shape
Interp: Sinus tachycardia

4–12

Rhythm: Totally irregular
Rate: 45
Atrial: P waves: one P before each QRS; normal; consistent
AV Cond: PRI: 0.20 second; same for whole strip
Vent: QRS: 0.10 second; same shape
Interp: Sinus dysrhythmia (sinus brady-dysrhythmia, due to very slow rate)

4–13

Rhythm: Regular
Rate: 108
Atrial: P waves: one P before each QRS; normal; consistent
AV Cond: PRI: 0.14 second; same for whole strip
Vent: QRS: 0.08 second; same shape
Interp: Sinus tachycardia

4–14

Rhythm: Regular
Rate: 68
Atrial: P waves: one P before each QRS; normal; consistent
AV Cond: PRI: 0.14 second; same for whole strip
Vent: QRS: 0.12 second; same shape
Interp: Normal sinus rhythm

4–15

Rhythm: Regular
Rate: 115
Atrial: P waves: one P before each QRS; normal; consistent
AV Cond: PRI: 0.18 second; same for whole strip
Vent: QRS: 0.08 second; same shape
Interp: Sinus tachycardia (large T wave)

4–16

Rhythm: Regular
Rate: 60
Atrial: P waves: one P before each QRS; normal; consistent
AV Cond: PRI: 0.12 second; same for whole strip
Vent: QRS: 0.09 second; same shape
Interp: Normal sinus rhythm

4–17

Rhythm: Regular
Rate: 66
Atrial: P waves: one P before each QRS; flattened; consistent
AV Cond: PRI: 0.14 second; same for whole strip
Vent: QRS: 0.08 second; same shape
Interp: Normal sinus rhythm

4–18

Rhythm: Regular
Rate: 50
Atrial: P waves: one P before each QRS; wide and inverted, but consistent across strip
AV Cond: PRI: 0.16 second; same for whole strip
Vent: QRS: 0.10 second; same shape
Interp: Sinus bradycardia

4–19

Rhythm: Regular
Rate: 108
Atrial: P waves: one P before each QRS; normal; consistent
AV Cond: PRI: 0.16 second; same for whole strip
Vent: QRS: 0.06 second; same shape
Interp: Sinus tachycardia

4–20

Rhythm: Regular
Rate: 68
Atrial: P waves: one P before each QRS; diphasic and wide; consistent in shape
AV Cond: PRI: 0.10 second; same for whole strip
Vent: QRS: 0.10 second; same shape (elevated ST segment)
Interp: Sinus rhythm (with an elevated ST segment)

CHAPTER 5

5–1

Rhythm: Totally irregular
Rate: Approx. 95
Atrial: P waves: chaotic, irregular base line; "f" waves
AV Cond: PRI: not measured
Vent: QRS: O.08 second; same shape
Interp: Uncontrolled atrial fibrillation

5–2

Rhythm: Basically regular interrupted by one premature ectopic
Rate: 56
Atrial: P waves: one P before each QRS; normal shape for the basic rhythm; P wave before the ectopic is more peaked than others; incomplete compensatory pause after ectopic
AV Cond: PRI: basic rhythm = 0.14 second; ectopic = 0.12 second
Vent: QRS: 0.08 second; same shape for all beats
Interp: Sinus bradycardia with one PAC

5-3

Rhythm: Slightly irregular
Rate: 36
Atrial: P waves: change shape from beat to beat; one complex without a P wave
AV Cond: PRI: 0.20 second where present
Vent: QRS: 0.10 second; same shape
Interp: Slow wandering pacemaker

5-4

Rhythm: Regular P to P interval; regular R to R interval
Rate: Atrial = 300; ventricular = 150
Atrial: P waves: sawtooth pattern; more Ps than QRSs; 2:1 ratio
AV Cond: PRI: not measured
Vent: QRS: 0.08 second; shape distorted on some complexes due to P waves
Interp: Uncontrolled atrial flutter; 2:1 ratio

5-5

Rhythm: Totally irregular
Rate: Approx. 150
Atrial: P waves: chaotic, irregular baseline; "f" waves
AV Cond: PRI: not measured
Vent: QRS: 0.10 second; slight variation in size
Interp: Uncontrolled atrial fibrillation

5-6

Rhythm: Basically regular with one premature ectopic
Rate: 75
Atrial: P waves: one P wave before each QRS; same shape for basic rhythm; P wave before ectopic has different shape; incomplete compensatory pause after ectopic
AV Cond: PRI: 0.20 second for basic rhythm; 0.14 for ectopic
Vent: QRS: 0.06 second; ectopic has slightly different shape but same duration
Interp: Sinus rhythm with one PAC

5-7

Rhythm: Regular P to P interval; totally irregular R to R
Rate: Atrial = 300; ventricular = approx. 90
Atrial: P waves: sawtooth pattern; more P waves than QRSs; variable ratio
AV Cond: PRI: not measured
Vent: QRS: 0.08 second; same shape
Interp: Controlled atrial flutter with variable ratio

5–8

Rhythm: Basically regular with two premature ectopic beats
Rate: Approx. 58
Atrial: P waves: one P wave before each QRS; same shape for basic rhythm; P waves before ectopics have different shapes
AV Cond: PRI: basic rhythm = 0.12 second; ectopics = 0.18 second
Vent: QRS: 0.08 second; same shape
Interp: Sinus dysrhythmia with two PACs

5–9

Rhythm: Totally irregular
Rate: Approx. 120
Atrial: P waves: generally chaotic, irregular baseline ("f" waves); some sawtooth P waves present
AV Cond: PRI: not measured
Vent: QRS: 0.06 second; shape varies slightly due to the effect of the P waves
Interp: Uncontrolled atrial fibrillation/flutter

5–10

Rhythm: Regular P to P interval; totally irregular R to R
Rate: Atrial = 300; ventricular = approx. 65
Atrial: P waves: sawtooth pattern; more P waves than QRSs; variable ratio
AV Cond: PRI: not measured
Vent: QRS: 0.10 second; varies slightly in shape due to effect of P waves
Interp: Controlled atrial flutter with variable ratio

5–11

Rhythm: Regular except for last beat
Rate: 150 overall
Atrial: P waves: normal diphasic P wave before last QRS (sinus beat); F waves before all other QRSs are abnormal-shaped—large and peaked; one hidden in QRS
AV Cond: PRI: 0.18 second last beat—others not measured
Vent: QRS: 0.08 second; same shape
Interp: Atrial flutter with 2 : 1 conduction changing to atrial fibrillation

5–12

Rhythm: Regular P to P intervals; regular R to R intervals
Rate: Atrial = 300; ventricular = 150
Atrial: P waves: sawtooth pattern; every other P wave partially hidden in T wave—appears inverted; more P waves than QRSs; 2 : 1 ratio
AV Cond: PRI: not measured
Vent: QRS: 0.08 second; same shape
Interp: Uncontrolled atrial flutter in 2 : 1 ratio

5–13

Rhythm: Regular
Rate: 215
Atrial: P waves: difficult to see; partially hidden in the T wave of the preceding QRS complex; abnormal-shaped
AV Cond: PRI: unable to measure due to hidden P waves
Vent: QRS: 0.08 second; same shape
Interp: Atrial tachycardia

5–14

Rhythm: Regular P to P interval where measurable; slightly irregular R to R intervals
Rate: Atrial (where measurable = 375; ventricular = 93
Atrial: P waves: combination of sawtooth P waves and a chaotic, irregular baseline
AV Cond: PRI: not measured
Vent: QRS: 0.08 second; shape varies slightly
Interp: Controlled atrial fibrillation/flutter (coarse atrial fibrillation)

5–15

Rhythm: Totally irregular; Ashman's pattern
Rate: Approx. 40
Atrial: P waves: no distinct P waves; uneven, flattened baseline
AV Cond: PRI: not measured
Vent: QRS: 0.1 second; same shape
Interp: Slow atrial fibrillation (flat-line type)

5–16

Rhythm: Slightly irregular
Rate: Approx. 60
Atrial: P waves: change shape from beat to beat; some are inverted; some upright and normal; one P wave for each QRS
AV Cond: PRI: 0.014 second where present; varies slightly as P waves change shape
Vent: QRS: 0.1 second; same shape
Interp: Wandering pacemaker

CHAPTER 6

6–1

Rhythm: Regular
Rate: 28
Atrial: P waves: not visible; hidden in QRS complexes
AV Cond: PRI: not measured
Vent: QRS: 0.08 second; same shape
Interp: Slow junctional escape rhythm

6–2

Rhythm: Totally irregular
Rate: Approx. 30
Atrial: P waves: normal before first three beats; no visible P wave with the fourth beat
AV Cond: PRI: 0.24 second with first three beats; not measured with fourth beat
Vent: QRS: 0.06 second; same shape
Interp: Sinus dysrhythmia (slow), with a sinus arrest and one junctional escape beat

6–3

Rhythm: Regular
Rate: 65
Atrial: P waves: after the QRS complexes
AV Cond: PRI: not measured
Vent: QRS: 0.10 second; same shape
Interp: Accelerated junctional rhythm

6–4

Rhythm: Regular
Rate: 94
Atrial: P waves: not visible; hidden in QRS complexes
AV Cond: PRI: not measured
Vent: QRS: 0.08 second; same shape
Interp: Accelerated junctional rhythm

6–5

Rhythm: Totally irregular
Rate: Approx. 28
Atrial: P waves: normal before first two beats; after the QRS complex of the third beat
AV Cond: PRI: 0.18 second before first two beats; not measured with the third beat
Vent: QRS: 0.08 second; same shape
Interp: Sinus bradycardia with one junctional escape beat

6—6

Rhythm: Regular
Rate: 75
Atrial: P waves: after the QRS complexes on top of T waves
AV Cond: PRI: not measured
Vent: QRS: 0.08 second; same shape
Interp: Accelerated junctional rhythm

6—7

Rhythm: Slightly irregular with a pause
Rate: 43
Atrial: P waves: flattened before first three beats; after the fourth beat
AV Cond: PRI: 0.20 second before first three beats; not measured in fourth beat
Vent: QRS: 0.10 second; last beat is a slightly different shape but measures the same duration
Interp: Sinus bradycardia with a junctional escape beat

6—8

Rhythm: Regular
Rate: 75
Atrial: P waves: come after the QRS complexes in T waves
AV Cond: PRI: not measured
Vent: QRS: 0.08 second; same shape
Interp: Accelerated junctional rhythm

6—9

Rhythm: Slightly irregular with one late ectopic escape beat
Rate: Approx. 40
Atrial: P waves: normal P waves before the first four beats; P wave hidden in the QRS complex of the last beat
AV Cond: PRI: 0.14 second on normal beats; not measured on ectopic
Vent: QRS: 0.08 second; same shape
Interp: Sinus bradycardia with a sinus arrest and a junctional escape beat

6—10

Rhythm: Regular
Rate: 75
Atrial: P waves: hidden in QRS complexes
AV Cond: PRI: not measured
Vent: QRS: 0.08 second; same shape
Interp: Accelerated junctional rhythm

CHAPTER 7

7-1

Rhythm: Slightly irregular
Rate: 300+
Aatrial: P waves: not present
AV Cond: PRI: not measured
Vent: QRS: 0.20 second—wide, ventricular configuration; change shape a little; difficult to distinguish T wave from QRS complex
Interp: Ventricular flutter (rapid ventricular tachycardia)

7-2

Rhythm: Slightly irregular
Rate: 80
Atrial: P waves: not present
AV Cond: PRI: not measured
Vent: QRS: 0.60+ second; wide, rounded
Interp: Agonal rhythm

7-3

Rhythm: Basically regular interrupted by 4 premature ectopics
Rate: 130
Atrial: P waves: one P wave before each nonectopic QRS complex; no P waves before ectopic beats
AV Cond: PRI: 0.14 second with nonectopics; not measured with ectopic beats
Vent: QRS: 0.08 second in nonectopic beats; 0.14+ second in 4 premature ectopics in a row; QRS complexes are all in the same direction
Interp: Sinus tachycardia with a run of 4 (unifocal) PVCs

7-4

Rhythm: Basically regular with one wide premature ectopic beat that does not interrupt the underlying rhythm
Rate: 75
Artial: P waves: one P wave before each nonectopic QRS complex; no P wave before ectopic beat
AV Cond: PRI: 0.20 second in nonectopic beats; not measured with ectopic
Vent: QRS: 0.08 second in nonectopic beats; 0.18+ second in ectopic, wide with ventricular configuration
Interp: Sinus rhythm with one interpolated PVC

7–5

Rhythm: Regularly irregular in repetitive pattern of one normal beat followed by one wide ectopic
Rate: Approx. 75
Atrial: P waves: one flattened P wave before each nonectopic QRS complex; no P waves before ectopic beats
AV Cond: PRI: 0.18 second with nonectopic beats; not measured with ectopic beat
Vent: QRS: 0.06 second in nonectopic beats; 0.14+ second in ectopics, wide with ventricular configuration
Interp: Sinus rhythm with bigeminal PVCs

7–6

Rhythm: Totally irregular
Rate: Undetermined
Atrial: P waves: none visible
AV Cond: PRI: not measured
Vent: QRS: irregular, small, chaotic undulations
Interp: Fine ventricular fibrillation

7–7

Rhythm: Regular
Rate: 167
Atrial: P waves: not present
AV Cond: PRI: not measured
Vent: QRS: 0.20+ second, wide with ventricular configuration; difficult to distinguish T waves from QRS complexes
Interp: Ventricular tachycardia

7–8

Rhythm: Bascially regular interrupted by multiple premature ectopics
Rate: 107
Atrial: P waves: one small, inverted P wave for each nonectopic QRS complex; no P waves before ectopic beats
AV Cond: PRI: 0.16 second in nonectopic beats; not measured with ectopic
Vent: QRS: 0.08 second in the nonectopic; 0.18+ second in the ectopic; wide with ventricular configuration; all in the same direction; three in a row and two separate
Interp: Sinus tachycardia with a run of 3 (unifocal) PVCs and two other PVCs

7–9

Rhythm: Slightly irregular
Rate: 48
Atrial: P waves: not present
AV Cond: PRI: not measured
Vent: QRS: 0.22+ second, wide in ventricular configuration
Interp: Ventricular escape rhythm

7–10

Rhythm: Regularly irregular in a repetitive pattern of one normal beat followed by one premature wide ectopic beat
Rate: Approx. 70
Atrial: P waves: one peaked P wave before each nonectopic beat; no P waves before ectopic beats
AV Cond: PRI: 0.14 second in nonectopic beats; not measured with ectopics
Vent: QRS: 0.08 second in the nonectopic; 0.18+ second in the ectopic, wide in ventricular configuration
Interp: Sinus rhythm with bigeminal PVCs

7–11

Rhythm: Basically regular interrupted by 4 premature wide ectopic beats in a row
Rate: 110
Atrial: P waves: one P wave before each nonectopic beat; no P waves with ectopics
AV Cond: PRI: 0.16 second in nonectopic beats; not measured with ectopic beats
Vent: QRS: 0.06 second in nonectopic beats; 0.14 to 0.20+ second in ectopic beats, wide in ventricular configuration; R waves of ectopic beats go in different directions with one small, atypical beat
Interp: Sinus rhythm with coupled, multifocal PVCs and one fusion beat

7–12

Rhythm: Regularly irregular with a repetitive pattern of four normal beats followed by one wide premature ectopic beat
Rate: 125
Atrial: P waves: one P wave before each nonectopic QRS complex; no P waves before the ectopic QRS complexes
AV Cond: PRI: 0.16 second in nonectopic beats; not measured in ectopics
Vent: QRS: 0.06 second in nonectopics; 0.14+ second in ectopics, wide in ventricular configuration
Interp: Sinus tachycardia with frequent PVCs (Although this is a pattern of PVCs, there is no name for it.)

7–13

Rhythm: Irregular
Rate: Approx. 20
Artrial: P waves: none present
AV Cond: PRI: not measured
Vent: QRS: 9.48+ second, wide and rounded
Interp: Agonal rhythm

7–14

Rhythm: Totally irregular
Rate: 30 for strip
Atrial: P waves: not present
AV Cond: PRI: not measured
Vent: QRS: 0.20+ second; wide in ventricular configuration, then no electrical, activity with an isoelectric line
Interp: Ventricular tachycardia going into an asystole

7–15

Rhythm: Slightly irregular
Rate: 180
Atrial: P waves: not present
AV Cond: PRI: not measured
Vent: QRS: 0.20+ second; wide in ventricular configuration; difficult to distinguish T waves from QRS complexes
Interp: Ventricular tachycardia

7–16

Rhythm: Regularly irregular in a repetitive pattern of three normal beats followed by a wide, premature ectopic
Rate: 115
Atrial: P waves: one P wave before each nonectopic QRS complex: no P waves before ectopics
AV Cond: PRI: 0.16 second in nonectopic beats; not measured with ectopics
Vent: QRS: 0.08 second in nonectopic; 0.20+ second in ectopic beats; wide in ventricular configuration
Interp: Sinus tachycardia with quadrigeminal PVCs

7–17

Rhythm: Slightly irregular
Rate: 33
Atrial: P waves: not present
AV Cond: PRI: not measured
Vent: QRS: 0.16+ second; wide in ventricular configuration
Interp: Ventricular escape rhythm

7–18

Rhythm: Regular
Rate: 214
Atrial: P waves: not present
AV Cond: PRI: not measured
Vent: QRS: 0.22+ second; wide in ventricular configuration; difficult to distinguish T waves from QRS complexes
Interp: Fast ventricular tachycardia

7–19

Rhythm: Totally irregular
Rate: Approx. 50
Atrial: P waves: not present
AV Cond: PRI: not measured
Vent: QRS: 0.44+ second; wide and rounded; irregular
Interp: Agonal rhythm

7–20

Rhythm: Basically regular interrupted by premature ectopics
Rate: 107
Atrial: P waves: one P wave before each nonectopic QRS complex; no P waves before ectopics
AV Cond: PRI: 0.16 second in nonectopic beats; 0.18+ second in ectopics; wide in ventricular configuration; group of these that go in different directions
Interp: Sinus tachycardia with one PVC and a run of three multifocal PVCs

CHAPTER 8

8–1

Rhythm: Regular
Rate: 79
Atrial: P waves: one P wave before each QRS complex; normal shape
AV Cond: PRI: 0.30 second, consistent
Vent: QRS: 0.12 second, same shape
Interp: Sinus rhythm with a first degree AV block (and BBB)

8–2

Rhythm: Regular P to P interval; regular R to R interval
Rate: Atrial = 60; ventricular = 30
Atrial: P waves: 2 P waves for each QRS complex; normal
AV Cond: PRI: 0.24 second; same in all conducted beats
Vent: QRS: 0.08 second; same shape
Interp: Classic second degree AV block with a long PRI and 2:1 ratio

8–3

Rhythm: Regular P to P interval; irregular R to R interval
Rate: Atrial = 68; ventricular = approx. 50
Atrial: P waves: more P waves than QRS complexes; normal
AV Cond: PRI: 0.20 to 0.44 second; gets progressively longer until there is a P wave without a QRS complex after it
Vent: 0.08 second; same shape
Interp: SR with AV Wenckebach

8–4

Rhythm: Regular P to P interval; regular R to R interval
Rate: Atrial = 94; ventricular = 58
Atrial: P waves: more P waves than QRS complexes; peaked
AV Cond: PRI: varies; inconsistent; no pattern
Vent: QRS: 0.16 second; same shape
Interp: Third degree AV block with accelerated ventricular escape rhythm

8–5

Rhythm: Regular
Rate: 115
Atrial: P waves: one P wave before each QRS complex; normal
AV Cond: PRI: 0.28 second; consistent
Vent: QRS: 0.12 second; same shape
Interp: Sinus tachycardia with first degree AV block (and BBB)

8–6

Rhythm: Regular P to P interval; regular R to R interval
Rate: Atrial = 125; ventricular = 42
Atrial: P waves: three P waves for each QRS complex; some P waves hidden in the T waves; normal shape
AV Cond: PRI: 0.16 second; consistent in conducted beats
Vent: QRS: 0.10 second; same shape
Interp: Classic second degree AV block in 3:1 ratio (advance block, type II)

8–7

Rhythm: Regular
Rate: 55
Atrial: P waves: one P wave before each QRS complex; normal
AV Cond: PRI: 0.24 second; consistent
Vent: QRS: 0.10 second; same shape
Interp: Sinus rhythm with first degree AV block

8–8

Rhythm: Regular P to P interval; irregular R to R interval
Rate: Atrial = 88; ventricular = approx. 70
Atrial: P waves: more P waves than QRS complexes; normal
AV Cond: PRI: 0.20 to 0.28; gets progressively longer until a P wave is not followed by a QRS complex; repeats pattern
Vent: QRS: 0.08 seconds; same shape
Interp: SR with AV Wenckebach (2:1 type I block)

8–9

Rhythm: Regular P to P; slightly irregular R to R interval
Rate: Atrial = 125; ventricular = approx. 70
Atrial: P waves: more P waves than QRS complexes; diphasic
AV Cond: PRI: variable; inconsistent; no pattern
Vent: QRS: 0.10 second; same shape
Interp: SR with third degree AV block and a junctional escape rhythm

8–10

Rhythm: Regular P to P interval; regular R to R interval
Rate: Atrial = 94; ventricular = 47
Atrial: P waves: two P waves per QRS complex; normal
AV Cond: PRI: 0.24 second; consistent where conducted
Vent: QRS: 0.08 second; same shape
Interp: Classic second degree AV block with long PRI in 2:1 ratio

8–11

Rhythm: Regular P to P interval; regular(?) R to R interval
Rate: Atrial = 90; ventricular = 30
Atrial: P waves: more P waves than QRS complexes; some hidden in the QRS complexes or T waves
AV Cond: PRI: 0.64 second where present; probably too long to be conducted
Vent: QRS: 0.10 second; same shape
Interp: Third degree AV block with slow junctional escape rhythm (advanced type II block)

8–12

Rhythm: Regular P to P interval; irregular R to R interval
Rate: Atrial = 125; ventricular = approx. 45
Atrial: P waves: more P waves than QRS complexes; normal; some hidden in T waves
AV Cond: PRI: 0.16 second; consistent where conducted
Vent: QRS: 0.12 second; same shape
Interp: Classic second degree AV block with a variable ratio (2 : 1 and 3 : 1) (advance block, type II)

8–13

Rhythm: Regular P to P interval; irregular R to R interval
Rate: Atrial = 79; ventricular = approx. 70
Atrial: P waves: more P waves than QRS complexes; diphasic
AV Cond: PRI: 0.28 to 0.44 second; gets progressively longer until there is a P wave without a QRS complex; repeats pattern
Vent: QRS: 0.08 second; same shape
Interp: SR with AV Wenckebach

8–14

Rhythm: Regular P to P interval; irregular R to R interval
Rate: Atrial = 45; ventricular = approx. 30(?)
Atrial: P waves: more P waves than QRS complexes; normal
AV Cond: PRI: variable; inconsistent; no pattern
Vent: QRS: 0.16 second; same shape
Interp: SB with third degree AV block and a ventricular escape pattern (high grade AV Block)

8–15

Rhythm: Irregular
Rate: 88
Atrial: P waves: one P wave for each QRS complex; normal
AV Cond: PRI: 0.32 second; consistent
Vent: QRS: 0.06 second; same shape
Interp: Sinus dysrhythmia (or WP) with first degree AV block

8–16

Rhythm: Regular P to P interval; regular(?) R to R interval
Rate: Atrial = 100; ventricular = 20(?)
Atrial: P waves: more P waves than QRS complexes; peaked
AV Cond: PRI: 0.22 second; consistent where conducted
Vent: QRS: 0.12 second; same shape
Interp: Classic second degree AV block with long PRI in a 6:1 ratio (SR with advanced block, type II)

CHAPTER 9

9–1

Rhythm: Regular
Rate: 250
Atrial: P waves: no clear identifiable P waves
AV Cond: PRI: not measured
Vent: QRS: 0.08 second; same shape
Interp: Supraventricular tachycardia

9–2

Rhythm: Regular
Rate: 188
Atrial: P waves: no clear identifiable P waves
AV Cond: PRI: not measured
Vent: QRS: 0.08 second; same shape
Interp: Supraventricular tachycardia

9–3

Rhythm: Totally irregular
Rate: Approx. 45
Atrial: P waves: normal before first three, fifth and seventh QRS complexes; none before the fourth and sixth QRS complexes.
AV Cond: PRI: 0.18 second where present
Vent: QRS: 0.08 second; same shape
Interp: Sinus bradycardia with junctional escape beats (Sick Sinus syndrome)

9–4

Rhythm: Slightly irregular
Rate: 150
Atrial: P waves: no clear identifiable P waves
AV Cond: PRI: not measured
Vent: QRS: 0.06 second; same shape
Interp: Supraventricular tachycardia (possibly atrial fib.)

9–5

Rhythm: Regular
Rate: 214
Atrial: P waves: no clear identifiable P waves
AV Cond: PRI: not measured
Vent: QRS: 0.08 second; same shape
Interp: Supraventricular tachycardia

9–6

Rhythm: Irregular overall
Rate: Approx. 105 overall (tachycardia = 140; bradycardia = 30?)
Atrial: P waves: normal before first nine QRS complexes; no P waves before the last two QRS complexes
AV Cond: PRI: 0.16 second where present
Vent: QRS: 0.06 second; same shape for all beats
Interp: Tachy-brady syndrome

CHAPTER 10

10–1

Rhythm: Regular
Rate: 52
Atrial: P waves: no P waves before the QRS complexes; last four QRS complexes have P waves after them
AV Cond: PRI: not measured
Vent: QRS: 0.16 second; rsR' configuration; positive direction; same shape
Interp: Junctional escape rhythm with a right bundle branch block

10–2

Rhythm: Totally irregular; some Ashman's pattern
Rate: Approx. 110
Atrial: P waves: none visible; straight line baseline
AV Cond: PRI: not measured
Vent: QRS: 0.18 second; monophasic configuration; negative direction; same shape
Interp: Uncontrolled atrial fibrillation with a left bundle branch block pattern

10–3

Rhythm: Regular
Rate: 71
Atrial: P waves: normal shape; one P wave before each QRS
AV Cond: PRI: 0.18 second; consistent across the strip
Vent: QRS: 0.14 second; monophasic configuration; negative direction; same shape
Interp: Sinus rhythm with a left bundle branch block

10-4

Rhythm: Regular
Rate: 79
Atrial: P waves: flattened; difficult to see; one P wave before each QRS complex
AV Cond: PRI: 0.18 second; consistent across the strip
Vent: QRS: #1-2-6-7 = 0.08 second; negative direction; #3-4-5-8-9 = 0.14 second; rR' configuration; positive direction
Interp: Sinus rhythm with an intermittent right bundle branch block

10-5

Rhythm: Regular
Rate: 65
Atrial: P waves: one P wave before each QRS complex
AV Cond: PRI: 0.14 second; consistent
Vent: QRS: 0.16 second; Rr' notched configuration; positive direction; same shape
Interp: Sinus rhythm with a right bundle branch block

10-6

Rhythm: Totally irregular
Rate: Approx. 60
Atrial: P wave: not visible; flat line baseline
AV Cond: PRI: not measured
Vent: QRS: #1-2-3-5-6-7 = 0.20 second; monophasic configuration; positive direction; #4 = 0.16 second; monophasic configuration; negative direction
Interp: Controlled atrial fibrillation with alternating bundle branch block (predominantly RBBB)

10-7

Rhythm: Regular
Rate: 83
Atrial: P wave: diphasic shape; one P wave before each QRS
AV Cond: PRI: 0.22 second; consistent across the strip
Vent: QRS: 0.14 second; RSR' configuration; positive direction; same shape
Interp: Sinus rhythm with a first degree AV block and a right bundle branch block

10–8

Rhythm: Totally irregular
Rate: Approx. 67
Atrial: P wave: no distinct P waves; uneven, chaotic atrial wave forms
AV Cond: PRI: not measured
Vent: QRS: 0.20 second; Ss' with notch configuration; negative direction; same shape
Interp: Controlled atrial fibrillation with a left bundle branch block

10–9

Rhythm: Slightly irregular
Rate: 115
Atrial: P waves: diphasic; one P wave before each QRS complex
AV Cond: PRI: 0.16 second; consistent across the strip
Vent: QRS: 0.20 second; monophasic configuration; positive direction; same shape
Interp: Sinus tachycardia with a right bundle branch block

10–10

Rhythm: Irregular
Rate: 80
Atrial: P waves: upright; irregular P to P intervals; variable shape and size; more P waves than QRS complexes
AV Cond: PRI: variable; inconsistent
Vent: QRS: 0.18 second; srS' configuration; negative direction; same shape
Interp: Chaotic atrial rhythm with a left bundle branch block

10–11

Rhythm: Regular
Rate: 65
Atrial: P waves: normal; one P wave before each QRS complex
AV Cond: PRI: 0.24 second; consistent across the strip
Vent: QRS: 0.16 second; monophasic configuration; negative direction; same shape
Interp: Sinus rhythm with a first degree AV block and a left bundle branch block

10–12

Rhythm: Regular
Rate: 65
Atrial: P waves: normal; one P wave before each QRS complex
AV Cond: PRI: 0.24 second; consistent across the strip
Vent: QRS: 0.18 second; Rsr' configuration; positive direction; same shape
Interp: Sinus rhythm with a right bundle branch block

CHAPTER 12

12–1

Rhythm: Regular spike to spike; regular R to R
Rate: 71
Atrial: P waves: none; pacemaker spike before each QRS complex
AV Cond: PRI: not measured; pacemaker spikes are less than 0.04 second before the QRS complexes
Vent: QRS: 0.14 second; negative deflection; same shape
Interp: Normal pacing rhythm

12–2

Rhythm: Regular spike to spike; regular R to R
Rate: 71
Atrial: P waves: none; pacemaker spike before each QRS complex
AV Cond: PRI: not measured; pacemaker spikes are less than 0.04 second before the QRS complexes
Vent: QRS: 0.16 second, negative deflection; two QRS complexes are smaller than the others and positively deflected with pacemaker before them
Interp: Pacing rhythm with two fusion beats

12–3

Rhythm: Regular spike to spike; irregular R to R
Rate: 71 pacemaker rate; approx. 50 ventricular
Atrial: P waves; present without QRS complexes after P waves; pacemaker spikes present, some without QRS complexes after them
AV Cond: PRI: not measured; where pacemaker spikes are before QRS complexes, they are less than 0.04 second
Vent: QRS: 0.16 second; negative deflection except for one small positive QRS complex
Interp: Intermittent capture pacing rhythm with one fusion beat (underlying rhythm probably complete heart block with ventricular asystole)

12–4

Rhythm: Regular spike to spike; regular R to R
Rate: 70
Atrial: P waves: small P wave present in T waves—may be a retrograde P wave; positively deflected spike before each QRS complex
AV Cond: PRI: not measured; pacemaker spikes are less than 0.04 second before the QRS complexes
Vent: QRS: 0.18 second; negative; same shape
Interp: Normal pacemaker rhythm

12–5

Rhythm: Totally irregular spike to spike and R to R
Rate: Approx. 170
Atrial: P waves: none; pacemaker spikes fall randomly throughout the pattern with QRS complexes after them
AV Cond: PRI: not measured
Vent: QRS: 0.16+ second; varied shapes; some positive, some negative
Interp: Ventricular tachycardia with noncapture pacemaker

12–6

Rhythm: Regular spike to spike and R to R
Rate: 63 for pacemaker; 63 for ventricles
Atrial: P waves: no intrinsic P waves; pacemaker spikes in groups of two at preset intervals; no wave complexes after pacemaker spikes
AV Cond: PRI: not measured
Vent: QRS: 0.08 second; same shape
Interp: Noncapture dual chamber pacemaker pattern (underlying rhythm probably a junctional escape rhythm)

12–7

Rhythm: Regular spike to spike; irregular R to R; one premature QRS complex
Rate: 71 for pacemaker; approx. 40 for ventricular
Atrial: P waves: none; some pacemaker spikes have QRS complexes after them, some do not
AV Cond: PRI: not measured; where pacemaker spikes have a QRS after them, interval is less than 0.04 second
Vent: QRS: 0.18 second; negative; same shape
Interp: Intermittent capture pacemaker pattern with one PVC

12–8

Rhythm: Regular
Rate: 65
Atrial: P waves; one P wave after each pacemaker spike; one spike before each QRS complex
AV Cond: PRI: (AVI) 0.16 second between the atrial spike and the ventricular spike; consistent
Vent: QRS: 0.14 second; negative; same shape
Interp: Normal dual chamber pacemaker pattern

INDEX

Page numbers followed by *f* indicate figures; *t* following a page number indicates tabular material; *b* following a page number indicates boxed material.

A

AAI. *See* Atrial demand pacemaker
Absorbocarpine. *See* Pilocarpine hydrochloride
Accessory atrioventricular (AV) connections. *See* Kent bundles
Accessory pathways. *See* Bypass mechanisms
Acetylcholine
   effect of, 8t, 21
Adrenalin. *See* Epinephrine hydrochloride
Adrenergic system. *See* Sympathetic nervous system
Agonal rhythm, 334, 355
   conversion to ventricular fibrillation, 318, 348
   criteria for, 179
   definition of, 178–179, 179f
   examples of, 179f, 182, 187, 190, 287, 307, 311, 336, 344, 345, 376, 379, 380
Alternating bundle branch block, 236, 237f
Alupent. *See* Metaproterenol sulfate
Amiodarone hydrochloride (Cordarone)
   for premature ventricular contractions, 161
ANS. *See* Autonomic nervous system
APCs (atrial premature contractions). *See* Premature atrial contractions
Aramine. *See* Metaraminol bitartrate
Artane. *See* Trihexyphenidyl hydrochloride
Arteries, 3f
Artifact
   definition of, 43

intentional, 44
   pacemaker, 44f
   standardization in, 44f
interference
   from 60-cycle current, 46f, 46–47
   from loose electrodes or breakage, 45, 45f
   from muscle tremors, 45, 45f
   from patient movements, 46, 46f
   from stray current, 47
Artificial pacemaker(s)
classification of
   by catheter insertion, 264–265
   by catheter type, 263
   by pulse generator type, 265–266
definitions in, 266–268
dual chamber, 273–275
ICHD code in, 265t, 265–266, 268–269
malfunctioning
   with intermittent capture, 316, 348
permanent
   demand, 268
   fixed rate, 268
   indications for, 260, 262
single chamber
   atrial demand, 271–272, 272f, 273
   ventricular demand, 270f, 270–271, 271f
temporary
   example of, 262f
   indications for, 262–263
Ashman's pattern, 118, 118f
Asystole
   causes of, 180
   criteria for, 181
   examples of, 179f
      with conversion to agonal rhythm, 301, 341